Clinical Dermatology:
Diagnosis and Therapy

Clinical Dermatology: Diagnosis and Therapy

Editor: Heidi Mueller

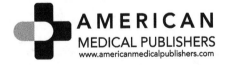

AMERICAN
MEDICAL PUBLISHERS
www.americanmedicalpublishers.com

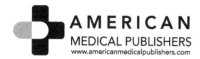

Cataloging-in-Publication Data

Clinical dermatology : diagnosis and therapy / edited by Heidi Mueller.
   p. cm.
Includes bibliographical references and index.
ISBN 978-1-63927-064-4
1. Dermatology. 2. Skin--Diseases. 3. Skin--Diseases--Etiology. 4. Skin--Diseases--Diagnosis.
5. Skin--Diseases--Treatment. I. Mueller, Heidi.
RL72 .D47 2021
616.5--dc23

American Medical Publishers,
41 Flatbush Avenue,
1st Floor, New York,
NY 11217, USA

ISBN 978-1-63927-064-4 (Hardback)

Contents

Permissions

List of Contributors

Index

Preface

Dermatology is a medical field which deals with the diagnosis and treatment of skin diseases. It is also concerned with the management of some cosmetic problems of skin, nails and hair. The sub-fields of dermatology that deal with the problems and diseases of the skin are cosmetic dermatology, immunodermatology and Mohs surgery. Cosmetic dermatology can also include cosmetic procedures such as liposuction, face lifts and blepharoplasty. Immunodermatology is concerned with the treatment of immune-mediated skin diseases such as lupus, bullous pemphigoid, and other disorders. It is also used in the diagnosis and treatment of several diseases such as those which affect gastrointestinal and respiratory tracts. Mohs surgery focuses on the excision of skin cancers by using a tissue-sparing technique. It requires an in-depth knowledge of both pathology and surgery. This book contains some path-breaking studies in the field of dermatology. It presents researches and studies performed by experts across the globe. Those with an interest in this field would find this book helpful.

Various studies have approached the subject by analyzing it with a single perspective, but the present book provides diverse methodologies and techniques to address this field. This book contains theories and applications needed for understanding the subject from different perspectives. The aim is to keep the readers informed about the progresses in the field; therefore, the contributions were carefully examined to compile novel researches by specialists from across the globe.

Indeed, the job of the editor is the most crucial and challenging in compiling all chapters into a single book. In the end, I would extend my sincere thanks to the chapter authors for their profound work. I am also thankful for the support provided by my family and colleagues during the compilation of this book.

Editor

In-House Preparation and Standardization of Herbal Face Pack

Rashmi Saxena Pal*, Yogendra Pal and Pranay Wal

Department of Pharmacy, PSIT, NH-2, Bhauti, Kanpur (U.P), 209305, India

Abstract:

Background:

Since the ancient times, there has been awareness among people regarding the use of plants for the essential needs of a healthy and beautiful skin. Cosmetics are the products used to clean, beautify and promote attractive appearance. Cosmetics designed *via* incorporating natural sources such as herbs have been proven very fulfilling, in coping up with the present needs of different skin types.

Objective:

As due to increased pollution, allergy, microbes etc, human skin has become more sensitive and prone to faster aging. An attempt has been made to synthesize a pack ideal for all skin types. After the synthesis, all the parameters have been calculated in order to meet up the quality standards.

Materials and Methods:

The constituents were extracted from herbal ingredients such as Multani mitti, green tea, saffron, gram flour, turmeric, shwet chandan and milk powder. They were purchased from the local area and were dried separately, grinded, passed through sieve no 40, mixed homogenously and then evaluated for parameters including organoleptic, physicochemical, rheological features, phytochemical, stability, and irritancy examination.

Results:

The dried powders of combined pack showed good flow property which is suitable for a face pack. Organoleptic evaluation showed that the pack is smooth and pleasant smelling powder. Rheological findings justified the flow properties of the pack as it was found to be free flowing and non-sticky in nature. The results proved that the formulation was stable on all aspects. Irritancy test showed the negative. Stability tests performed revealed the inert nature of the pack.

Conclusion:

Thus, in the present work, we formulated a pack, which can be easily made with the easily available ingredients. It showed all the benefits of a face pack and further optimization studies are required on its various parameters to find its useful benefits on the human beings.

Keywords: Skin, Herbal face pack, Preparation, Standardization, Synthesis, Ingredients.

---

1. INTRODUCTION

Since the ancient era, people are aware of the use of plants for the essential needs of a healthy and beautiful skin. Cosmetics are the products used to clean, beautify and promote attractive appearance [1]. Skin of the face is the major part of the body, which is a mirror, reflecting the health of an individual. A balanced nutrition containing amino acids,

---

* Address correspondence to this author at the Department of Pharmacy, PSIT, Kanpur - Agra - Delhi National Highway - 2, Bhauti, Kanpur, Uttar Pradesh 209305, India, E-mail: rashmisaxenapal@gmail.com

lipids and carbohydrates are required for the skin to keep it clear, glossy and healthy. In ancient times, women were very conscious about their beauty and took special care of their specific skin types [2]. Even today, people especially in rural areas, and hilly regions go for the natural remedies like plants extracts for various cosmetics purposes like neem, aloe vera, tulsi, orange peel, rose *etc.* Herbal cosmetics are the products which are used to purify and beautify the skin. The main advantage of using herbal cosmetic is that it is pure and does not have any side effects on the human body. Men have rough skin and when they don't take sufficient care, then the skin turns dark due to overexposure to the sun, other pollutants etc [3]. In this article we have formulated homemade face pack to whiten, lighten and brighten the skin naturally for men and women. This face pack has natural skin lightening property and can be easily prepared at home [4]. Face packs with natural constituents are rich in vital vitamins that are essential for the health and glow of the skin. These substances have been proven to be beneficial for skin in many ways. Natural facial packs are easy to use. They increase the circulation of the blood within the veins of the face, thereby increasing the liveliness of the skin [5]. A good herbal face pack must supply necessary nutrients to the skin, available in the form of free-flowing powder applied facially for the external purpose. It should penetrate deep down the subcutaneous tissues to deliver the required nutrients. Every type of skin is specific for the requirement of skin pack. Nowadays different types of packs are available separately for the oily, normal and dry skin. Face packs are used to increase the fairness and smoothness of the skin. It reduces wrinkles, pimples, acne and dark circles of the skin [6]. Face packs which are recommended for oily skin prone to acne, blackheads, usually control the rate of sebum discharge from sebaceous glands and fight the harmful bacteria present inside acne lesion. The leftover marks of skin can be reduced by incorporation of fine powders of sandalwood, rose-petals and dried orange peels. Herbal face packs are nowadays being used on a large scale, due to the various benefits of them over chemical based packs. They are non-toxic, non-allergic and non-habit forming. They are natural in every aspect, having larger shelf lives. They have no added preservatives. They can be easily formulated and stored over a larger span of time. Present research article deals with the formulation and characterization of cosmetic herbal face pack made from natural constituents.

2. MATERIALS AND METHODS

The crude drugs used in this study were procured from the nearby local area. All the ingredients were washed, shade dried and powdered finely for further use. The following ingredients were used for the preparation of this polyherbal face pack formulation [7].

2.1. Multani Mitti OR Fuller's Earth

Fig. (**1**) multani mitti which helps to remove the impurities in the form of dead skin cells. It helps to make the skin radiant. It has been proven best for the irritation-prone skin. Its soothing action calms the skin, cures the inflammation caused due to elevated phlogistic agents. It is perfect for oily skin. It removes the dirt and excess of oil by acting as a perfect adsorbent. It provides fresh, radiant and glowing skin [8].

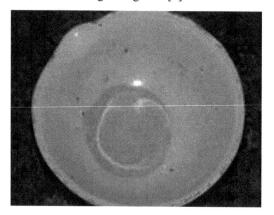

Fig. (1). Multani mitti.

2.2. Haridra (Curcuma Longa)

Haridra in Fig. (2) has been used in this preparation due to its blood purifying property and helps in wound healing, because of its antiseptic action. It cures the skin diseases occurring due to blood impurities. It is a very good anti-inflammatory and anti-allergic agent. The phytoconstituents, mainly terpenoids present in it helps to lighten the skin tone. Haridra delays the signs of aging like wrinkles, improves skin elasticity. It cures pigmentation, uneven skin tone and dull skin [9].

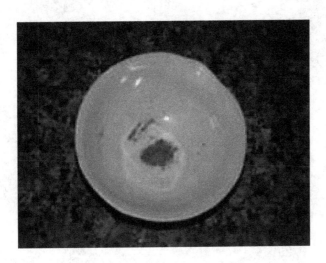

Fig. (2). Turmeric.

2.3. ShwetChandan (Santalum Album)

White Sandalwood powder in Fig. (3) is used to cure various skin allergies. It has cooling and soothing action. It protects the skin from environmental pollution and keeps it glowing, fair and healthy. Sandalwood possesses antimicrobial properties, therefore it is used to cure various skin problems and also removes scars, acne etc [10].

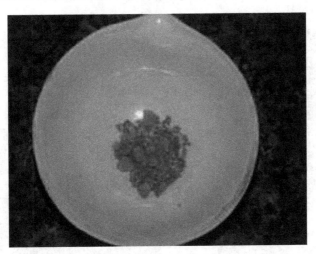

Fig. (3). Santalum album.

2.4. Green Tea

Belonging to the family Theaceae, green tea in Fig. (4) due to its rich phytoconstituents, serves for numerous therapeutic benefits. It slows down aging, reduces inflammation and provides a healthy glow [11].

2.5. Gram Flour

Gram flour, commonly known as Besan in Fig. (**5**), has been used extensively since the olden times for its beauty-enhancing benefits. It mainly acts as a tonic for the skin as it helps to clean and exfoliate it. Gram flour is nothing but a pulse flour obtained from grinded chickpeas. It is very beneficial for skin as well as hair. It is used to decrease tanning of the skin, also reduces the oiliness of skin, thus proving as a good anti-pimple agent. It lightens the skin tone, therefore used as an instant fairness agent [12].

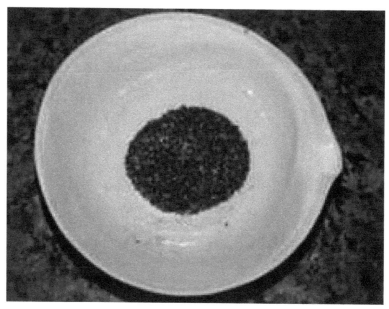

Fig. (4). Green tea.

2.6. Saffron

Mainly consists of dried stigmas and upper parts of styles of plant known as Crocus sativus in Fig. (**5**), belonging to the family Iridaceae. It is rich in carotenoid glycosides, mainly containing terpenoids. It lightens the skin tone and provides fair and glowing skin [13].

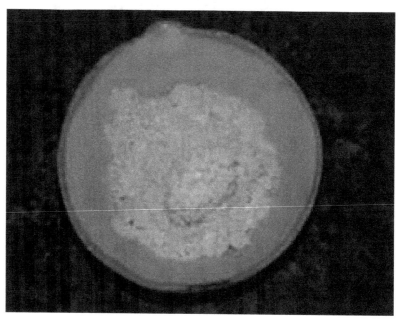

Fig. (5). Gram fluor.

2.7. Milk Powder

It is very beneficial for skin, as it provides nourishment for dry, rough skin for the longer duration. Milk cream either in the form of powdered raw milk in Fig. (6) or milk as such provides a brilliant shine to skin. This is beneficial in hydrating the face deeply and makes skin youthful, lustrous and flawless. It bleaches the skin to remove dark spots, pigmentation, acne *etc.* This pack also removes blackheads, whiteheads, and other skin imperfections naturally. This facial pack helps in fading sun tan [14].

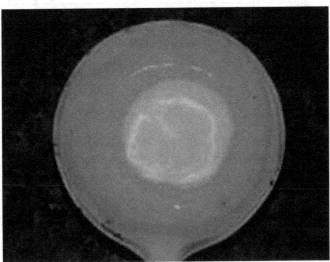

Fig. (6). Milk powder.

2.8. The composition of Face Pack

The powdered constituents were sieved using #40 mesh and mixed homogenously in Fig. (7) for uniform formulation. It was then kept in a moisture-proof container in a cool place for the purpose of standardization of various parameters [15 - 17] (Table 1).

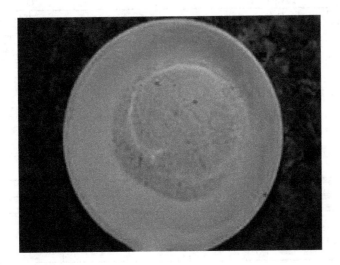

Fig. (7). Prepared face pack.

Table 1. Composition of Herbal face pack.

S.No	Constituent	Percentage
1.	Gram flour	40
2.	Multani mitti	20

(Table 1) contd.....

S.No	Constituent	Percentage
3.	Shwet Chandan	10
4.	Milk powder	10
5.	Turmeric	5
6.	Green tea	10
7.	Saffron	5

3. APPLICATION OF FACE PACK

The pack should be applied daily on wet face, forming a paste of it in water with optimum thickness. It should be applied evenly on the face with the help of a brush. It should be left for 15 minutes for complete drying. Then it should be removed with the help of a wet sponge.

4. USES OF FACE PACK

- Softens the skin, removes the dryness as it is rich in hydrating agents as milk powder.
- Brightens the skin tone due to the presence of shwet Chandan, turmeric, and saffron.
- Cleanses the skin, due to the presence of gram flour as it clears the skin by removing the dirt particles adhered to it.
- Clarifies the skin by fighting the problems of acne and blemishes, by the removal of excess oil from the face due to the presence of Multani mitti.
- Contains antiseptic action to deal with the minor cuts, marks due to the presence of turmeric.
- Exfoliates skin by removing the dead cells, which also prevents early aging due to the presence of green tea.

5. MORPHOLOGICAL EVALUATION

It refers to the evaluation of the pack by its color, odor, appearance, touch, *etc*. The external characters of the samples were examined based on the method described by Siddiqui *et al* [18] (Table **2**).

Table 2. Morphological evaluation.

S.No	Parameter	Observation
1.	Color	Pale yellow
2.	Odor	Pleasant
3.	Appearance	Smooth, fine

6. PHYSICOCHEMICAL EVALUATION

Physicochemical parameters were determined, including the determination of extractive value, ash value, pH and moisture content [19] (Table **3**).

Table 3. Physicochemical evaluation.

S.No	Parameter	Observation
1.	L.O.D	5%
2.	pH	Neutral
3.	Ash value	4.5
4.	Extractive value(aq.)	8.7

7. DETERMINATION OF RHEOLOGICAL PROPERTIES OF THE PREPARED PACK

Physical parameters like Untapped (Bulk) density, tapped density, the angle of repose, Hausner's ratio, and Carr's index were observed and calculated for the formulation. Bulk density refers to the adjustment of particles or granules to pack themselves collectively. The formula for determination of bulk density (D) is $D = M/V$ where M is the mass of particles and V the total volume occupied by them. The volume of packing can be determined in a graduated cylinder. 100 grams of weighed formulation powder was taken and slowly added to the cylinder with the aid of a funnel. The initial volume was observed firstly and the sample was then tapped until no further volume reduction occurred. The bulk density value was obtained from the initial volume and after tapping the volume reduced, from which tapped density was calculated. The angle of repose is used to quantify the flow properties of powder because it influences cohesion among the different particles. The fixed funnel cone method employs the calculation of height (H) above the glass paper that is placed on a flat tabular surface. The pack was carefully poured through the funnel till the peak of the conical heap just touched the tip of the funnel. Here, R denotes the radius of the conical heap, tan a = H/R or a = arc tan H/R, where 'a' is the angle of repose.Hausner's ratio is associated with interparticle friction and predicts powder flow properties. The Hausner's ratio is calculated as D /D' where D is the tapped density and D, the bulk density. Carr's index helps to measure powder flow from bulk density [20, 21] (Table **4**).

Table 4. Rheological evaluation.

S.No	Parameter	Observation
1.	Tapped density	0.83 gm/ml
2.	Untapped density	0.58gm/ml
3.	Angle of Repose	15
4.	Hausner'sr ratio	1.43
5.	Carr's index	30.1%

8. PHYTOCHEMICAL SCREENING

The aqueous extract of the herbal face pack was evaluated for the presence of different phytoconstituents as per the standard procedures [22] (Table **5**).

Table 5. Phytochemical evaluation.

S.No	Phytoconstituents	Presence
1.	Carbohydrates	+
2.	Alkaloids	+
3.	Glycosides	+
4.	Tannins	-
5.	Volatile oil	-

9. IRRITANCY TEST

Mark an area (1sq.cm) on the dorsal surface of the left hand. Definite quantities of prepared face packs were applied to the specified area and time was noted. Irritancy, redness, and swelling were checked and reported for regular intervals up to 24 hours if any [23] (Table 7).

Table 6. Irritancy evaluation.

S.No	Parameter	Observation
1.	Irritation	-
2.	Redness	-
3.	Swelling	-

10. STABILITY TEST

Stability testing of the prepared formulation was conducted by storing at different temperature conditions for the period of one month. The packed glass vials of formulation stored at different temperature conditions viz.., Room temperature and 35°C were evaluated for the physical parameters like Color, Odor, pH, texture, and smoothness [1] (Table 7).

Table 7. Stability evaluation:

S.No	Parameter	Room temperature	35C
1.	Color	No change	No change
2.	Odor	No change	No change
3.	pH	6.62	6.65
4.	Texture	fine	fine
5.	Smoothness	smooth	smooth

11. RESULTS

Organoleptic evaluation showed that the pack is smooth and pleasant smelling powder. Physicochemical parameters reflected that the moisture content was as minimal as 5%. pH was found neutral to suit the requirements of all the skin types. Ash value and extractive values were found within the limits. Rheological findings justified the flow properties of the pack as it was found to be free-flowing and non-sticky in nature. The results proved that the formulation was stable in all aspects. It is rich in the major phytoconstituents such as carbohydrates, alkaloids, and glycosides which act as true nourisher for the skin. Irritancy test showed negative results for irritancy, redness and swelling as the herbals in their natural form without addition of chemicals were found to be compatible with the skin proteins. Stability tests performed at different temperatures over a period of one month revealed the inert nature of the pack in the terms of color, odor, appearance, texture, and pH.

12. DISCUSSIONS

From the above observations, it has been notified that since the formulation is made up of naturally occurring dried herbal ingredients, there are almost negligible chances of the deterioration of the formulation, as there is no moisture containing the element in raw as well as processed form. The formulation was kept for one month at room temperature to observe the changes in its color, odor, texture and appearance. The pH was also noticed before and after one month. The formulation was found to be stable. It can be easily used at any temperature, at any place. Since it is a herbal formulation, it takes time to show the results. However, the use provides smooth and clear skin within 4-5 days. Its continuous use shows superb effects such as flawless, radiant and clear skin. Since natural ingredients are non-toxic, non-habit forming, they take time but remove the defects from roots. Since no chemical, preservative, artificial color or perfume has been added in the pack, the chances of its degradation are almost negligible. This leads to an increased shelf life with stable ingredients.

CONCLUSION

An herbal face pack is used to rejuvenate the muscles, maintain the elasticity of the skin, remove adhered dirt particles and improve the blood circulation. The benefits of herbal based cosmetics are their nontoxic nature. It nourishes the facial skin. This face pack supplies vital nourishment to the skin. It helps in the elimination of acne, pimple, scars, and marks. Face pack exfoliates skin and provides a soothing, calming and cooling effect on the skin. They restore the natural glow of skin in the optimum time period. Frequent uses of natural face packs improve skin texture and complexion. Pollution and harsh climates badly affect the skin and these effects can be countered by the regular usage of face packs. They help to retain the elasticity of skin cells, thereby controlling premature aging of the skin. Wrinkles, fine lines, and loosening of skin can be effectively controlled by using natural face. In this work, we found excellent properties of the face packs and further studies are needed to be performed to ascertain more useful benefits of face packs as cosmetics. Natural remedies are accepted nowadays with open hands as they are safer with fewer side effects than the chemical based products. Herbal formulations are required in large amounts to fulfill the needs of the growing world market. It is an effective attempt to formulate the herbal face pack containing different powders of different plants with multiple therapeutic benefits.

HUMAN AND ANIMAL RIGHTS

No Animals/Humans were used for studies that are base of this research.

CONFLICT OF INTEREST

The authors declare no conflict of interest, financial or otherwise.

ACKNOWLEDGEMENTS

Declared none.

REFERENCES

[1] Rani S, Hiremanth R. Formulation & Evaluation of Poly-herbal Face wash gel. World J Pharm Pharm Sci 2015; 4(6): 585-8.

[2] Sowmya KV, Darsika CX, Grace F, Shanmuganathan S. Shanmuganathan S.Formulation & Evaluation of Poly-herbal Face wash gel. 4(6): 585-588.. World J Pharm & Pharma sci 2015; 4(6): 585-8.

[3] Ashawat MS, Banchhor M. Herbal Cosmetics Trends in skin care formulation. Pharmacogn Rev 2009; 3(5): 82-9.

[4] Kanlayavattanakul M, Lourith N. Therapeutic agents and herbs in topical application for acne treatment. Int J Cosmet Sci 2011; 33(4): 289-97.
[http://dx.doi.org/10.1111/j.1468-2494.2011.00647.x] [PMID: 21401650]

[5] Chanchal D, Swarnlata S. Herbal photoprotective formulations, and their evaluation. Open Nat Prod J 2009; 2: 71-6.
[http://dx.doi.org/10.2174/1874848100902010071]

[6] Mithal BM, Saha RN. A Hand book of cosmetics. 2nd ed. Delhi: Vallabh Prakashan 2004.

[7] Kumar KK, Sasikanth K, Sabareesh M. NDorababu. Formulation and Evaluation Of DiacereinCream. Asian J Pharm Clinical Research 2011; 4(2): 93-8.

[8] Rajapet M. Amazing Benefits Of Multani Mitti For Face, Skin, And Health Cited on Dec 2016, available at http://www.stylecraze.com/articles/ benefits-of-multani-mitti-for-face/#gref 2016.

[9] Mieloch M, Witulska M. Evaluation of Skin Colouring Properties of Curcuma Longa Extract. Int. J Pharm Sci 2014; 76(4): 374-8.

[10] Bhat KV, Balasundaran M, Balagopalan M. Identification of Santalum album and Osyrislanceolata through morphological and biochemical characteristics and molecular markers to check adulteration (Final Report of the project KFRI 509/06) Available from: http://wwwdocskfriresin/KFRI-RR/KFRI-RR307pdf

[11] Sadowska-Bartosz I, Bartosz G. Effect of Antioxidants Supplementation on Aging and Longevity. J BioMed Research International 2014; (2014): 1-17.

[12] Tadimalla TR. 23 benefits of chickpea flour/gram flour/besan for skin, hair & health, Available from http://www.stylecraze.com/articles/ benefits-of-besangram-flour-for-skin-and-hair/#gref. cited 19 June 2017

[13] Kokate CK, Purohit AP, Gokhale SB. Textbook of Pharmacognosy. 49th ed. Pune: NiraliPrakashan 2014.

[14] Sinha NK. Beauty And Skin Benefits Of Milk Powder: Milk Powder Home Made Facial Mask Recipes, available from http://nutankumarisinha.expertscolumn.com/article/ 10-beauty-and-skin-benefits-milk-powder-milk-powder-home-made-facial-mask-r. 2017.http://nutankumarisinha.expertscolumn.com/article/10-beauty-and-skin-benefits-milk-powder-milk-powder-home-made-facial-mask-r Cited 20 June

[15] Basic tests for pharmaceutical dosage formsSecondedition. AITBS publisher 1998.

[16] Baby AR, Zague V, Maciel CP. Kaneko TM,Consiglieri VO, Velasco MVR. Development Of Cosmetic Mask Formulations. J Rev Bras Cienc Farm 2004; 40(1): 159-61.

[17] Wilkinson JB, Moore RJ. Harry's Cosmetology 7 th Edition. London: Longman Group 1982.

[18] MA Siddhiqui. Format for the pharmacopoeial analytical standards of compound formulation, workshop on standardization of Unani drugs, Central Council for Research in UnaniMedicine. New Delhi. 1995.

[19] World Health Organisation. Pharmaceuticals Unit: Quality control methods for medicinal plant materials:1992: Available from: http://www.who.int/iris/handle/10665/63096

[20] Lachman L, Lieberman HA, Kanig JL. The Theory and practice of Industrial pharmacy. 3rd ed. Mumbai: Verghese Publishing House 1987.

[21] Aulton ME. Pharmaceutics, The science of dosage forms design. 2nd ed. New Delhi: Churchill Livingstone 2002.

[22] Khandelwal KR. Practical Pharmacognosy. 12th ed. Pune: NiraliPrakashan 2004.

[23] Mandeep S, Shalini S, Sukhbir LK, Ram KS, Rajendra J. Preparation and Evaluation of Herbal Cosmetic Cream. Pharmacologyonline 2011; 1258-64.

2

Sensitizing Capacities and Cross-Reactivity Patterns of some Diisocyanates and Amines using the Guinea-Pig Maximization Test: Can *p*-phenylenediamine be used as a Marker for Diisocyanate Contact Allergy?

Haneen Hamada[*], Erik Zimerson, Magnus Bruze, Marléne Isaksson and Malin Engfeldt

Department of Occupational and Environmental Dermatology, Lund University, Skåne University Hospital, Malmö, Sweden

Abstract:

Background:

Isocyanates are mainly considered respiratory allergens but can also cause contact allergy. Diphenylmethane-4,4′-diamine (4,4′-MDA) has been considered a marker for diphenylmethane-4,4′-diisocyanate (4,4′-MDI) contact allergy. Furthermore, overrepresentation of positive patch-test reactions to *p*-phenylenediamine (PPD) in 4,4′-MDA positive patients have been reported.

Objectives:

To investigate the sensitizing capacities of toluene-2,4-diisocyanate (2,4-TDI) and PPD and the cross-reactivity of 4,4′-MDA, 2,4-TDI, dicyclohexylmethane-4,4′-diamine (4,4′-DMDA), dicyclohexylmethane-4,4′-diisocyanate (4,4′-DMDI), 4,4′-MDI and PPD.

Methods:

The Guinea Pig Maximization Test (GPMT) was used.

Results:

PPD was shown to be a strong sensitizer (p<0.001). Animals sensitized to PPD showed cross-reactivity to 4,4′-MDA (p<0.001). Animals sensitized to 4,4′-MDA did not show cross-reactivity to PPD. 8 animals sensitized to 2,4-TDI were sacrificed due to toxic reactions at the induction site and could thus not be fully evaluated.

Conclusion:

PPD was shown to be a strong sensitizer. However, it cannot be used as a marker for isocyanate contact allergy. On the other hand, positive reactions to 4,4′-MDA could indicate a PPD allergy. The intradermal induction concentration of 2,4-TDI (0.70% w/v) can induce strong local toxic reactions in guinea-pigs and should be lowered.

Keywords: Guinea Pig Maximization Test, PPD, Cross-reactivity, Sensitization, Diphenylmethane-4,4′-diamine, 4,4′-MDA.

1. INTRODUCTION

Diisocyanates are reactive compounds used in the production of polyurethane (PUR). PUR products are widely used and can be found in applications stretching from rigid and flexible foams to coatings, elastomers (rubber) and adhesives [1]. Diisocyanates are mainly associated with airborne occupational exposure which can lead to negative effects on the

---

* Address correspondence to this author at the Department of Occupational and Environmental Dermatology, Lund University, Skåne University Hospital, Jan Waldenströms gata 18, 205 02 Malmö, Sweden; Tel: +46(0)40331759; E-mail: haneen.hamada@med.lu.se

respiratory tract and cause airway disorder and asthma [2 - 5]. However, they can also cause contact allergy and lately the importance of the dermal exposure as possible route to isocyanate asthma has been discussed in several papers [3, 6, 7]. Allergic contact dermatitis caused by isocyanates is mainly considered to be an occupational problem and consumers are rarely exposed to isocyanates.

There are several commercially available patch-test preparations that can be used for the establishment of isocyanate contact allergy. The most common is diphenylmethane-4,4′-diisocyanate (4,4′-MDI) since it represents the most commonly used isocyanate within industry. However, patch-test preparations of 4,4′-MDI have been shown to be inadequate [8]. Therefore, the structurally related amine, diphenylmethane-4,4′-diamine (4,4′-MDA), has been suggested as a marker for 4,4′-MDI allergy [9, 10] since several reports show that workers exposed to MDI react positively to 4,4′-MDA but not to 4,4′-MDI [9 - 11]. This was confirmed in a recent animal study where the cross-reactivity patterns of 4,4′-MDI, 4,4′-MDA, dicyclohexylmethane-4,4′-diisocyanate (4,4′-DMDI) and dicylohexylmethane-4,4′-diamine (4,4′-DMDA) were investigated [12]. There are also reports of concomitant positive reactions to 4,4′-MDA and p-phenylenediamine (PPD) [13, 14].

The aim of this study was to investigate the sensitizing capacity of PPD and its cross-reactivity to 4,4′-MDI, 2,4-TDI, PPD, 4,4′-DMDI, 4,4′-MDA and 4,4′-DMDA using the guinea-pig maximization test (GPMT). All investigated substances are specified in Table 1.

Table 1. All the investigated substances including the positive control are listed together with some common synonyms, their CAS-number, their classification according to the CLP regulation[§§], their log $P_{o/w}$ as well as the purity of each investigated substance as stated by the manufacturers.

Name[§]	Synonyms	CAS-no	Structure	Harmonized Classification[§§]			log $P_{o/w}$	Purity* (%)
				Class and Category Code	Hazards Statement Code	Specific Concentration Limits		
Diphenylmethane-4,4′-diisocyanate	4,4′-MDI; 4,4′-Diisocyanatodiphenylmethane; 4,4′-Methylenebis(phenyl isocyanate); 4,4′-Methylenediphenyl diisocyanate	101-68-8		Skin Sens. 1 Resp. Sens. 1 Carc. 2	H317 H334 H351	Resp. Sens. 1; H334: C ≥ 0.1%	5.22	98%
Diphenylmethane-4,4′-diamine	4,4′-MDA; 4,4′-Methylenedianiline; 4,4′-Dimethylenediamine; 4,4′-Diaminodiphenyl methane;	101-77-9		Carc. 1B Muta. 2 Skin Sens. 1	H350 H341 H317		1.59	>98%
Dicyclohexylmethane-4,4′-diisocyanate	4,4′-DMDI; 4,4′-HMDI; Methylene bis(4-cyclohexylisocyanate); 4,4′-Methylenedicyclohexyl diisocyanate; Hydrogenated MDI;	5124-30-1		Resp. Sens. 1 Skin Sens. 1	H334 H317	Resp. Sens. 1; H334: C ≥ 0.5% Skin Sens. 1; H317: C ≥ 0.5%	6.11	91%
Dicyclohexylmethane-4,4′-diamine	4,4′-DMDA; 4,4′-HMDA; 4,4′-Diaminodicyclohexylmethane; 4,4′-Methylenebis(cyclohexylamine),	1761-71-3		Classification not harmonized but notified classification as below** Skin Sens. 1	H317		3.26	95%
p-Phenylenediamine	PPD; 1,4-diaminobenzene; benzene-1,4-diamine; para-phenylenediamine;	106-50-3		Skin Sens. 1	H317		0.43	98%
Toluene-2,4-diisocyanate	2,4-TDI; 4-methyl-m-phenylene diisocyanate; 2,4-diisocyanato-1-methylbenzene;	584-84-9		Skin Sens. 1 Resp. Sens. 1 Carc. 2	H317 H334 H351	Resp. Sens. 1; H334: C ≥ 0.1%	3.74	95%

[§] Name as used in this article; [§§] Classification as found in Annex VI of Regulation (EC) No 1272/2008 on the classification, labelling and packaging of substances and mixtures (CLP Regulation); * as stated on the package, other isomers of the substances can occur ; **Most commonly notified self-classification in ECHA's database (https://echa.europa.eu/information-on-chemicals/cl-inventory-database/-/discli/notification-details/66995/968242; last visited 2017-03-06).

2. MATERIALS AND METHODS

2.1. Chemicals

4,4′-MDI, 2,4-TDI, 4,4′-DMDI, PPD, and 4,4′-DMDA were obtained from Sigma-Aldrich Chemie GmbH (Steinheim, Germany) and 4,4′-MDA, which was obtained from TCI Europe N.V. (Zwijrdecht, Belgium). Vehicles were acetone of analytical grade obtained from Scharlau Chemie S.A. (Sentemenat, Spain), ethanol from Kemetyl AB

(Haninge, Sweden), liquid paraffin from Apoteksbolaget (Stockholm, Sweden), and propylene glycol from VWR International S.A.S. (Fontenay-sous-Bois, France). Sodium lauryl sulphate (SLS) and N,N-dimethylacetamide 99% were bought from Sigma-Aldrich Co (St. Louis, MO, USA), 2-methylol phenol (2-MP) 97% from Acros Organics (Geel, Belgium), and Imject® Freund's complete adjuvant (FCA) from Thermo Scientific (Rockford, IL, USA).

2.2. Materials

The used materials for the study were the following; Comprilan® 6 cm, elastic compression band was obtained from BSN medical GmbH (Hamburg, Germany), Al-test® from Imeco AB (Södertälje, Sweden), filter papers number 3 from Munktell Filter AB (Grycksbo, Sweden), and 1 ml syringes with injection needle 0.4×20 mm from Codan Triplus AB (Kungsbacka, Sweden). Adhesives bandages were purchased from Durapore™ 3M Health Care (St. Paul, MN, USA) and the plastic adhesive tape from Acrylastic, Biersdorf AG (Hamburg, Germany)

2.3. Ethics

The study was approved by the Lund ethical committee on animal experiments, Lund, Sweden, and conducted in accordance with ethical standards (approval No. M 340-12).

2.4. Guinea-Pig Maximization Test

The GPMT was performed according to the original description [15 - 17], which is also the method described in the OECD test guideline 406 that can be used to classify skin sensitizers according to the Globally Harmonized System of Classification and Labelling of Chemicals (GHS) [18]. Some modifications of the original method were made, e.g. statistical calculations were used to evaluate potency, furthermore non-irritant epidermal induction concentrations were used and blind readings and a positive control group was introduced in order to be able to standardize the test and objectify the evaluation of the patch test reactions [19 - 21]. The background for introducing these modifications is specified elsewhere [12, 22]. In Fig. (1) the GPMT in this study is described in detail.

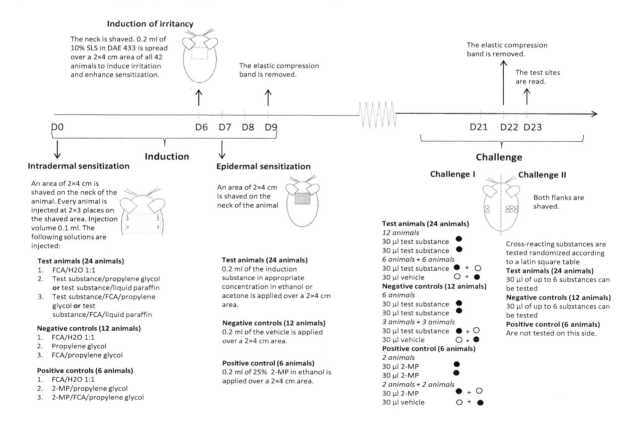

Fig. (1). Schematic figure of the performance of a sensitization series in the guinea pig maximization test in which one substance is evaluated in terms of its sensitizing capacity and cross-reactivity to the investigated substances. SLS= sodium lauryl sulphate; DAE 433= N,N-dimethylacetamide; FCA= Freund's Complete adjuvant; 2-MP= 2-Methylol phenol.

2.5. Animals

Female albino guinea-pigs weighing 400 g (±25 g) of the Hartley-Dunkin strain (HP Lidköpings Kaninfarm, Lidköping, Sweden) were used.

2.6. Topical Irritancy

Before sensitization and cross-reactivity patterns can be assessed, the topical irritancy thresholds have to be determined in order to assure that the chosen test concentrations do not give rise to irritant reactions. This was done by applying different concentrations of each of the investigated substances intended for induction as a closed patch test for 2 days on both the neck and the flank of one side of four animals pre-treated with FCA. In order to maximize the number of test concentrations that could be evaluated the animals were first tested on one side of the body and then on the other side. Concentrations that did not cause irritation were chosen for topical induction and elicitation (Table **2**).

Table 2. Summary of the sensitization and cross-reactivity rates of *p*-phenylenediamine, toluene-2,4-diisocyanate, diphenylmethane-4,4′-diisocyanate, dicyclohexylmethane-4,4′-diisocyanate and their corresponding amines diphenylmethane-4,4′-diamine, dicyclohexylmethane-4,4′-diamine using the Guinea Pig maximization test.

	Sensitization Series I	Sensitization Series II	Sensitization Series III	Sensitization Series IV	Sensitization Series V	Sensitization Series VI
Induction Intradermal and Epidermal concentrations	*p*-phenylenediamine (PPD) 0.43% p.g 0.43% EtOH	Toluene-2,4-diisocyanate (2,4-TDI) 0.70% p.o 0.70% ac	Diphenylmethane-4,4′-diisocyanate (4,4′-MDI) 1.0% p.o 1.0% ac	Diphenylmethane-4,4′-diamine (4,4′-MDA) 0.79 p.g 0.79% EtOH	Dicyclohexylmethane-4,4′-diisocyanate (4,4′-DMDI) 1.0% p.o 1.0% ac	Dicyclohexylmethane 4,4′-diamine (4,4′-DMDA) 0.84 p.g 0.84% EtOH
Challenge I Test concentration	0.43% EtOH C = 1/12 T = 20/24 V = 0/12 Pos = 5/6 p < 0.001	0.70% ac C = 2/12 T = 6/16 V = 1/4 Pos = 5/6 p = 0.22*	**	**	**	**
Challenge II PPD	0.43% EtOH C = 1/12 T = 18/24 p < 0.001	0.43% EtOH C = 3/12 T = 1/16 p = 0.20	0.43% EtOH C = 1/12 T = 1/24 p > 0.3	0.43% EtOH C = 1/12 T = 2/24 p > 0.3	0.43% EtOH C = 1/12 T = 0/24 p > 0.3	0.43% EtOH C = 1/12 T = 0/24 p > 0.3
2,4-TDI	0.70% ac C = 0/12 T = 1/24 p > 0.3	0.70% ac C = 2/12 T = 6/16 p = 0.22	0.70% ac C = 1/12 T = 2/24 p > 0.3	0.70% ac C = 0/12 T = 3/24 p = 0.28	0.70% ac C = 4/12 T = 1/24 p > 0.3	0.70% ac C = 1/12 T = 0/24 p > 0.3
4,4′-MDI	1.0% ac C = 2/12 T = 2/24 p > 0.3	1.0% ac C = 1/12 T = 2/16 p > 0.3	**	**	**	**
4,4′-MDA	0.79% EtOH C = 3/12 T = 21/24 p < 0.001	0.79% EtOH C = 5/12 T = 6/16 p > 0.3	**	**	**	**
4,4′-DMDI	1.0% ac C = 0/12 T = 2/24 p > 0.3	1.0% ac C = 3/12 T = 8/16 p = 0.17	**	**	**	**
4,4′-DMDA	0.84% EtOH C = 0/12 T = 6/24 p = 0.070	0.84% EtOH C = 3/12 T = 6/16 p > 0.3	**	**	**	**

p.o = liquid paraffin; p.g = propylene glycol; EtOH = ethanol; ac = acetone
C = negative control animals (in total 12); T = test animals (in total 24); V = reactions to the vehicle in test animals (in total 12); pos = positive control animals (in total 6)
* = 8 animals sacrificed due to strong toxic reactions. P-value not significant.
** presented elsewhere [13].

2.7. Concentrations

Equimolar concentrations were used for the tested substances. The concentrations used for induction and challenge are given in Table **2**.

2.8. Induction

24 test animals, 12 control animals and 6 positive control animals were used for induction for each sensitization series (Table **2**).

Day 0: All animals were shaved on the neck and thereafter 3 intradermal injections in a row on each side of the shoulder were given, thus 6 injections in total. For the test animals the following injections were made in duplicate: 1)

0.1 ml of 40% FCA in water (w/v); 2) 0.1 ml of the test substance (w/v) in propylene glycol or liquid paraffin; 3) 0.1 ml of a mixture of the test substance and FCA in propylene glycol or liquid paraffin in which the concentration for test substance was the same as in 2) and the concentration of FCA was the same as in 1). For 1) and 2) the vehicle varied depending upon if the sensitizing substance was an isocyanate or an amine since isocyanates can react with propylene glycol which normally is the vehicle of choice. For sensitization series II, III and V liquid paraffin was used and for sensitization and for series I, IV and VI propylene glycol was used (Table **2**). For the control animals, the following injections were made in duplicate: 1) 0.1 ml of 40% FCA in water (w/v); 2) 0.1 ml propylene glycol; 3) 0.1 ml of 40% FCA in propylene glycol (w/v). For the positive control animals, the following injections were made in duplicate: 1) 0.1 ml of 40% FCA in water (w/v); 2) 0.1 ml of 25% 2-MP in propylene glycol (w/v); 3) 0.1 ml of 25% 2-MP and 40% FCA in water (w/v).

Day 6: All animals were shaved on the neck and thereafter they underwent a pretreatment of the 2×4 cm area intended for topical induction in order to induce irritancy. The area was treated with 0.2 ml of a preparation consisting of 10% SLS (w/v) in dimethyl acetamide/acetone/99.5% ethanol (DAE) 4:3:3 (v/v/v).

Day 7: All animals were shaved on the neck and thereafter epidermal induction was made in the test animals and the positive controls animals by applying 0.2 ml of the sensitizing substance in acetone or ethanol, depending upon the nature of the sensitizing substance on a 2×4 cm piece of filter paper placed on adhesives bandages. The patches were covered with impermeable plastic adhesive tape and held in place by adhesive bandages. The patches were left on for 48 hours. The control animals were patch tested with the vehicle alone but in the same manner as the test animals and the positive controls.

2.9. Challenge

The challenge procedure consists of two parts; challenge I in which the sensitization rate of the test substance used in the induction is assessed and challenge II in which cross-reactivity to other substances is assessed. Challenge I and II are performed at the same time but on different flanks of the animal; challenge I is performed on the left flank and challenge II on the right.

Day 21: All animals were shaved on their left flank and the test animals and control animals were also shaved on their right flank.

Challenge I (left flank, 2 patches) was performed by challenging 12 test animals with the induction substance in acetone or ethanol, depending on whether it was an isocyanate or an amine, on both the cranial and caudal patch. 6 + 6 test animals were challenged with the induction substance on either the cranial or the caudal patch, and the vehicle (acetone or ethanol) alone on the other patch. 6 of the control animals were tested with the induction substance on both patches and 3 + 3 animals were patch tested with the induction substance on either the cranial or the caudal patch, and the vehicle alone on the other patch. 2 of the positive control animals were tested with 2-MP on both the patches and 2+2 animals were patch tested with 2-MP on either the cranial or the caudal patch, and the vehicle alone on the other patch. Al-test® on Durapore™ adhesive band was used for patch testing. 30 µl test solution was applied. The patches were covered with impermeable plastic adhesive tape and held in place by adhesive bandages.

Challenge II (right flank, 6 patches) was performed on 24 test animals and 12 negative control animals by patch testing with putative cross-reacting substances. The distribution of the positions of the test substance was based on a Latin square table. In this article, cross-reactions to 4,4′-MDI, 4,4′-MDA, 4,4′-DMDI, 4,4′-DMDA in animals sensitized to PPD and 2,4-TDI, respectively, are presented. The results of the investigation of sensitizing capacity of PPD and 2,4-TDI are also presented. The sensitizing capacities of 4,4′-MDI, 4,4′-MDA, 4,4′-DMDI and 4,4′-DMDA as well as the cross-reactivity between the four substances are described elsewhere [12].

2.10. Evaluation

Day 23: The minimum criterion for a positive reaction was a confluent erythema. All tests were evaluated blindly 24 hours after the patch tests had been removed, i.e. 48 hours after test application. First, the left flanks of all the animals were read and thereafter, still blindly and without knowing the test outcome of the left side, the right flanks were read on all animals except the positive controls.

2.11. Statistics

The proportion of positive animals within the test group was compared to the proportion of positive animals in the control group. Among the animals challenged with the induction substance on both the cranial and caudal patches (12 test animals and 6 negative control animals) only one of the patches, chosen in advance, was included.

Statistical significance for the sensitizing capacity and cross-reactivity was calculated with one-sided Fisher's exact test. When significant values ($p < 0.05$) were obtained with Fisher's exact test the compound was considered a sensitizer or showing cross-reactivity to other compounds based upon set criterion ($p < 0.001$ strong, $p < 0.01$ moderate, $p < 0.05$ weak). Indicated cross-reactivity was defined $0.050 \le p < 0.3$.

3. RESULTS

Six different sensitization series were performed at different occasions during a period stretching from May 2013 to September 2015. The results regarding sensitization to PPD and 2,4-TDI as well as the cross-reactivity patterns for each of these series are given in Table **2**. For all the sensitization series equimolar concentrations were tested. In Fig. (**2**), the sensitizing capacity as well as cross-reactivity patterns for the sensitization series are presented.

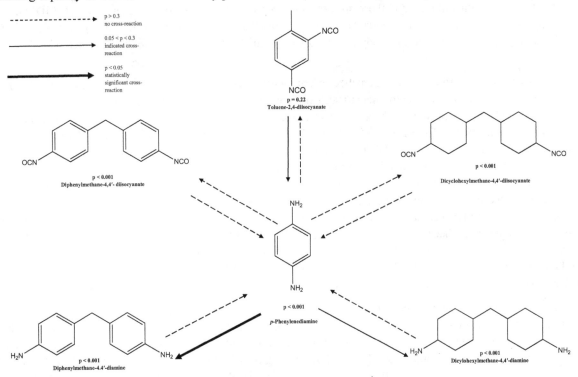

Fig. (2). PPD sensitizing capacity and cross-reactivity to diisocyanates and their corresponding amines using GPMT. The figure shows the sensitizing capacity and cross-reactivity pattern of all the investigated substances.. All the depicted substances were used separately for induction and challenge. The arrows point from the induction substance towards the substance investigated for cross-reactivity.

3.1. Sensitizing Capacity

PPD was shown to be a strong sensitizer ($p < 0.001$). The sensitizing capacity of 2,4-TDI ($p = 0.22$) was based on a test group of 16 test animals instead of 24 since 8 test animals had to be sacrificed due to oozing wounds at the intradermal injection site whose capacity to dry and form crusts was considered to deviate from what was stated in the ethical approval (Table **2**).

3.2. Cross-Reactivity

The cross-reaction patterns between the investigated substances when tested equimolar are presented in Fig. (**2**). Animals sensitized to PPD showed cross-reactivity to 4,4′-MDA ($p < 0.001$). The cross-reactivity did not go in both directions, i.e. animals sensitized to 4,4′-MDA did not show cross-reactivity to PPD. Since 8 animals in the 2,4-TDI induction series (series II, Table **2**) were sacrificed statistically significant cross-reactivity patterns could not be fully evaluated.

4. DISCUSSION

4.1. Sensitizing Capacity

The exposure to diisocyanates is usually highest in settings where PUR products are produced industrially. However, exposure in do-it-yourself settings has also been reported [23 - 25, 26]. The main exposure route for isocyanates is through inhalation [27], and can also occur when PUR products are heated at high temperatures as this leads to degradation of PUR resulting in release of isocyanates, amines and aminoisocyanates [28]. Dermal exposure has been suggested to contribute to respiratory problems and in animal models it has been shown that dermal sensitization could trigger respiratory response when isocyanates are inhaled [29 - 32].

Contact allergy to isocyanates has been considered a minor problem compared to the respiratory issues and, additionally, much less reported in literature. It has been suggested that the strict rules of handling of isocyanates to avoid respiratory problems have contributed to minimize contamination of skin and thus contact allergy [33]. However, isocyanates do cause contact allergy and there are especially reports describing contact allergy to 4,4'-MDI and 4,4'-DMDI. Many of these reports have also shown simultaneous positive reactions to the corresponding amines, 4,4'-MDA and 4,4'-DMDA [13, 34 - 39]. In a recent study it was shown that all 4 are sensitizers when investigated with the GPMT [12].

2,4-TDI has been shown to be a strong sensitizer when investigated with the local lymph node assay (LLNA) [40], and has also been described to cause active sensitization in humans following patch testing with 1% 2,4-TDI in pet [40, 41]. Additionally, TDI has been found to be a strong sensitizer both in mouse ear swelling test (MEST) [42] and in the Buehler test on guinea-pigs [43]. LLNA, MEST and Buehler tests are methods that do not involve intradermal injections of allergens as done in the GPMT, in which the allergens are injected intradermally to induce sensitization. In the present study, it could not be statistically significantly shown that 2,4-TDI is a sensitizer based upon our set criteria, when using Fisher's exact test on the results from the remaining 16 animals. Therefore,it was not possible to fully evaluate the substance since 8 animals were sacrificed due to oozing wounds at the site of the intradermal injection and whose capacity to dry and form crusts was considered to deviate from what was stated in the ethical approval. However, if the sacrificed animals had been positive, the results of 2,4-TDI would have been statistically significant and would have indicated that 2,4-TDI is a moderate skin sensitizer. Notably, based upon the 16 animals that could be read (Table 2) 2,4-TDI fulfil the criteria for classification as subcategory 1B skin sensitizer according to GHS and the CLP regulation since ≥30% to ≤ 60% of the test animals responded at > 0.1% to ≤1.0% intradermal induction dose.

In the present study the sensitizing capacity of PPD was also studied. PPD is an ingredient in hair dyes and is considered a potent contact sensitizer. It is usually used to detect hair dye allergy [38, 39, 44]. In this study it was shown to be a strong sensitizer ($p < 0.001$). This is in accordance with other studies in which PPD has been shown to be a strong sensitizer in both LLNA and GPMT [46 - 48]. According to GHS and the CLP regulation PPD can be classified as a subcategory 1A skin sensitizer i. e strong sensitizer, since ≥60% of the test animals responded to > 0.1% to ≤ 1% intradermal induction dose.

4.2. Cross-Reactivity

4,4'-MDA has been suggested to be a marker of 4,4'-MDI allergy [9, 10] which was supported when investigating their cross-reactivity pattern with GPMT [12]. In this context, the term cross-reactivity refers to when an individual initially sensitized to one chemically defined substance (A) reacts to a second chemically defined substance (B) that he or she has not been in previous contact with. The first compound is the primary sensitizer while the other is the secondary sensitizer [48]. Cross-reactivity can occur because A and B are structurally similar, or because A is metabolized to a compound that is similar to B and vice versa, or because A and B are both metabolized into similar compounds [49]. Cross-reactivity does not need to go in both directions, i.e if A is a primary sensitizer giving rise to reaction to the secondary sensitizer B it does not automatically mean that a primary sensitization to B also give rise to a reaction to A.

Studies have also reported concurrent reactions between 4,4'-MDA and PPD [13]. One study showed that one third of the 4,4'-MDA positive patients also reacted to PPD [14]. A study presenting clinical patch-test data indicated that "para-amino" compounds could cross-react with each other. Patients positive to PPD were also positive to 4,4'-MDA and other para-amino compounds that are similar in structure [50]. Cross-reactivity has also been reported between PPD and azo dyes [51]. In the present study guinea pigs sensitized to PPD, showed cross-reactivity to 4,4'-MDA which indicates that 4,4'-MDA can be used for detection of PPD contact allergy which supports earlier findings [13]. The

Sensitizing Capacities and Cross-Reactivity Patterns of some Diisocyanates and Amines...

17

cross-reactivity between 4,4′-MDA and PPD should be taken into consideration if 4,4′-MDA is used as a marker for 4,4′-MDI and it should be considered that a positive reaction to 4,4′-MDA could also be a sign of hair dye habits and not only isocyanate exposure. Since no cross-reactivity could be found between 4,4′-MDI and PPD, one can assume that, individuals with hair dye allergy can work with isocyanates. However, it is noteworthy that in many plastic applications, such as PUR production and epoxy applications, 4,4′-MDA at least has been used as a hardener. Thus, nothing in the results from this study suggests that 4,4′-MDI sensitized individuals have a higher risk to develop eczema when dying their hair. However, we cannot draw any conclusions on whether 2,4-TDI sensitized individuals are more likely to develop eczema from hair dyes containing PPD since the result could not be fully evaluated due to the sacrifice of 8 animals which resulted in non-significant p-value. However, it should be noted that an indicated cross-reactivity to PPD was seen in animals sensitized with 2,4-TDI ($p=0.20$). It is possible that significant results had been seen if all the sacrificed animals had been positive. In a study by Tanaka et al, cross-reactivity between MDI and 2,4-TDI was indeed shown in MEST [52].

In the present study there was also an indicated cross-reactivity to 4,4′-DMDA ($p=0.069$) in animals sensitized to PPD. In this study all substances were tested equimolar to each other in order to be able to compare the sensitizing capacities between the investigated substances. However, the GPMT is a method that is defined by maximization which, according to the original method, means that the animals are sensitized with the highest non-irritating concentration of the test substance regardless of the equimolarity. If the substances in this study had been tested according to the original method it is possible that statistically significant numbers of reactions had been seen for 4,4′-DMDA in the animals sensitized to PPD. This, together with the fact that the previous GPMT-study [12] showed cross-reactivity to 4,4′-DMDA in animals sensitized to 4,4′-MDA and an indicated cross-reactivity in the reversed situation highlights the need of further studies to investigate the cross-reactivity patterns between the investigated amines and other structurally close substances such as 2,4-TDA, Disperse Orange 3 and other azo-dyes.

CONCLUSION

PPD was shown to be a strong sensitizer. PPD-sensitized animals showed cross-reactivity to 4,4′-MDA. However, PPD cannot be used as a marker for isocyanate contact allergy. Our results indicate that allergy to 4,4′-MDA can indicate sensitization to either PPD or 4,4′-MDI or to both. Our results do not support the suspicion that PPD allergic individuals should avoid working with isocyanates since no cross-reactivity between PPD and 4,4′- MDI could be shown. The intradermal induction concentration of 2,4-TDI (0.70% w/v) can induce strong local reactions in guinea-pigs and should be lowered.

AUTHOR CONTRIBUTIONS

All authors have participated sufficiently to take public responsibility for the work.

FUNDING

Swedish Research Council for Health, Working Life and Welfare.

HUMAN AND ANIMAL RIGHTS

The work is approved by the swedish/european ethical comitee of animal testing.

CONFLICT OF INTEREST

The authors declare no conflict of interest, financial or otherwise.

ACKNOWLEDGEMENTS

The authors thank Monica Andersson, Lena Persson and Lotta Thorsson for skilful technical assistance and the Swedish Research Council for Health, Working Life and Welfare for providing funds.

REFERENCES

[1]   Eckert H. Chemistry and technology of isocyanates. In: Von H. Ulrich, Ed. Angewandte Chemie. New York: John Wiley and Sons; 1997;109(21):2487

[2]   Redlich CA. Skin exposure and asthma: Is there a connection? Proc Am Thorac Soc 2010; 7(2): 134-7.
        [http://dx.doi.org/10.1513/pats.201002-025RM] [PMID: 20427586]

[3]   Redlich CA, Karol MH. Diisocyanate asthma: Clinical aspects and immunopathogenesis. Int Immunopharmacol 2002; 2(2-3): 213-24.
        [http://dx.doi.org/10.1016/S1567-5769(01)00174-6] [PMID: 11811926]

[4]   Kimber I, Dearman RJ, Basketter DA. Diisocyanates, occupational asthma and IgE antibody: Implications for hazard characterization. J Appl Toxicol 2014; 34(10): 1073-7.
        [http://dx.doi.org/10.1002/jat.3041] [PMID: 25059672]

[5]   Bernstein JA. Overview of diisocyanate occupational asthma. Toxicology 1996; 111(1-3): 181-9.
        [http://dx.doi.org/10.1016/0300-483X(96)03375-6] [PMID: 8711734]

[6]   Bello D, Herrick CA, Smith TJ, et al. Skin exposure to isocyanates: Reasons for concern. Environ Health Perspect 2007; 115(3): 328-35.
        [http://dx.doi.org/10.1289/ehp.9557] [PMID: 17431479]

[7]   Liljelind I, Norberg C, Egelrud L, Westberg H, Eriksson K, Nylander-French LA. Dermal and inhalation exposure to methylene bisphenyl isocyanate (MDI) in iron foundry workers. Ann Occup Hyg 2010; 54(1): 31-40.
        [PMID: 19783835]

[8]   Frick M, Zimerson E, Karlsson D, et al. Poor correlation between stated and found concentrations of diphenylmethane-4,4'-diisocyanate (4,4'-MDI) in petrolatum patch-test preparations. Contact Dermat 2004; 51(2): 73-8.
        [http://dx.doi.org/10.1111/j.0105-1873.2004.00404.x] [PMID: 15373847]

[9]   Estlander T, Keskinen H, Jolanki R, Kanerva L. Occupational dermatitis from exposure to polyurethane chemicals. Contact Dermat 1992; 27(3): 161-5.
        [http://dx.doi.org/10.1111/j.1600-0536.1992.tb05246.x] [PMID: 1451461]

[10]   Goossens A, Detienne T, Bruze M. Occupational allergic contact dermatitis caused by isocyanates. Contact Dermat 2002; 47(5): 304-8.
        [http://dx.doi.org/10.1034/j.1600-0536.2002.470509.x] [PMID: 12534536]

[11]   Frick M, Björkner B, Hamnerius N, Zimerson E. Allergic contact dermatitis from dicyclohexylmethane-4,4'-diisocyanate. Contact Dermat 2003; 48(6): 305-9.
        [http://dx.doi.org/10.1034/j.1600-0536.2003.00123.x] [PMID: 14531868]

[12]   Hamada H, Bruze M, Zimerson E, Isaksson M, Engfeldt M. Sensitization and cross-reactivity patterns of contact allergy to diisocyanates and corresponding amines: investigation of diphenylmethane-4,4'-diisocyanate, diphenylmethane-4,4'-diamine, dicyclohexylmethane-4,4'-diisocyanate, and dicylohexylmethane-4,4'-diamine. Contact Dermat 2017; 77(4): 231-41.
        [http://dx.doi.org/10.1111/cod.12809] [PMID: 28555927]

[13]   Engfeldt M, Goossens A, Isaksson M, Zimerson E, Bruze M. The outcome of 9 years of consecutive patch testing with 4,4'-diaminodiphenylmethane and 4,4'-diphenylmethane diisocyanate. Contact Dermat 2013; 68(2): 98-102.
        [http://dx.doi.org/10.1111/j.1600-0536.2012.02158.x] [PMID: 22928981]

[14]   Liippo J, Lammintausta K. Contact sensitization to 4,4'-diaminodiphenylmethane and to isocyanates among general dermatology patients. Contact Dermat 2008; 59(2): 109-14.
        [http://dx.doi.org/10.1111/j.1600-0536.2008.01375.x] [PMID: 18759878]

[15]   Magnusson B. Identification of contact sensitizers by animal assay. Contact Dermat 1980; 6(1): 46-50.
        [http://dx.doi.org/10.1111/j.1600-0536.1980.tb03894.x] [PMID: 7398258]

[16]   Magnusson B, Kligman AM. The identification of contact allergens by animal assay. The guinea pig maximization test. J Invest Dermatol 1969; 52(3): 268-76.
        [http://dx.doi.org/10.1038/jid.1969.42] [PMID: 5774356]

[17]   Magnusson B, Kligman AM. Allergic contact dermatitis in the guinea pig; Identifications of contact allergens. Springfield, Ill: Charles Thomas 1970.

[18]   Globally Harmonized System of Classification and Labelling of Chemicals (GHS). 6th ed. New York Geneva: United Nations; 2016.

[19]   Bruze M. Contact sensitizers in resins based on phenol and formaldehyde. Acta Derm Venereol Suppl (Stockh) 1985; 119: 1-83.
        [PMID: 2934936]

[20]   Malinauskiene L, Zimerson E, Bruze M, Ryberg K, Isaksson M. Sensitizing capacity of Disperse Orange 1 and its potential metabolites from azo reduction and their cross-reactivity pattern. Contact Dermat 2013; 69(1): 40-8.
        [http://dx.doi.org/10.1111/cod.12078] [PMID: 23782357]

[21]   Wahlberg JE, Boman A. Guinea pig maximization test. Curr Probl Dermatol 1985; 14: 59-106.
       [http://dx.doi.org/10.1159/000411607] [PMID: 3905272]

[22]   Bruze M. Relevance of sensitization studies in guinea pigs. Acta Derm Venereol Suppl (Stockh) 1988; 135: 21-3.
       [PMID: 3163454]

[23]   Belsito DV. Common shoe allergens undetected by commercial patch-testing kits: Dithiodimorpholine and isocyanates. Am J Contact Dermat
       2003; 14(2): 95-6.
       [http://dx.doi.org/10.1097/01634989-200306000-00010] [PMID: 14749029]

[24]   Krone CA. Diisocyanates and nonoccupational disease: A review. Arch Environ Health 2004; 59(6): 306-16.
       [PMID: 16238165]

[25]   Militello G, Sasseville D, Ditre C, Brod BA. Allergic contact dermatitis from isocyanates among sculptors. Dermatitis 2004; 15(3): 150-3.
       [http://dx.doi.org/10.2310/6620.2004.04013] [PMID: 15724350]

[26]   Verschoor L, Verschoor AH. Nonoccupational and occupational exposure to isocyanates. Curr Opin Pulm Med 2014; 20(2): 199-204.
       [http://dx.doi.org/10.1097/MCP.0000000000000029] [PMID: 24366354]

[27]   Streicher RP, Reh CM, Key-Schwartz RJ, Schlecht PC, Cassinelli ME, O'Connor PF. Determination of airborne isocyanate exposure:
       Considerations in method selection. AIHAJ 2000; 61(4): 544-56.
       [http://dx.doi.org/10.1080/15298660008984567] [PMID: 10976685]

[28]   Karlsson D, Spanne M, Dalene M, Skarping G. Airborne thermal degradation products of polyurethene coatings in car repair shops. J Environ
       Monit 2000; 2(5): 462-9.
       [http://dx.doi.org/10.1039/b004562o] [PMID: 11254051]

[29]   Erjefält I, Persson CG. Increased sensitivity to toluene diisocyanate (TDI) in airways previously exposed to low doses of TDI. Clin Exp
       Allergy 1992; 22(9): 854-62.
       [http://dx.doi.org/10.1111/j.1365-2222.1992.tb02831.x] [PMID: 1330235]

[30]   Karol MH, Stadler J, Underhill D, Alarie Y. Monitoring delayed-onset pulmonary hypersensitivity in guinea pigs. Toxicol Appl Pharmacol
       1981; 61(2): 277-85.
       [http://dx.doi.org/10.1016/0041-008X(81)90418-X] [PMID: 7324069]

[31]   Kimber I. The role of the skin in the development of chemical respiratory hypersensitivity. Toxicol Lett 1996; 86(2-3): 89-92.
       [http://dx.doi.org/10.1016/0378-4274(96)03678-8] [PMID: 8711782]

[32]   Rattray NJ, Botham PA, Hext PM, et al. Induction of respiratory hypersensitivity to diphenylmethane-4,4'-diisocyanate (MDI) in guinea pigs.
       Influence of route of exposure. Toxicology 1994; 88(1-3): 15-30.
       [http://dx.doi.org/10.1016/0300-483X(94)90108-2] [PMID: 8160196]

[33]   Björkner B, Frick M, Pontén A, Zimerson E. Plastic Materials. 4th ed. Berlin, Heidelberg: Springer-Verlag 2011; pp. 583-622.

[34]   Emmett EA. Allergic contact dermatitis in polyurethane plastic moulders. J Occup Med 1976; 18(12): 802-4.
       [http://dx.doi.org/10.1097/00043764-197612000-00006] [PMID: 136505]

[35]   Frick M, Isaksson M, Björkner B, Hindsén M, Pontén A, Bruze M. Occupational allergic contact dermatitis in a company manufacturing
       boards coated with isocyanate lacquer. Contact Dermat 2003; 48(5): 255-60.
       [http://dx.doi.org/10.1034/j.1600-0536.2003.00107.x] [PMID: 12868966]

[36]   Malten KE. 4,4' diisocyanato dicyclohexyl methane (Hylene W): A strong contact sensitizer. Contact Dermat 1977; 3(6): 344-6.
       [http://dx.doi.org/10.1111/j.1600-0536.1977.tb03705.x] [PMID: 146591]

[37]   White IR, Stewart JR, Rycroft RJ. Allergic contact dermatitis from an organic di-isocyanate. Contact Dermat 1983; 9(4): 300-3.
       [http://dx.doi.org/10.1111/j.1600-0536.1983.tb04395.x] [PMID: 6225609]

[38]   Yazar K, Boman A, Lidén C. Potent skin sensitizers in oxidative hair dye products on the Swedish market. Contact Dermat 2009; 61(5):
       269-75.
       [http://dx.doi.org/10.1111/j.1600-0536.2009.01612.x] [PMID: 19878241]

[39]   Yazar K, Boman A, Lidén C. p-Phenylenediamine and other hair dye sensitizers in Spain. Contact Dermat 2012; 66(1): 27-32.
       [http://dx.doi.org/10.1111/j.1600-0536.2011.01979.x] [PMID: 22085034]

[40]   van Och FM, Slob W, de Jong WH, Vandebriel RJ, van Loveren H. A quantitative method for assessing the sensitizing potency of low
       molecular weight chemicals using a local lymph node assay: employment of a regression method that includes determination of the
       uncertainty margins. Toxicology 2000; 146(1): 49-59.
       [http://dx.doi.org/10.1016/S0300-483X(00)00165-7] [PMID: 10773362]

[41]   Le Coz CJ, El Aboubi S, Ball C. Active sensitization to toluene di-isocyanate. Contact Dermat 1999; 41(2): 104-5.
       [http://dx.doi.org/10.1111/j.1600-0536.1999.tb06239.x] [PMID: 10445695]

[42]   Gad SC, Dunn BJ, Dobbs DW, Reilly C, Walsh RD. Development and validation of an alternative dermal sensitization test: The mouse ear
       swelling test (MEST). Toxicol Appl Pharmacol 1986; 84(1): 93-114.
       [http://dx.doi.org/10.1016/0041-008X(86)90419-9] [PMID: 3715870]

[43]   Zissu D, Binet S, Limasset JC. Cutaneous sensitization to some polyisocyanate prepolymers in guinea pigs. Contact Dermat 1998; 39(5):
       248-51.

[http://dx.doi.org/10.1111/j.1600-0536.1998.tb05918.x] [PMID: 9840262]

[44]   Young E, Svedman C, Zimerson E, Engfeldt M, Bruze M. Is p-phenylenediamine (PPD) a better marker of contact allergy to PPD-based hair dyes than its salt PPD dihydrochloride? Contact Dermat 2016; 75(1): 59-61.
        [http://dx.doi.org/10.1111/cod.12572] [PMID: 27264294]

[45]   Warbrick EV, Dearman RJ, Lea LJ, Basketter DA, Kimber I. Local lymph node assay responses to paraphenylenediamine: Intra- and inter-laboratory evaluations. J Appl Toxicol 1999; 19(4): 255-60.
        [http://dx.doi.org/10.1002/(SICI)1099-1263(199907/08)19:4<255::AID-JAT573>3.0.CO;2-S] [PMID: 10439339]

[46]   Yamano T, Shimizu M. Skin sensitization potency and cross-reactivity of p-phenylenediamine and its derivatives evaluated by non-radioactive murine local lymph node assay and guinea-pig maximization test. Contact Dermat 2009; 60(4): 193-8.
        [http://dx.doi.org/10.1111/j.1600-0536.2008.01500.x] [PMID: 19338586]

[47]   Søsted H, Basketter DA, Estrada E, Johansen JD, Patlewicz GY. Ranking of hair dye substances according to predicted sensitization potency: Quantitative structure-activity relationships. Contact Dermat 2004; 51(5-6): 241-54.
        [http://dx.doi.org/10.1111/j.0105-1873.2004.00440.x] [PMID: 15606648]

[48]   Benezra C, Maibach H. True cross-sensitization, false cross-sensitization and otherwise. Contact Dermat 1984; 11(2): 65-9.
        [http://dx.doi.org/10.1111/j.1600-0536.1984.tb00928.x] [PMID: 6488781]

[49]   Lepoittevin JP. Molecular Aspects in Allergic and Irritant Contact Dermatitis. 5th ed. Berlin, Heidelberg: Springer 2011; pp. 91-110.
        [http://dx.doi.org/10.1007/978-3-642-03827-3_4]

[50]   Uter W, Lessmann H, Geier J, Becker D, Fuchs T, Richter G. The spectrum of allergic (cross-)sensitivity in clinical patch testing with 'para amino' compounds. Allergy 2002; 57(4): 319-22.
        [http://dx.doi.org/10.1034/j.1398-9995.2002.1o3314.x] [PMID: 11906362]

[51]   Di Prisco MC, Puig L, Alomar A. Contact dermatitis due to para-phenylenediamine (PPD) on a temporal tattoo with henna. Cross reaction to azoic dyes. Invest Clin 2006; 47(3): 295-9.
        [PMID: 17672289]

[52]   Tanaka K, Takeoka A, Nishimura F, Hanada S. Contact sensitivity induced in mice by methylene bisphenyl diisocyanate. Contact Dermat 1987; 17(4): 199-204.
        [http://dx.doi.org/10.1111/j.1600-0536.1987.tb02713.x] [PMID: 2827956]

3

Higher Risk of Future Cardiovascular Events Among Patients with Psoriatic Arthritis Compared to Psoriatic Patients between the Ages of 30-50

Magdalena Krajewska–Włodarczyk[1], Agnieszka Owczarczyk-Saczonek[2,*] and Waldemar Placek[2]

[1]Department of Rheumatology of Municipal Hospital in Olsztyn, Olsztyn, Poland
[2]Department of Dermatology, Sexually Transmitted Diseases and Clinical Immunology, The University of Warmia and Mazury in Olsztyn, Olsztyn, Poland

Abstract:

Introduction:

Psoriasis and Psoriatic Arthritis (PsA) are chronic diseases with a number of complications that, among others, may include alterations in the cardio-vascular system.

Methods:

The aim of this study was to evaluate the risk of Cardiovascular Diseases (CVD) in patients with psoriasis and psoriatic arthritis between the ages of 30-50. The research covered 95 outpatients and inpatients: 51 with plaque psoriasis (23 women and 28 men) and 44 with psoriasis and psoriatic arthritis (16 women and 28 men). The risk of cardio-vascular incident was evaluated with the use of the Framingham algorithm covering the age, total cholesterol, HDL cholesterol, blood pressure, the habit of smoking and diabetes. The 10-year risk of the occurrence of a cardio-vascular incident was higher in patients with psoriatic arthritis than in patients with plaque psoriasis (9,9% *vs*6,2%). A high risk of cardio-vascular events was observed in 35% men with psoriatic arthritis in comparison to 11% men with only psoriasis. In patients with plaque psoriasis, the increase in the risk of cardio-vascular incident was connected with the late beginning of psoriasis; whereas in the group of patients with psoriatic arthritis, the risk of cardio-vascular incident was connected with the intensification of psoriatic lesions.

Conclusion:

The patients with psoriasis, especially men with psoriatic arthritis, certainly require special medical care in terms of cardio-vascular diseases prevention.

Key words: Cardiovascular Diseases, Psoriatic Arthritis, Psoriatic Patients, Psoriasis, Chronic Diseases, Cholesterol

1. INTRODUCTION

Psoriasis and Psoriatic Arthritis (PsA) are chronic diseases of complex pathogenesis and heterogeneous clinical course with a number of complications which may include Cardiovascular Diseases (CVD). The latest epidemiological studies prove that metabolic disorders (insulin resistance, atherogenic dyslipidemia, hypertension) often co-exist with cardiovascular diseases in psoriatic patients, especially with a severe course of the disease [1,2]. The newest European consensus regarding the prevention of CVD in 2012 was developed by the European Society of Cardiology, among others, and includes psoriasis to the diseases which carry an increased risk of the development of CVD [3]. Age, gender, smoking, hypertension, hyperlipidemia or type 2 diabetes are traditional risk factors, and obviously influence the progress of CVD. However, this also occurs in patients with psoriasis and psoriatic arthritis.

* Address correspondence to this author at the Department Dermatology, Sexually Transmitted Diseases and Clinical Dermatology, The University of Warmia and Mazury, Al. Wojska Polskiego 30, 10-900 Olsztyn, Poland; E-mail: aganek@wp.pl

Various scales were elaborated and validated for the evaluation of the total cardiovascular risk, as well as the development of the risk of defined manifestations of cardiovascular diseases (*e.g.* stroke, coronary artery disease) or death during the course of the disease. The Framingham algorithm is a multifactorial algorithm including age, gender, hypertension, total cholesterol, HDL cholesterol, diabetes and the habit of smoking that estimates a 10-year risk of the occurrence of myocardial infraction or death due to cardiovascular reasons [4]. The patients with a defined high risk (*i.e.* 10-year risk > 20%) should constitute a group requiring intensive preventive action in the area of modifiable risk factors (hypertension, dyslipidemia, diabetes t.2). The simplicity of this algorithm enables it to be used in everyday practice and the height of the estimated risk may be a starting point in making a decision about the introduction, the type and intensity of the actions within the prevention of CVD. So far, single reports concerning a higher risk than the general population for a serious cardio-vascular incident or death in patients with psoriasis, based on the Framingham algorithm have been issued [5]. Our research is the first study that is attempting to compare the estimated risk with the Framingham algorithm risk of cardiovascular incidents in patients with psoriasis or psoriatic arthritis.

2. AIM OF THE STUDY

The main aim of this study was an evaluation of the risk of developing CVD in patients with psoriasis and psoriatic arthritis between the ages of 30-50.

3. MATERIALS AND METHODS

This study covered 95 people: 51 with plaque psoriasis (23 women and 28 men) and 44 with psoriasis and psoriatic arthritis (16 women and 28 men) between the ages of 30-50, treated in the Department of Dermatology and the Department of Rheumatology of Municipal Hospital in Olsztyn. The studies were performed in the years 2011-2013. Patients with chronic and severe inflammatory diseases other than psoriasis and psoriatic arthritis, such as malignancies, or severe cardiovascular incidents (myocardial infarction or stroke) were excluded.

In every patient, the following anthropometric parameters were evaluated: body mass index – BMI, waist circumference, and blood pressure. During dermatological examination, the severity of psoriasis was estimated with a PASI score (*Psoriasis Area Severity Index*), a BSA score (*Body Surface Area*) and an influence on the quality of life score - DLQI (*Dermatology Life Quality Index*). On these bases, the degree of the severity of psoriasis was evaluated, based on the latest findings of a group of experts known as EuCOTT from 2011 [6]. The group with mild psoriasis included the patients whose PASI, BSA and DLQI score was ≤ 10 points. Severe psoriasis included the patients with a PASI or BSA score > 10 points and a DLQI > 10 points.

The laboratory tests for lipids (HDL, total cholesterol, triglycerides) and glucose were performed 12 hours after the last meal (fasting). A metabolic syndrome was recognized based on expert opinion from 2009 using the modified criteria developed by the IDF (International Diabetes Federation). Abdominal obesity (defined as a waist circumference for Europeans ≥ 94 cm for men, ≥ 80 cm for women) was not a preliminary criterion for the diagnosis, but was one of them. A metabolic syndrome was recognized if 3 out of 5 criteria were fulfilled (abdominal obesity, triglycerides ≥ 150 mg/dl or current treatment for hypertriglyceridemia; HDL < 40 mg/dl for men and < 50 mg/dl for women; blood glucose ≥ 100 mg/dl or pharmacotherapy for hyperglycemia and blood pressure with a systolic ≥ 130 and/or a diastolic ≥ 85 mm Hg or hypotensive pharmacotherapy) [7]. The risk of the development of cardio-vascular diseases was evaluated with the use of the Framingham algorithm including age, total cholesterol, HDL cholesterol, blood pressure, the habit of smoking and diabetes. The evaluation calculator available on the website was used [8].

Smoking was included when a patient reported smoking any amount of tobacco during the 30 days preceding the clinical assessment.

For calculations, the data analysis software system STATISTICA version 9.1 (StatSoft, Inc., 2010) was used. The results were presented as the arithmetic mean, standard deviation and median. For comparative analysis among the groups, the Student's t-test, U Mann test and Kruskal–Wallis test were used. The differences were treated as being statistically significant at $p < 0,05$.

4. RESULTS

The groups of patients with plaque psoriasis and psoriatic arthritis were not different as far as age, the onset and duration of psoriasis, BMI or waist circumference. No vital differences in the level of systolic and diastolic blood pressures were found (Tables **1** and **2**). In patients with psoriatic arthritis, a significantly higher level of cholesterol and triglycerides in comparison to patients without arthritis was revealed (Table **3**). No essential differences in the parameters of glucose were found. Analyzing the qualitative occurrence of traditional factors of the risk of ischemic heart disease in the group of people with arthritis showed that lipid disorders (hypertriglyceridermia, hypercholesterolemia, decreased HDL), and hypertension were more frequently present; whereas, hyperglycemia or a smoking habit were observed less frequently than in the group without joint involvement. A metabolic syndrome was present in 36,1% of patients with psoriatic arthritis (woman 23% and men 43.4%). In the group with psoriasis, however, the metabolic syndrome was present in 25% of patients (women and men had similar levels: 22% *vs.* 27%) (Table **4**). Among patients with arthritis with severe psoriasis (according to the criteria of EuCOTT), lower levels of HDL cholesterol, higher levels of LDL cholesterol and higher values of systolic and diastolic blood pressure were observed in comparison with the group with psoriatic arthritis without severe skin involvement (Table **5**). In patients with severe psoriasis without arthritis, we observed lower levels of HDL cholesterol (p=0.03) than in patients with mild psoriasis. Cardiac risk was estimated with the Framingham algorithm. Among all patients, the average risk was 7.3%. The risk of cardio-vascular incident grew with the age (p=0.043) and the time of psoriasis onset (p=0.03). In the group with psoriatic arthritis, the risk was 9.9% on average and it was significantly higher than in the group with psoriasis 6.2%, (p=0.04). Ten men with psoriatic arthritis (35%), 3 men with psoriasis (11%) and no woman had a high risk of CVD. The intensification of psoriatic lesions in patients with psoriatic arthritis was connected with a high risk of heart attack or death due to cardiac reasons (according to the Framingham algorithm). In patients with psoriatic arthritis and severe psoriasis, the risk was estimated at 13% *vs.* 6.1% in the patients with psoriatic arthritis with mild skin lesions (Table **5**). In patients with psoriasis without joint involvement, grouped according to the severity of skin lesions, no significant differences in the estimated risk were found.

Table 1. Anthropometric parameters and blood pressure in the group of patients with PsA and psoriasis (PsO). The results are presented respectively as an average, standard deviation and median.

–	PsA Patients	PsO Patients	p
BMI (kg/m²)	28,2±4,6; 28,4	26,4±2,6;25,5	0,209
Waist circumference (cm)	93±15,4; 90,5	87,1±13,2;86	0,057
RR systolic (mmHg)	130,5±14,7;130	128,5±19,2;122	0,18
RR diastolic (mmHg)	98.5±12.3;94	94.7±11.8;89	0,52

Table 2. The characteristics of the groups of patients with PsA and psoriasis (PsO). The results are presented respectively as an average, standard deviation and median.

–	PsA Patients (n=44)	PsO Patients (n=51)	p
Age (in years)	**40,72± 5,87;41,0**	**38,4±6,19;38**	0,06
Sex (f/m)	16/28	23/28	0,39
Duration of psoriasis (in years)	15,3±10,3;14,5	13,1±8,3;12,0	0,42
Age of psoriasis recognition (in years)	25,3±10,7;26,0	24,7±10,1;22,0	0,77
Patients with severe psoriasis	21 (48%)	18 (35%)	0,09

Table 3. Lipid profile and glucose concentration in the group of patients with PsA and psoriasis (PsO). The results are presented respectively as an average, standard deviation and median.

–	PsA Patients	PsO Patients	p
Cholesterol (mg/dl)	214,05±47,2;194	185,4±39,06;186	0,006
TG (mg/dl)	155,8±50,4;154	134,3±84,2;106	0,019
HDL (mg/dl)	49,7±12,2;49	56,2±18,0;55	0,13
LDL (mg/dl)	135,3±42,6;126,4	110,7±37,1;108	0,14
Glc (mg/dl)	88,2±10,8;87	88,3±8,6;86	0,78

Table 4. The qualitative occurrence of traditional risk factors of cardiovascular disease.

–	PsA Patients	PsO Patients	p
Metabolic syndrome	36.1%	25%	0.044
Metabolic syndrome (women)	23%	22%	0.86

(Table 4) contd.....

–	PsA Patients	PsO Patients	p
Metabolic syndrome (men)	43.4%	27%	0.027
Hypertrigliceridemia	45%	33%	0.036
Hypercholesterolemia	48%	35%	0.041
Hypertension arterialis	50%	33%	0.034
Lower HDL	48%	29%	0.029
Hyperglycemia	9%	17%	0.043
Habit of smoking	18%	10%	0.046

Table 5. The differences in the lipid profile, glucose concentration, blood pressure and the estimated risk of cardio-vascular diseases in patiens with psoriatic arthritis grouped according to the severity of skin lesions.

–	PsA patients with severe psoriasis	PsA patients with mild psoriasis	p
Cholesterol (mg/dl)	234,02±49,7;201	198,5±41,1;195	0.06
TG (mg/dl)	167,4±54,7;163	154,8±64.6;149	0.07
HDL (mg/dl)	44,7±16,2;44	51,9±20.0;52	0.022
LDL (mg/dl)	149,3±44,9;142	129.9±47.1;116	0.032
Glc (mg/dl)	97.5±12.9;89	89.9±10.6;87	0.08
RR systolic (mmHg)	139.9±17.8;138	128.1±8.7;131	0.041
RR diastolic (mmHg)	101.1±11.4;100	89.5±7.9;88	0.034
Risk of CVD	13%	6.1%	0.042

5. DISCUSSION

The co-existence of metabolic disorders, CVD and psoriasis is more often noticed and documented [1, 2, 9 - 13]. According to the hypothesis of 'psoriatic march', psoriasis is a chronic systemic inflammatory disease. It intensifies the metabolically induced inflammation (*metainflammation*) and causes resistance to insulin, contributing to the dysfunction of endothelium cells and the acceleration of the development of atherosclerosis. As a result, it leads to myocardial infarction or stroke [10]. The latest data suggest that psoriasis may be connected to an increased risk of CVD development, regardless of the occurrence of traditional risk factors [2, 12 - 16]. The results of other studies do not confirm the correlation between the intensification of psoriatic lesions, evaluated with a PASI and a BSA score, and the time of duration of psoriasis with the increased risk of CVD calculated from the Framingham algorithm [5]. The presence of a metabolic syndrome was observed in a much larger percentage of patients with psoriasis in comparison to people without psoriasis [17 - 19]. In the course of psoriatic arthritis, the metabolic syndrome occurred in as many as 58,1% of cases [20]. Significantly more frequently, the metabolic syndrome was present in patients with psoriatic arthritis (38%) when compared with the control group (18%) and with the groups of patients with rheumatoid arthritis (20%) and ankylosing spondylitis (11%) [21]. In 30 - 50% of patients with psoriatic arthritis and with atherosclerotic lesions present in vessels, neither classic risk factors nor clinical manifestation of CVD were found [22 - 25]. In our study, the groups of patients with psoriatic arthritis and psoriasis did not differ significantly in terms of age, BMI or waist circumference. Despite the lack of vital anthropometric differences, among the patients with psoriatic arthritis one could observe the following diseases more often than in the group without arthritis: hypertriglyceridemia (45% *vs*33%), hypercholesterolemia (48% *vs*35%), lower level of HDL cholesterol (48% *vs*29%), and hypertension (50% *vs*33%); whereas disorders of carbohydrate metabolism were less frequently observed (9% *vs*17%). A metabolic syndrome was also more frequently diagnosed among patients with psoriatic arthritis than in patients with psoriasis (36% *vs*25%). A special group was comprised of men with arthritis – a metabolic syndrome was present in more than 40% of people studied. The results of our study were similar to the results recorded by other authors [20, 21, 23 - 25]. In order to limit the influence of age, hormonal and postmenopausal disorders or co-existing diseases on the risk of the occurrence of CVD, the study covered people between 30 and 50 years of age. Despite the narrow age span, the 10-year risk of CVD, evaluated by the Framingham algorithm, increased together with the age of all the patients (p<0,001). Among the patients with arthritis, there was also a connection between the increase of the evaluated risk and the later beginning of psoriasis (p=0,04). It may suggest an initiating influence of certain metabolic disorders on the origin and development of psoriasis and partially confirm the results of the studies conducted by Naldi and co-authors [26]. The correlation between the intensification of psoriatic lesions evaluated with a PASI, BSA and DLQI score (according to the criteria of EuCOTT) with the increase of the risk of cardiovascular incident occurrence or death was also evaluated. Among the patients with psoriasis, after grouping in terms of the severity of skin lesions, no essential differences were found; whereas a significant increase in the estimated risk was seen in patients with arthritis and severe psoriasis in relation to the patients with psoriatic arthritis and mild skin lesions (13% vs 6,1%). This specific 'psoriatic syndrome' in patients with arthritis, especially in such a young group, seems to be especially important. In our own research, only about 30% of patients with dyslipidemia received medication to correct the lipid profile before the study; similarly, less than 40% of people with hypertension were using medication to control the condition before the study.

In the case of psoriasis, the increased morbidity of cardiovascular diseases in comparison with the general population is well documented. This increase in the frequency of morbidity is obviously caused by conventional risk factors, including: atherosclerosis, hypertension, diabetes, obesity, lipid disorders, non-alcoholic steatohepatitis, the habit of smoking and also, among others, the increase of CRP and inflammatory cytokine concentration [25, 27 - 30]. Systemic inflammation stimulates insulin resistance, a condition in which insulin contributes to the creation of atherosclerotic plaques. It accelerates the disorder of endothelium functions, leading to atherosclerosis and finally to the symptoms of coronary artery disease and myocardial infarction [31 - 33]. Polachek et al. found that patients with PsA had a 43% higher risk of having (or developing) cardiovascular diseases compared to non-psoriatic individuals while the risk of developing an incident cardiovascular event was 55% higher in PsA patients compared with the general population. Furthermore, the risk of each of the individual cardiovascular outcomes was increased, including myocardial infarction (68%), cerebrovascular diseases (22%) and heart failure (31%) in PsA patients compared with the general population [34]. According to carotid ultrasound data, PsA patients have a high prevalence of subclinical atherosclerosis. In a recent study carotid IMT was significantly higher in patients with PsA adjusted for age and tobacco smoking than in controls [35]. Among the patients with psoriatic arthritis, an important factor seems to be the limitation of physical activity caused by pain and disability, which is sometimes significant. In people with psoriasis and PsA, in addition to the factors mentioned above, one may add an essential psychological condition, which includes a type of depression caused in particular by stigmatization due to the skin disease. The connection between psoriasis and psoriatic arthritis with CVD seems to be very complex and multifactorial. Despite the young age of the respondents, the 10-year risk of cardiovascular incident occurrence evaluated in our study was greater in the patients with psoriatic arthritis than in the patients with plaque psoriasis. The patients with psoriasis, especially with psoriatic arthritis, undoubtedly constitute a group of people requiring special medical care in terms of CVD prevention, which requires various clinicians from different specializations [36]. This may include the cooperation of dermatologists, rheumatologists, cardiologists and general practitioners.

CONCLUSION

The 10- year risk of cardiovascular incident was higher for patients with psoriatic arthritis than plaque psoriasis. In patients with plaque psoriasis, the increase in the risk of cardio-vascular incident was connected with the late beginning of psoriasis; whereas in the group of patients with psoriatic arthritis the risk of cardio-vascular incident was connected with the intensification of psoriatic lesions. The highest risk was observed in the group of men with psoriatic arthritis suggesting the special need for risk factor monitoring of these patients.

HUMAN AND ANIMAL RIGHTS

No Animals were used in this research. All human research procedures followed were in accordance with the ethical standards of the committee responsible for human experimentation (institutional and national), and with the Helsinki Declaration of 1975, as revised in 2008.

CONFLICT OF INTEREST

The authors declare no conflict of interest, financial or otherwise.

ACKNOWLEDGEMENTS

Declared none.

REFERENCES

[1]   Kimball AB, Szapary P, Mrowietz U, *et al*. Underdiagnosis and undertreatment of cardiovascular risk factors in patients with moderate to severe psoriasis. J Am Acad Dermatol 2012; 67(1): 76-85.
        [http://dx.doi.org/10.1016/j.jaad.2011.06.035] [PMID: 22018756]

[2]   Mehta NN, Azfar RS, Shin DB, Neimann AL, Troxel AB, Gelfand JM. Patients with severe psoriasis are at increased risk of cardiovascular mortality: Cohort study using the general practice research database. Eur Heart J 2010; 31(8): 1000-6.
        [http://dx.doi.org/10.1093/eurheartj/ehp567] [PMID: 20037179]

[3]   Perk J, De Backer G, Gohlke H, *et al*. European Guidelines on cardiovascular disease prevention in clinical practice (version 2012): The Fifth Joint Task Force of the European Society of Cardiology and Other Societies on Cardiovascular Disease Prevention in Clinical Practice (constituted by representatives of nine societies and by invited experts). Atherosclerosis 2012; 223(1): 1-68.
        [http://dx.doi.org/10.1016/j.atherosclerosis.2012.05.007] [PMID: 22698795]

[4]   D'Agostino RB Sr, Vasan RS, Pencina MJ, *et al*. General cardiovascular risk profile for use in primary care: The Framingham Heart Study. Circulation 2008; 117(6): 743-53.
        [http://dx.doi.org/10.1161/CIRCULATIONAHA.107.699579] [PMID: 18212285]

[5]   Gisondi P, Farina S, Giordano MV, Girolomoni G. Usefulness of the framingham risk score in patients with chronic psoriasis. Am J Cardiol 2010; 106(12): 1754-7.
        [http://dx.doi.org/10.1016/j.amjcard.2010.08.016] [PMID: 21055711]

[6]   Mrowietz U, Kragballe K, Reich K, *et al*. Definition of treatment goals for moderate to severe psoriasis: A European consensus. Arch Dermatol Res 2011; 303(1): 1-10.
        [http://dx.doi.org/10.1007/s00403-010-1080-1] [PMID: 20857129]

[7]   Alberti KG, Eckel RH, Grundy SM, *et al*. Harmonizing the metabolic syndrome. Circulation 2009; 120(16): 1640-5.
        [http://dx.doi.org/10.1161/CIRCULATIONAHA.109.192644] [PMID: 19805654]

[8]   http://cvdrisk.nhlbi.nih.gov/calculator.as. (access from 20th September 2017).

[9]   Alexandroff AB, Pauriah M, Camp RD, Lang CC, Struthers AD, Armstrong DJ. More than skin deep: Atherosclerosis as a systemic manifestation of psoriasis. Br J Dermatol 2009; 161(1): 1-7.
        [http://dx.doi.org/10.1111/j.1365-2133.2009.09281.x] [PMID: 19500102]

[10]   Boehncke WH, Boehncke S, Tobin AM, Kirby B. The 'psoriatic march': A concept of how severe psoriasis may drive cardiovascular comorbidity. Exp Dermatol 2011; 20(4): 303-7.
        [http://dx.doi.org/10.1111/j.1600-0625.2011.01261.x] [PMID: 21410760]

[11]   Eder L, Chandran V, Cook R, Gladman DD. The risk of developing diabetes mellitus in patients with psoriatic arthritis: A cohort study. J Rheumatol 2017; 44(3): 286-91.
        [http://dx.doi.org/10.3899/jrheum.160861] [PMID: 28148695]

[12]   Reich K. The concept of psoriasis as a systemic inflammation: Implications for disease management. J Eur Acad Dermatol Venereol 2012; 26(Suppl. 2): 3-11.
        [http://dx.doi.org/10.1111/j.1468-3083.2011.04410.x] [PMID: 22356630]

[13]   Shaharyar S, Warraich H, McEvoy JW, *et al*. Subclinical cardiovascular disease in plaque psoriasis: Association or causal link? Atherosclerosis 2014; 232(1): 72-8.
        [http://dx.doi.org/10.1016/j.atherosclerosis.2013.10.023] [PMID: 24401219]

[14]   Bonanad C, González-Parra E, Rivera R, *et al*. Clinical, diagnostic, and therapeutic implications in psoriasis associated with cardiovascular disease. Actas Dermosifiliogr 2017.

[15]   Garg N, Krishan P, Syngle A. Atherosclerosis in psoriatic arthritis: A multiparametric analysis using imaging technique and laboratory markers of inflammation and vascular function. Int J Angiol 2016; 25(4): 222-8.
        [http://dx.doi.org/10.1055/s-0036-1584918] [PMID: 27867287]

[16]   Mehta NN, Yu Y, Pinnelas R, *et al*. Attributable risk estimate of severe psoriasis on major cardiovascular events. Am J Med 2011; 124(8): 775.e1-6.
        [http://dx.doi.org/10.1016/j.amjmed.2011.03.028] [PMID: 21787906]

[17]   Sommer DM, Jenisch S, Suchan M, Christophers E, Weichenthal M. Increased prevalence of the metabolic syndrome in patients with moderate to severe psoriasis. Arch Dermatol Res 2006; 298(7): 321-8.
        [http://dx.doi.org/10.1007/s00403-006-0703-z] [PMID: 17021763]

[18]   Gisondi P, Tessari G, Conti A, *et al*. Prevalence of metabolic syndrome in patients with psoriasis: a hospital-based case-control study. Br J Dermatol 2007; 157(1): 68-73.
        [http://dx.doi.org/10.1111/j.1365-2133.2007.07986.x] [PMID: 17553036]

[19]   Cohen AD, Sherf M, Vidavsky L, Vardy DA, Shapiro J, Meyerovitch J. Association between psoriasis and the metabolic syndrome. A cross-sectional study. Dermatology (Basel) 2008; 216(2): 152-5.

[http://dx.doi.org/10.1159/000111512] [PMID: 18216477]

[20] Raychaudhuri SK, Chatterjee S, Nguyen C, Kaur M, Jialal I, Raychaudhuri SP. Increased prevalence of the metabolic syndrome in patients with psoriatic arthritis. Metab Syndr Relat Disord 2010; 8(4): 331-4.
[http://dx.doi.org/10.1089/met.2009.0124] [PMID: 20367239]

[21] Mok CC, Ko GT, Ho LY, Yu KL, Chan PT, To CH. Prevalence of atherosclerotic risk factors and the metabolic syndrome in patients with chronic inflammatory arthritis. Arthritis Care Res (Hoboken) 2011; 63(2): 195-202.
[http://dx.doi.org/10.1002/acr.20363] [PMID: 20890981]

[22] Gonzalez-Juanatey C, Llorca J, Amigo-Diaz E, Dierssen T, Martin J, Gonzalez-Gay MA. High prevalence of subclinical atherosclerosis in psoriatic arthritis patients without clinically evident cardiovascular disease or classic atherosclerosis risk factors. Arthritis Rheum 2007; 57(6): 1074-80.
[http://dx.doi.org/10.1002/art.22884] [PMID: 17665475]

[23] Gonzalez-Juanatey C, Llorca J, Miranda-Filloy JA, et al. Endothelial dysfunction in psoriatic arthritis patients without clinically evident cardiovascular disease or classic atherosclerosis risk factors. Arthritis Rheum 2007; 57(2): 287-93.
[http://dx.doi.org/10.1002/art.22530] [PMID: 17330278]

[24] Radner H, Lesperance T, Accortt NA, Solomon DH. Incidence and prevalence of cardiovascular risk factors among patients with rheumatoid arthritis, psoriasis, or psoriatic arthritis. Arthritis Care Res (Hoboken) 2017; 69(10): 1510-8.
[http://dx.doi.org/10.1002/acr.23171] [PMID: 27998029]

[25] Tam LS, Shang Q, Li EK, et al. Subclinical carotid atherosclerosis in patients with psoriatic arthritis. Arthritis Rheum 2008; 59(9): 1322-31.
[http://dx.doi.org/10.1002/art.24014] [PMID: 18759318]

[26] Naldi L, Parazzini F, Peli L, Chatenoud L, Cainelli T. Dietary factors and the risk of psoriasis. Results of an Italian case-control study. Br J Dermatol 1996; 134(1): 101-6.
[http://dx.doi.org/10.1111/j.1365-2133.1996.tb07846.x] [PMID: 8745893]

[27] Kimhi O, Caspi D, Bornstein NM, et al. Prevalence and risk factors of atherosclerosis in patients with psoriatic arthritis. Semin Arthritis Rheum 2007; 36(4): 203-9.
[http://dx.doi.org/10.1016/j.semarthrit.2006.09.001] [PMID: 17067658]

[28] Han C, Robinson DW Jr, Hackett MV, Paramore LC, Fraeman KH, Bala MV. Cardiovascular disease and risk factors in patients with rheumatoid arthritis, psoriatic arthritis, and ankylosing spondylitis. J Rheumatol 2006; 33(11): 2167-72.
[PMID: 16981296]

[29] Nas K, Karkucak M, Durmus B, et al. Comorbidities in patients with psoriatic arthritis: A comparison with rheumatoid arthritis and psoriasis. Int J Rheum Dis 2015; 18(8): 873-9.
[http://dx.doi.org/10.1111/1756-185X.12580] [PMID: 26173043]

[30] Tam LS, Tomlinson B, Chu TT, et al. Cardiovascular risk profile of patients with psoriatic arthritis compared to controls--the role of inflammation. Rheumatology (Oxford) 2008; 47(5): 718-23.
[http://dx.doi.org/10.1093/rheumatology/ken090] [PMID: 18400833]

[31] Giollo A, Dalbeni A, Cioffi G, et al. Factors associated with accelerated subclinical atherosclerosis in patients with spondyloarthritis without overt cardiovascular disease. Clin Rheumatol 2017; 36(11): 2487-95.
[http://dx.doi.org/10.1007/s10067-017-3786-3] [PMID: 28889188]

[32] Gisondi P, Girolomoni G. Cardiometabolic comorbidities and the approach to patients with psoriasis. Actas Dermosifiliogr 2009; 100(Suppl. 2): 14-21.
[http://dx.doi.org/10.1016/S0001-7310(09)73373-3] [PMID: 20096157]

[33] Santilli S, Kast DR, Grozdev I, et al. Visualization of atherosclerosis as detected by coronary artery calcium and carotid intima-media thickness reveals significant atherosclerosis in a cross-sectional study of psoriasis patients in a tertiary care center. J Transl Med 2016; 14(1): 217.
[http://dx.doi.org/10.1186/s12967-016-0947-0] [PMID: 27448600]

[34] Polachek A, Touma Z, Anderson M, Eder L. Risk of Cardiovascular Morbidity in Patients With Psoriatic Arthritis: A Meta-Analysis of Observational Studies. Arthritis Care Res (Hoboken) 2017; 69(1): 67-74.
[http://dx.doi.org/10.1002/acr.22926] [PMID: 27111228]

[35] Ibáñez-Bosch R, Restrepo-Velez J, Medina-Malone M, Garrido-Courel L, Paniagua-Zudaire I, Loza-Cortina E. High prevalence of subclinical atherosclerosis in psoriatic arthritis patients: a study based on carotid ultrasound. Rheumatol Int 2017; 37(1): 107-12.
[http://dx.doi.org/10.1007/s00296-016-3617-x] [PMID: 27885376]

[36] Agca R, Heslinga SC, Rollefstad S, et al. EULAR recommendations for cardiovascular disease risk management in patients with rheumatoid arthritis and other forms of inflammatory joint disorders: 2015/2016 update. Ann Rheum Dis 2017; 76(1): 17-28.
[http://dx.doi.org/10.1136/annrheumdis-2016-209775] [PMID: 27697765]

4

Topical 1% Propranolol in Liposomal Gel: A New Adjuvant Tool for Chronic Leprosy Ulcers

Ayman Abdelmaksoud[1], Domenico Bonamonte[2], Giuseppe Giudice[3], Angela Filoni[2] and Michelangelo Vestita[2,3,*]

[1]Dermatology and Leprology Hospital, Elsamanoudy street, 5, Mansoura, Egypt.

[2]Section of Dermatology, Department of Biomedical Science and Human Oncology, University of Bari, 11, Piazza Giulio Cesare, Bari, 70124, Italy

[3]Unit of Plastic and Reconstructive Surgery, Department of Emergency and Organ Transplantation, University of Bari, 11, Piazza Giulio Cesare, Bari, 70124, Italy

Abstract:

Objective:

To evaluate the effects of 1% topical propranolol in liposomal gel in 3 patients with plantar ulcers.

Methods:

We enrolled 3 patients with 3 ulcers who had completed the WHO recommended treatment regimen. The ulcers were cleaned with sterile normal saline, and 1% topical propranolol in liposomal gel was applied 2 times/day for 3 months, or less if complete healing was reached before. Assessment of ulcer re-epithelization was recorded at baseline, 6 weeks, and 3 and 6 months after initiation of treatment.

Results:

Response in the form of granulation tissue formation started by the second week. Substantial reduction in size subsequently continued over the next 3 months. Two of the 3 patients showed complete healing of the ulcers at the 6 months follow up. In the 3rd patient, the ulcer showed only modest signs of healing. Surprisingly, in all patients, the sensory function was restored, particularly in terms of pain. Some motor functional recovery at the ulcer site and surrounding tissue was also documented.

Conclusion:

To the best of our knowledge, this is the first trial of topical propranolol for the treatment of trophic ulcers of leprosy. This may represent a promising adjuvant therapy for leprosy ulcers, including ulcers of older age. Further studies are warranted with a larger number of patients and a longer period of follow up to determine the ideal candidates and to identify clinical factors predictive of response.

Keywords: Liposomal gel, Chronic, Leprosy, Ulcers, Topical proranolol, Mycobacterium tuberculosis.

1. INTRODUCTION

Leprosy is a chronic infectious disease caused by a close relative of *Mycobacterium tuberculosis*, *Mycobacterium leprae* (*M. leprae*) [1]. Non-healing chronic trophic foot ulcers are a major problem and a major cause of handicap in patients with leprosy. Approximately 30% of patients with leprosy develop nerve damage. The involvement of

* Address correspondence to this author at the Section of Dermatology, Department of Biomedical Science and Human Oncology, University of Bari, 11, Piazza Giulio Cesare, Bari, 70124, Italy; Tel: +39-80-5592024; E-mail: michelangelovestita@gmail.com

peripheral nerves in the extremities in leprosy often results in a trophic ulcer. Trophic, or neuropathic, ulcer is a common complication of an anesthetic foot. The term plantar, trophic, or perforating ulcer was introduced in 1959. It was defined as a chronic ulceration of the anesthetic foot, situated in well-defined areas overlying bony prominences, resistant to local and/or systemic therapy, and characterized by a marked tendency to recur. The majority of neuropathic ulcers occur on the plantar surface of the feet, with approximately 70% on the forefoot. These ulcers are responsible for much of the morbidity associated with leprosy [2] and carry the potential of malignant transformation if recalcitrant, including squamous cell carcinoma and melanoma [3]. The chronicity of the ulcer is perpetuated by repeated inadvertent trauma or injury. Sensory loss, muscular paralysis, autonomic nerve damage, scar tissue formation, primary vascular insufficiency, and/or the direct action of *M. leprae* have been implicated in ulcer formation [4]. Despite relentless endeavors, neuropathic ulcers associated with leprosy continue to represent a treatment challenge. Conventional treatment of these wounds can be slow because of their chronic inflammatory state and the senescence of local reparative cells. Among the conventional treatment options, intralesional platelet rich-plasma [5] and topical phenytoin sodium zinc oxide paste have been shown to be successful [6]. Recently, three of the authors have tried, for the first time, topical β blocker therapy in the form of 1% propranolol under occlusion for a chronic plantar ulcer in an elderly man. Significant healing of the ulcers was noted 3 weeks later, with no side effects or recurrence at the 1-year follow up [7]. Herein, we report our application of 1% topical propranolol in liposomal gel for the treatment of chronic neuropathic ulcer of leprosy.

2. METHODS

We enrolled 3 patients with 3 ulcers (1 multi-neural leprosy and 2 borderline lepromatous variants) who had completed the WHO recommended treatment regimen and were in the follow-up period. All patients were thoroughly informed about the treatment and signed a written informed consent. All were undergoing a regular debridement of necrotic tissue and dressing of the ulcers. The patients had no comorbidities, except patient 3 who was also affected by type 2 diabetes. No systemic or intralesional therapies were given before or during the study. Bacterial cultures before and after treatment and radiography were performed in each case, with no evidence of active infection or findings of osteomyelitis. The morphological features of the ulcers were recorded, including size, site, depth, and presence of secondary infection. The ulcer was cleaned with sterile normal saline, and 1% topical propranolol in liposomal gel was applied 2 times/day for 3 months, or less if complete healing was reached before the end of 3 months. 1% propranolol liposomal gel was obtained using a reverse phase evaporation method, warranting a high encapsulation efficiency, up to 65%. The quantity of the drug used was directly proportional to the size of the ulcer (1 fingertip unit per 3 cm^2) to achieve a uniform application across ulcers of different sizes. The patients were instructed to apply the gel at the margin and the base of the ulcer with gentle massaging followed by protective dressing. The patients were instructed to avoid excessive walking and to wear suitable shoes made for the deformed leprosy foot. Regular follow up was arranged biweekly to ensure patients' adherence. Assessment of ulcer re-epithelization was recorded at baseline, 6 weeks, and 3 and 6 months after initiation of treatment (Table **1**).

Table 1. Clinical characteristics and outcomes.

Patient (Sex)	Duration of the Ulcers	Type of Leprosy	Comorbidities	Age	Ulcer Shape	Ulcer Size at Baseline	Ulcer Size at 6 Weeks	Ulcer Size at 3 Months	Ulcer Size at 6 Months	Bone Involvement	Sensitivity
Case 1 (Male)	10 ys	Multi-neural	None	65	Figurate	5*4.6*0.5 cm	1*1.5*0.5 cm	healed	healed	No	Improved
Case 2 (Male)	8 ys	Borderline lepromatous	None	62	Figurate	4.3*3*0.5 cm	1*0.5*0.3 cm	healed	healed	No	Improved
Case 3 (Female)	7 ys	Borderline lepromatous	Type 2 DM, stage IV melanoma	57	Figurate	10*4.5*0.5 cm	8*4*0.3 cm	7*4*0.2 cm	8*5*0.2 cm	No	Improved

3. RESULTS

The response in the form of granulation tissue formation started by the second week. Substantial reduction in size subsequently continued over the next 3 months. Two of the 3 patients showed complete healing of the ulcers at the end of the study, while 1 patient showed only minor improvement (Figs. **1**, **2**, **3**). Surprisingly, in all patients, good sensory function, up to 40%, was restored at the ulcers and in the surrounding tissue, particularly in terms of pain relief and reacquired sensation on the sole of the foot (tibial nerve sensitive fibers); some motor function, up to 25%, was also recovered, in terms of inversion and plantar flexion (tibial nerve motor fibers). None of the patients developed local or systemic adverse effects or relapsed to the pre-treatment state at 6-month follow up.

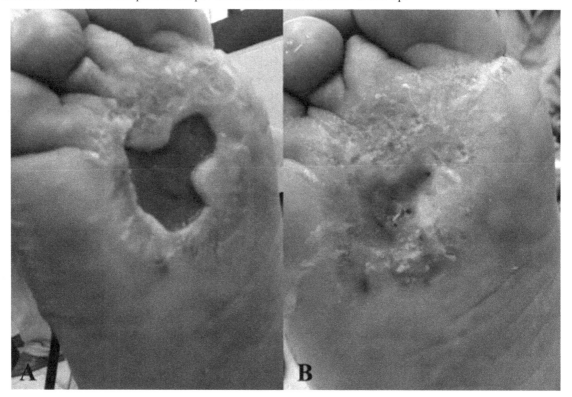

Fig. (1). Patient 1. **A**: Pre-treatment, **B**: After 3 months of 1% topical propranolol in liposomal gel.

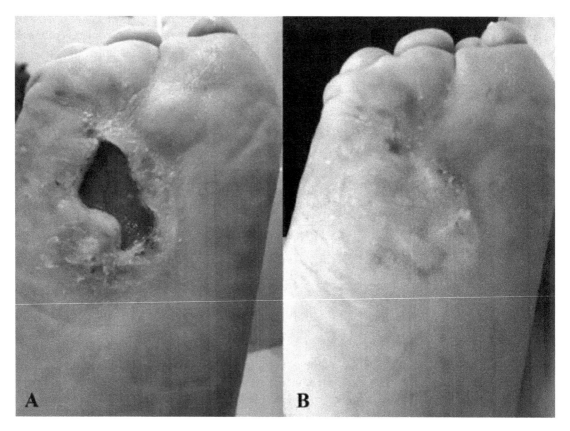

Fig. (2). Patient 2. **A**: Pre-treatment, **B**: After 3 months of 1% topical propranolol in liposomal gel.

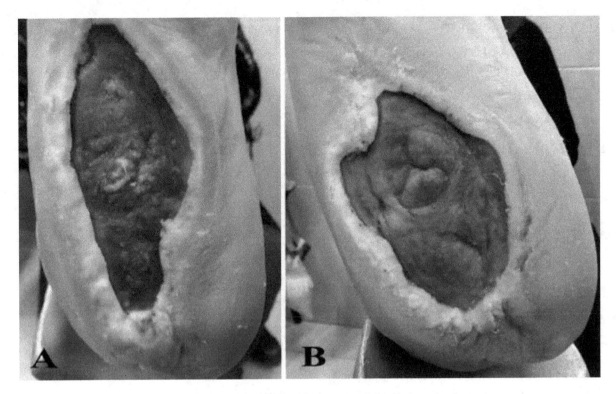

Fig. (3). Patient 3. **A**: Pre-treatment, **B**: After 3 months of 1% topical propranolol in liposomal gel.

4. DISCUSSION

β-adrenergic receptors are present on keratinocytes, fibroblasts, and melanocytes. High levels of circulating catecholamines, associated with burns or traumatic wounds, are known to impair wound healing. Catecholamines are produced endogenously by wounded keratinocytes. Propranolol has been shown to block the negative effect that catecholamines exert on wound healing [8]. Furthermore, it may enhance keratinocyte migration [9] and angiogenesis in wounds, regardless of the specific etiology [10 - 13]. Intriguingly, infection of Schwann cells with *M. leprae* results in demyelination, axonal dysfunction, and immunological granulomatous reaction in the nerve [14]. In vitro studies demonstrated the ability of *M. leprae* to induce demyelination. *M. leprae* interacts with ErbB2 receptors on the surface of myelinating Schwann cells and causes myelinated Schwann cells to dedifferentiation into an unmyelinated cell via an internal signaling process [15 - 17]. Recently, Sysa-Shah *et al.* [18] identified a novel activation loop in the heart (and in vitro systems) linking ErbB2 and β-adrenergic systems, where β-adrenergic receptor stimulation causes elevation and activation of ErbB2. Notably, antigen presenting Langerhans Cells (LC) are anatomically associated with peripheral nerves. Some neuropeptides have been shown to regulate LC antigen-presenting function. Pretreatment of epidermal cells with epinephrine or norepinephrine in vitro suppressed the ability of these cells to present antigen for elicitation of delayed-type hypersensitivity in previously immunized mice [19]. Given the know proprieties of beta-blockers in wound healing in general, we hypothesized that 1% topical propranolol not only counteracts the inhibitory effect of catecholamines on tissue reepithelization, but also the local inhibitory effect on *M. leprae*-presenting Langerhans cells. Further, it may interrupt linkage of the ErbB2 and β-adrenergic systems, preventing Schwann cell demyelination, and subsequently preventing further trophic ulceration. To our knowledge, this is the first trial of topical propranolol in trophic ulcers of leprosy. Though complete healing of the ulcers was not reached in all cases, the drug may be a potential adjuvant therapy for leprosy ulcers, even for those of older age. We can only speculate why patient 3 did not seem to respond to topical propranolol. Certainly, her comorbidity might have played a role, as type 2 diabetes is known to impair wound healing, even when controlled by medication therapy. However, definite data is lacking. Moreover, based on our experience in wound healing using topical β blockers [7, 11 - 13], we noticed that leprosy ulcers require more time to initiate a response and to complete healing when compared to other types of chronic wounds [12]. Further studies are warranted including a larger number of patients and a longer period of follow up to determine the ideal candidates and to identify clinical factors predictive of response.

HUMAN AND ANIMAL RIGHTS

No Animals were used in this research. All human research procedures followed were in accordance with the ethical standards of the committee responsible for human experimentation (institutional and national), and with the Helsinki Declaration of 1975, as revised in 2013.

CONFLICT OF INTEREST

The authors declare no conflict of interest, financial or otherwise.

ACKNOWLEDGEMENTS

Declared none.

REFERENCES

[1]   Grzybowski A, Sak J, Suchodolska E, Virmond M. Lepra: Various etiologies from miasma to bacteriology and genetics. Clin Dermatol 2015; 33(1): 3-7.
        [http://dx.doi.org/10.1016/j.clindermatol.2014.07.012] [PMID: 25432805]

[2]   Riyaz N, Sehgal VN. Leprosy: Trophic Skin Ulcers. Skinmed 2017; 15(1): 45-51.
        [PMID: 28270310]

[3]   Zhu J, Shi C, Jing Z, Liu Y. Nodular melanoma in trophic ulceration of a leprosy patient: A case study. J Wound Care 2016; 25(5): 250-3.
        [http://dx.doi.org/10.12968/jowc.2016.25.5.250] [PMID: 27169340]

[4]   World Health Organization. Disability Prevention and Rehabilitation. 1981.

[5]   Conde-Montero E, Horcajada-Reales C, Clavo P, Delgado-Sillero I, Suárez-Fernández R. Neuropathic ulcers in leprosy treated with intralesional platelet-rich plasma. Int Wound J 2016; 13(5): 726-8.
        [http://dx.doi.org/10.1111/iwj.12359] [PMID: 25196256]

[6]   Sehgal VN, Prasad PV, Kaviarasan PK, Rajan D. Trophic skin ulceration in leprosy: Evaluation of the efficacy of topical phenytoin sodium zinc oxide paste. Int J Dermatol 2014; 53(7): 873-8.
        [http://dx.doi.org/10.1111/ijd.12457] [PMID: 24601869]

[7]   Vestita M, Bonamonte D, Filoni A. Topical propranolol for a chronic recalcitrant wound. Dermatol Ther (Heidelb) 2016; 29(3): 148-9.
        [http://dx.doi.org/10.1111/dth.12328] [PMID: 26800510]

[8]   Romana-Souza B, Porto LC, Monte-Alto-Costa A. Cutaneous wound healing of chronically stressed mice is improved through catecholamines blockade. Exp Dermatol 2010; 19(9): 821-9.
        [http://dx.doi.org/10.1111/j.1600-0625.2010.01113.x] [PMID: 20629735]

[9]   Pullar CE, Rizzo A, Isseroff RR. beta-Adrenergic receptor antagonists accelerate skin wound healing: Evidence for a catecholamine synthesis network in the epidermis. J Biol Chem 2006; 281(30): 21225-35.
        [http://dx.doi.org/10.1074/jbc.M601007200] [PMID: 16714291]

[10]   Pullar CE, Le Provost GS, O'Leary AP, Evans SE, Baier BS, Isseroff RR. β2AR antagonists and β2AR gene deletion both promote skin wound repair processes. J Invest Dermatol 2012; 132(8): 2076-84.
        [http://dx.doi.org/10.1038/jid.2012.108] [PMID: 22495178]

[11]   Abdelmaksoud A, Filoni A, Giudice G, Vestita M. Classic and HIV-related Kaposi sarcoma treated with 0.1% topical timolol gel. J Am Acad Dermatol 2017; 76(1): 153-5.
        [http://dx.doi.org/10.1016/j.jaad.2016.08.041] [PMID: 27986137]

[12]   Vestita M, Filoni A, Bonamonte D, et al. Topical 0.5% Timolol for chronic refractory Wounds. An observational prospective study. Plast Reconstr Surg Glob Open 2017; 5: 21.
        [http://dx.doi.org/10.1097/01.GOX.0000526190.20003.08]

[13]   Vestita M, Maggio G, Filoni A, et al. Efficacy, safety and costs of 0.1% timolol gel in healing split-thickness skin grafts donor sites. A Case-Control Study. Surg Glob Open 2017; 5: 139-40.

[14]   Scollard DM. The biology of nerve injury in leprosy. Lepr Rev 2008; 79(3): 242-53.
        [PMID: 19009974]

[15]   Rambukkana A. Mycobacterium leprae-induced demyelination: A model for early nerve degeneration. Curr Opin Immunol 2004; 16(4):

511-8.
[http://dx.doi.org/10.1016/j.coi.2004.05.021] [PMID: 15245748]

[16]   Rambukkana A, Zanazzi G, Tapinos N, Salzer JL. Contact-dependent demyelination by *Mycobacterium leprae* in the absence of immune cells. Science 2002; 296(5569): 927-31.
[http://dx.doi.org/10.1126/science.1067631] [PMID: 11988579]

[17]   Franklin RJ, Zhao C. Tyrosine kinases: Maiming myelin in leprosy. Nat Med 2006; 12(8): 889-90.
[http://dx.doi.org/10.1038/nm0806-889] [PMID: 16892032]

[18]   Sysa-Shah P, Tocchetti CG, Gupta M, *et al.* Bidirectional cross-regulation between ErbB2 and β-adrenergic signalling pathways. Cardiovasc Res 2016; 109(3): 358-73.
[http://dx.doi.org/10.1093/cvr/cvv274] [PMID: 26692570]

[19]   Seiffert K, Hosoi J, Torii H, *et al.* Catecholamines inhibit the antigen-presenting capability of epidermal Langerhans cells. J Immunol 2002; 168(12): 6128-35.
[http://dx.doi.org/10.4049/jimmunol.168.12.6128] [PMID: 12055224]

5

Topical Antiacne Drugs Delivery Systems

Tesfaye Gabriel*

Department of Pharmaceutics and Social Pharmacy, School of Pharmacy, College of Health Sciences, Addis Ababa University, P. O. Box 1176, Addis Ababa, Ethiopia

Abstract:

Background:

Acne vulgaris (commonly called acne) is the most prevalent skin complication of different causes with a higher prevalence in adolescents. Topical administration is used as first-choice therapy in mild acne, whereas for moderate and severe acne, systemic administration is required in addition to topical therapy. Mechanisms by which treatments act are: normalizing shedding into the pore to prevent obstruction, destruction of *P.acnes*, suppression of inflammation, and hormonal management.

Objective:

This review focuses on the novel drug delivery systems displaying a strong ground for topical treatment of acne in order to enhance the therapeutic performance of the topical antiacne agents with improved patience compliance and a concomitant reduction in the side effects.

Method:

This literature review was obtained from electronic search on Pubmed, Google Scholars, Researchgate, Scimago, CABI, DOAJ, CiteFactor, GLOBAL HEALTH, Universal Impact Factor, Hinari among many others and also search was conducted on individual journals and manuals.

Conclusion:

Amongst various novel drug delivery systems, vesicular carriers like liposomes and niosomes, micro sponges, microemulsions, solid lipid nanoparticles, hydrogels, emulsifier-free formulations, fullerenes and aerosol foams have been reported as novel topical administration of antiacne drugs. Liposomes have been extensively explored and their ability to optimize and improve topical therapy has been proved by several clinical trials. Microemulsions, microsponges, solid lipid nanoparticles and hydrogels also exhibit a tremendous potential for commercialization.

Keywords: Anti-inflammatory effects, Hormonal manipulation, Hydrogels, Liposomes and niosomes, Micro sponges, Microemulsions, *P. acnes*, Solid lipid nanoparticles, Topical therapy.

1. INTRODUCTION

Skin is considered to be the largest organ consisting of three layers: the epidermis, the dermis, and the hypodermis [1]. The most outer non-living part of the epidermis, the stratum corneum (SC), is the key diffusional resistance to percutaneous absorption. The exceptional resistance properties of the SC can be ascribed to its unique structure and composition. The viable epidermis is situated beneath the SC and responsible for the generation of the SC. The dermis is directly adjacent to the epidermis and composed of a matrix of connective tissue, which renders the skin its elasticity

---

* Address correspondence to this author at the Department of Pharmaceutics and Social Pharmacy, School of Pharmacy, College of Health Sciences, Addis Ababa University, P. O. Box 1176, Addis Ababa, Ethiopia; E-mails: tesfu.gabriel@gmail.com, tesfaye.gabriel@aau.edu.et

and resistance to deformation [2, 3].

The outer layer of the skin forms an effective barrier to retain water within the body and keep exogenous compounds out of the body. As a result, the major problem in dermal and transdermal drug deliveries is the low penetration of drug compounds through the SC. Dermal drug delivery comprises the topical application of drugs for the local treatment of skin diseases. It requires the permeation of a drug through the outer skin layers to reach its site of action within the skin, with little or no systemic uptake. The application of drugs to the skin for systemic therapy is referred to as transdermal drug delivery. Hence, it is required that a pharmacologically potent drug reaches the dermis where it can be taken up by the systemic blood circulation. In either case, the drug has to cross the outermost layer of the skin, the SC [1].

1.1. The Viable Epidermis

The layers in the epidermis are: stratum basale, stratum spinosum, stratum granulosum, and SC [4]. The innermost layer of the epidermis, the stratum basale, consists of a single layer of columnar-shaped, undifferentiated stem cells. As the cells produced by the basal layer move upward, they alter morphologically as well as histochemically to form the outermost layer, the SC. Over a 4 to 5-week period the entire epidermis is renewed [5].

1.2. The SC

SC is considered to be the major diffusional resistance for different materials like water [2, 3]. It is about 10 to 20 A m in thickness when dehydrated but swells to several times this thickness when entirely humid [6]. It comprises 10 to 25 layers parallel to the corneocytes, as protein bricks embedded in a lipid mortar [7]. During the changeover of the mature keratinocyte into the corneocyte, profilaggrin that is released from the keratohyalin granules is dephosphorylated and transformed to filaggrin monomers. Filaggrin is converted into free amino acids and other derivatives, which contribute to the wetness of the SC [8].

1.3. Permeation Route Across the SC

Compounds could cross skin in two mechanisms: the transappendageal path and the transepidermal path. The transappendageal pathway is believed to be of less importance than the transepidermal route because of its relatively small area, approximately 0.1% of the total skin area [8]. However, some findings have revealed the possibility of specifically targeting certain compounds to the pilosebaceous structures [9, 10]. The success rate is mainly dependent on the lipophilicity of the permeant and the composition of the vehicle [11]. Due to the highly impermeable property of the cornified envelope, the tortuous intercellular route is proposed to be the key route for majority drug entities [12].

2. ACNE VULGARIS

The term *acne* is derived from the Greek *ἀκμή* refering to the occurrence of pustules and papules. Acne vulgaris (commonly called acne) is the most prevalent skin complication of different causes with a higher prevalence in adolescents.The majority of the acne sufferers exhibit mild to moderate acne initially, which progresses to the severe form in certain cases [13, 14]. For most people, acne diminishes over time and tends to disappear. However, some individuals will continue to suffer well into their thirties, forties and beyond [15]. The face and upper neck are most commonly influenced, but the chest, back and shoulders could possess acne too. Aside from scarring, its main effects are psychological, such as reduced self-esteem and depression or suicide [16].

2.1. Causes of Acne

Acne typically results from blockages in follicles. Enlargement of sebaceous glands and an increase in sebum production occur with increased androgen (DHEA-S) production at adrenarche. The microcomedo may enlarge to form an open comedo (blackhead) or closed comedo (whitehead). Whiteheads are the direct result of skin pores becoming clogged with sebum, naturally occurring oil, and dead skin cells. *Propionibacterium acnes* can cause inflammation, leading to inflammatory lesions (papules, infected pustules, or nodules) in the dermis around the microcomedo or comedo, which results in redness and may result in scarring or hyperpigmentation [17].

The main cause of acne is not well known. Notwithstanding, there are numerous related factors reported: hereditary, hormonal activity, for example, menstrual cycles and puberty, inflammation, skin irritation, anxiety, through expanded yield of hormones from the adrenal (anxiety) organs with some questions, hyperactive sebaceous organs, auxiliary to the hormone sources, amassing of dead skin cells, microbes in the pores, utilization of anabolic steroids, any drug comprising lithium, barbiturates or androgens, presentation to certain concoction mixes, for example, chlorinated dioxins and halogens and frequent use of amphetamines [18 - 20].

2.2. The Physical Effects of Acne

The impacts of acne - both physical and emotional - can last much longer than your breakouts. Indeed, even after sores have healed, they can leave lasting reminders. It's hard to avoid scars of acne. However, acne scars can be treated. Post-inflammatory hyperpigmentation and macules can be tackled with bleaching agent. Some superficial skin inflammation scarring can be treated with topical resurfacing agents, similar to Retinol, which is accessible in numerous over-the-counter preparation, and additionally in prescription only medicines, for example, Retin-A and Renova. Different types of scarring can be enhanced with microdermabrasion (at least 6-8 medications are normally required) or dermatologic surgery. It may not be conceivable to reestablish your skin to its pre-acne appearance - however in the event that your scars significantly affect your well-being, it merits considering [21].

3. TREATMENTS

Topical treatment is usually utilized as first-choice therapy in minor acne, though for severe and complicated acne, systemic treatment is vital along with topical treatment. However, it was reported that topical intralesional triamcinolone and lincomycin combination was effective to eliminate severe of nodulocystic lesions of acne. Currently, so many topical medications are accessible that influence the primary pathogenetic factors. Though topical treatment has an essential place in acne management, adverse reactions connected with different topical antiacne specialists and the undesirable physico-chemical attributes of some vital substances like tretinoin and benzoyl peroxide (BPO) influence their usefulness and compliance of patient [14].

Topical therapy is the most well-known and mainstream approach to treat acne and there are a number of treatments options (Table 1) often in combination to have a synergistic effect and target simultaneous various pathogenic components. Generally, topical monotherapy is suggested for mild and moderate acne [22].

Table 1. Overview of topical antiacne agents [14, 16].

Category	Drugs/Agents
Topical bactericidals	BPO, triclosan, or chlorhexidine gluconate
Topical antibiotics	Erythromycin, clindamycin, stievamycin, or tetracycline
Hormonal treatments	Oestrogen/progestogen, antiandrogen, Cyproterone, in combination with an oestrogen
Topical retinoids	Tretinoin, adapalene, and tazarotene, retinol
Alpha or Beta Hydroxy acids	Glycolic acid, lactic acid, mandelic acid, lipohydroxy acid, salicylic acid
Phototherapy	'Blue' and red light
Miscellaneous	Nicitinamide, sodium ascorbyl phosphate, pyruvic acid, sulfur

Chiou (2012) evaluated the contribution of vehicle (placebo) toward the reduction in total (inflammatory and non-inflammatory) lesion counts using 0.1% tretinoin, 0.1% adapalene, 5% dapsone, 1% clindamycin, a combination of benzoyl peroxide with adapalene or clindamycin, and a clindamycin-tretinoin combination and showed better significance of vehicle effects in topical therapy; in some cases this effect approached 90% [23].

Recently in US patent no. 8846646, Chiou (2014) has reported an effective and safe method for treating acne and rosacea by topically applying a therapeutically effective amount of propylene glycol alone or in combination with a therapeutically effective amount of salicylic acid or other anti-acne or anti-rosacea compounds in a dosage form to the area of skin lesion [24].

There are different formulations available for the acne management, but most of them are lacking any scientifically-proven responses. Successful treatments show little improvement within the first two weeks, instead taking a period of approximately three months to improve and start flattening out [16].

Treatments are believed to work in at least 4 different ways (with many of the best treatments providing multiple simultaneous effects): normalizing shedding into the pore to prevent blockage, eradicating *P. acnes*, anti-inflammatory responses and hormonal control.

Combination therapies can significantly diminish the extent and severity of acne in many cases, but have greater potential for side effects and need a greater degree of monitoring. Table 1 indicates different topical anticane agents and Table 2 shows cutaneous side-effects from topical acne treatments and potential drug delivery systems for agent delivery.

Table 2. Cutaneous side effects from topical antiacne agents and potential drug delivery [22].

Common Topical Acne Treatments	Cutaneous Side-effects	Drug Delivery
Retinoids (*e.g.*, adapalene, tazarotene, tretinoin)	Burning, peeling, erythema, dryness, photosensitivity	Microsponges, liposomes, nanoemulsions, aerosol foams
BPO	Dryness, erythema, peeling, hair and clothing discoloration	Polymers, fullerenes
Clindamycin phosphate	Erythema, dryness, allergic contact dermatitis	Aerosol foams, polymers, nanomemulsions
Erythromycin	Dryness, erythema, peeling, allergic contact dermatitis	Aerosol foams, polymers, nanomemulsions
Salicylic acid	Dryness, erythema, peeling	Polymers, microsponges

Another study by Lamel *et al.* (2015) revealed that clinical trial design, implementation, the biologic effects of vehicles, and natural disease progression influenced the patient responses in randomized controlled trials evaluating topical acne therapies for determination of efficacies of BPO [25].

4. DRUG DELIVERY SYSTEMS

Though topical treatment has an imperative role in acne treatment, side effects of different topical antiacne drugs and the unwanted physicochemical properties of certain important agents like tretinoin and BPO influence their use. Novel drug delivery can be used to improve the topical delivery of antiacne agents by promoting dermal localization and lowering their side effects. There are different advanced strategies like liposomes, niosomes, aspasomes microsponges, microemulsions, hydrogels and solid lipid nanoparticles to enhance the topical administration of antiacne agents [14].

4.1. Liposomes

Liposomes are often utilized as vehicles in pharmaceuticals and cosmetics for a modified drug delivery. They are considered to be spherical vesicles whose membrane comprises amphiphilic lipids that surround an aqueous core. Hydrophilic substances may be encapsulated in the aqueous core and lipophilic substances in the lipid bilayer so this enables the delivery of 2 types of substances once they are applied on the skin [26, 27].

The fundamental parts of liposomes are phospholipids (phosphatidylcholine, phophatidylethanolamine, phophatidylserine, dipalmitoyl phosphatidylcholine, and others), cholesterol, and water. Liposomes may differ considerably in terms of size and structure. One or more concentric bilayers emclose an aqueous core producing small or large unilamellar vesicles (SUV, LUV) or multilamellar vesicles (MLV), respectively [28, 29].

Liposomes are considered to be the first generation of novel drug delivery systems having diameters ranging from 80 nm to 100μm [14]. Due to their high degree of biocompatibility, liposomes have been used as advanced drug delivery systems for enclosing of molecules [28].

It was reported that Clindamycin hydrochloride multilamellar liposomes had been prepared using either lecithin and cholesterol or Hostaphat KW (Hoechst) and cholesterol acne management. *In vitro* diffusion studies on the Hostaphat liposomes exhibited a sustained release. Liposomal clindamycin lotion was much more effective in reducing the total number of comedones, papules and mainly pustules. Tretinoin, also known as all trans retinoic acid, is a successful antiacne drug used topically for reducing the size and number of comedones. Unfortunately, its poor aqueous solubility, photoliability, high instability in the presence of heat and light and skin irritating nature strongly limits its topical use. Moreover, tretinoin users experience side effects like erythema, peeling, burning at the application site and increased susceptibility to sunlight. In order to overcome these disadvantages and to improve its effectiveness after topical application, the use of liposomal formulations has been recommended [14].

Among liposomal formulations, positively charged liposomes exhibited enhanced tretinoin release and permeation as compared to negatively charged liposomes. Moreover, liposomal formulations improved tretinoin accumulation into newborn pig skin. Among liposomal formulations, the maximum accumulation values for tretinoin were found with negatively charged liposomes as compared to positively charged liposomes. Additionally, TEM analyses of the newborn pig skin-liposome interaction revealed that liposomes do not penetrate in the skin as intact structures and negatively charged liposomes strongly improved the hydration of pig skin. These reports suggested that the composition and charge of liposomes would play an important role in optimizing tretinoin delivery. Apart from the improved delivery, liposomal encapsulation of tretinoin is also expected to improve its photostability [28].

BPO is a successful topical agent in the treatment of acne. The key mechanism of action of BPO in acne is linked to its eradication property of *P. acnes* in the sebaceous follicle. Liposomal BPO gels exhibited a better stability profile with lower drug leakage as compared to BPO liposomal dispersions. The liposomal BPO gel showed a significant improvement in the therapeutic response (about 2-fold) at all times of evaluation when compared to the plain BPO gel [14, 30].

Combination therapy comprising of antiacne agents differing in mechanism of action is gaining importance in the effective management of acne. Topical retinoids combined with topical or oral antibiotics were reported to decrease acne lesions quicker and to a larger range than antimicrobial therapy alone [31].

Erythromycin and BPO have also been shown to possess synergism and can improve acne treatment. With this aim we have developed the combination gel containing liposome-encapsulated erythromycin and BPO. The *in vitro* skin permeation study indicated longer residence of erythromycin and BPO liposomes in the guinea pig skin [32].

The use of antiandrogen has received great attention in acne treatment ever since the sebaceous gland was found to be androgen sensitive. Cyproterone acetate (CPA) has been used since the early 1960s and denotes the first specific antiandrogen of clinical interest. It was reported that acne and hirsutism can be effectively managed with orally delivered CPA. However, oral administration of CPA is associated with side effects like lassitude, loss of libido, nausea and breast tenderness. Hence, a topical CPA formulation with the ability to deliver sufficient doses in order to target sebaceous glands with concomitant reduction in systemic CPA concentration would be an ideal approach in such a case. However, earlier trials conducted using topical CPA formulations were unsuccessful due to the lack of a suitable vehicle for transdermal delivery of CPA. Serum concentrations of CPA were ten-folds lesser after topical administration of CPA as compared to orally delivered CPA. Thus, liposomal CPA has opened a new avenue for effective acne treatment with reduced side effects [33].

Salicylic acid is widely used in the management of dry skin conditions and to minimize acne symptoms due to its keratolytic effect like sodium salycilate. However, users experience mild to strong irritation after application of salicylic acid. Since salicylic acid precipitates into a powder on the surface of the skin after solvent evaporation, it does not require neutralization. Hence, liposomal encapsulation can be an attractive approach for salicylic acid delivery. It was also shown that liposomal preparation of salicylic acid not only extended the salicylic acid release across the skin but also improved the retention of salicylic acid in the skin. Tea tree oil, a natural bioactive obtained from *Melaleuca alternifolia*, has also attained considerable interest in the topical treatment of acne due to its antibacterial properties. The study suggested that the liposomal approach would be a good option for improving the therapeutic efficacy of tea tree oil [14, 34, 35].

4.2. Niosomes

Niosomes are bilayer structures obtained from amphiphiles in aqueous media. Different kinds of surfactants are employed for niosomes formulation. Principally, they are analogous to liposomes. Niosome formation necessitates the existence of specific amphiphiles like polyoxyethylene alkyl ethers, sorbitan esters, polysorbate-cholesterol mixtures, crown ether derivatives, perfluoroalkyl surfactants, alkyl glycerol ethers and others, and aqueous solvent [28].

Niosomes represent second-generation vesicular carriers which have evolved as a substitute to liposomes largely because of their higher chemical stability, enhanced encapsulation efficiency, intrinsic skin penetration-enhancing properties and lower cost of production as compared to liposomes. Various nonionic surfactants like polyoxyethylene alkyl ethers and esters, glucosyl dialkyl ethers, poly glycerol alkyl ethers, crown ethers and sorbitan esters can be utilized to prepare niosomes. Charge inducers like dicetyl phosphate are intercalated in bilayers to incorporate electrostatic repulsions among the vesicles for improving the stability of vesicles. However, charge inducers used in the formulation should be biocompatible. The classification of niosomes, their methods of preparation and advantages in the dermal delivery are similar as described under liposomes [36, 37].

Although the utility of niosomes in dermal delivery for the enhanced delivery of topical agents was realized around a decade ago, their potential in the antiacne drugs administration was not very well studied yet. The potential of niosomes has been explored for delivering tretinoin. Manconi *et al.* have recently reported the utility of niosomes for encapsulating tretinoin in order to improve its photochemical stability. They prepared multilamellar, large unilamellar and small unilamellar niosomes by using sorbitan esters, polyoxyethylene lauryl ether, and a commercial mixture of octyl/decyl polyglucosides in the presence of cholesterol and dicetyl phosphate. Properties of niosomes are influenced by the surfactant composition and interaction [38, 39].

The photostability of tretinoin in either the 'free' or 'noisome-encapsulated' form was investigated by carrying out UV irradiation and artificial light irradiation. The integration of tretinoin in vesicles directed to a lessening of the photolysis of tretinoin and the photoprevention exhibited by the vesicles. Not all the studied vesicular formulations improved the stability of tretinoin in comparison with the stability of free tretinoin in methanol. Thus, niosomes can become interesting carriers for dermal delivery of antiacne agents and their ability needs to be explored to the fullest [40].

4.3. Aspasomes

Aspasomes are novel vesicular carriers recently investigated by Gopinath *et al.*, which are formed by using ascorbyl palmitate, cholesterol and dicetyl phosphate. Aspasomes can gain importance in acne therapy as the potential of ascorbic acid derivatives in acne treatment has been realized. They can be fabricated by the typical film hydration method. Aspasomes have been characterized by conventional techniques for bilayer formation and thermal behavior by differential scanning calorimetry (DSC) analysis. Their advantages in dermal delivery of therapeutic agents are similar to that of liposomes. Moreover, their inherent antioxidant potential can be complementary to the topical acne therapy [40].

4.4. Microsponges

Microsponges are biologically inactive, non-irritating, non-mutagenic, non-allergic, non-toxic, and non-biodegradable polymeric drug delivery systems, which exhibited great use in dermopharmaceuticals administration. Microsponges are also defined as porous microspheres, which are prepared by using cross-linked polymers like styrene-divinyl benzene by employing suitable polymerization techniques. Like a true sponge, a single Microsponge system comprises numerous interconnecting spaces within a noncollapsible structure with a large porous surface. These systems are produced mainly by suspension polymerization that leads to structures with an internal surface area ranging from 20 to 500 m^2 /g. Moreover, the generation of Microsponges of varying size (5-300 μm) is possible as the polymerization conditions can be varied over a wide range. A typical 25μm microsponge can have up to 250,000 pores, forming an entire pore volume of around 1 ml/g. Furthermore, release from the microsponge could be modulated by using various triggers or stimuli like pressure, change in temperature, change in pH, change in polarity and change in solubility. Microsponges mainly entrap the drug by sorption mechanisms [41].

The advantages that the microsponge offers in topical delivery are as follows: improved physical stability and better protection from environmental factors, reduction in side effects associated with the topical antiacne agents, sustained release of active agent thus prolonging the drug activity, ease of incorporation into formulations like gel, cream, liquid or powder, improved elegance and esthetic appeal, high drug payload, reduction in systemic absorption of the topical agents, and programmable and flexible delivery system since the release could be modulated by using various stimuli so as to tailor the release of active moiety on command. Microsponge technology has been successfully applied for improving tolerability of antiacne agents like BPO and tretinoin. Furthermore, tretinoin microsponges have reached commercialization and are currently marketed as Retin-A Micro®. Retin-A Micro consists of microsponges (based on methyl methacrylate/glycol dimethacrylate crosspolymers) of tretinoin incorporated in an aqueous gel. It is available in two strengths, namely 0.1 and 0.04% [14].

4.5. Emulsifier-free Formulations

They are also expanding for delivery of cosmetic and dermatologic formulations. Most skin care products are emulsions so during production they require the addition of surfactants ("emulsifiers"). Additionally, when the surfactant agents are spread on the skin, they emulsify and get rid of the natural lipids. Thus, the pharmaceutical factory is evolving them as substitutes to conventional preparations [22].

4.6. Microemulsions

Microemulsions are thermodynamically stable, isotropic, and transparent, low-viscosity colloidal dispersions comprising micro-domains of oil and/or water stabilized by an interfacial film of alternating surfactant and cosurfactant molecules. They contain swollen micellar (oil-in-water, O/W), reverse micellar (water-in-oil, W/O) and bicontinuous structures.

The advent of microemulsion-based gels (which amalgamate the advantages of microemulsions and gels) has helped in improving the patient compliance of microemulsions. Microemulsion-based gels are produced by using a suitable polymer that is capable of modifying the rheological behavior of microemulsions. However, it is essential to ensure that the polymer does not alter the desirable features of microemulsions. Several gelling agents have already been studied for their potential to form microemulsion-based gels [14].

Azelaic acid, a bioactive molecule utilized in managing acne and different skin complications, was first formulated in the form of microemulsions. Gasco *et al.* successfully achieved incorporation of azelaic acid into the microemulsion based on topically acceptable components like propylene glycol, decanol, dodecanol and polysorbate 20 and microemulsions were viscosized using Carbopol. An investigation of the *in vitro* diffusion profile of azelaic acid from marketed gel and microemulsion-based gel revealed that the microemulsion-based gels dramatically improved the transport of the azelaic acid across hairless mouse skin. Additionally, the effect of penetration enhancer like DMSO was studied on the permeation of azelaic acid from microemulsion-based gels. The permeation of azelaic acid increased with an increase in the DMSO content [14, 42].

4.7. Fullerenes

They are compounds made entirely of carbon that look like a hollow sphere. It was reported that when fullerenes come into touch with the skin, they migrate across the skin intercellularly. Hence, a fullerene could be employed to "trap" active substances and then release them into the epidermis upon skin application. Furthermore, fullerenes are considered to be possibly powerful antioxidants [22].

4.8. Hydrogels /Polymers

Hydrogels denote a novel drug delivery system comprising different applications. Their potential in peroral drug delivery and tissue engineering has been very well established and their potential in delivery of dermopharmaceuticals has been realized. Moreover, their biocompatibility and structural diversity have extended their utility for an array of applications. They are hydrophilic polymer linkages that exhibit the capacity of water absoprtion ranging from 10-20% up to thousands of times their dry weight in water [43].

Hydrogels produced in the form of sheets can appropriately be utilized in the dermal or transdermal administration of the active constituents. Moreover, by modulating the composition of the polymeric backbone and reaction conditions (in case of cross-linked hydrogels) hydrogels can be tailored to obtain desired physical properties and release profile. Owing to their versatility, hydrogels can be easily employed for localized delivery of antiacne agents especially the ones exhibiting the problem of skin irritation. In fact, the hydrogels exhibiting notable skin adhesion and moisturizer effect would be an ideal tactic for topical acne treatment.

Lee *et al.* [44] have successfully applied 'hydrogel technology' for improving dermal accumulation of an antiacne agent in order to avoid their percutaneous absorption. The investigation has not only revealed the potential of triclosan as an antiacne agent but also provided the platform technology for efficient topical delivery of various other antiacne agents. Lee *et al.* have designed peeloff-type adhesive hydrogel patches based on 2 matrix polymers, namely sodium polyacrylate and sodium carboxymethyl cellulose. The cross-linking of these negatively charged polymers was achieved by employing Al^{3+} ion generated in situ. They found that in order to obtain hydrogel in the patch form, the cross-linking reaction should be slow and the solidification of the hydrogel should not be completed before casting the fluidic gel as a thin film.

Hydrogel patches containing triclosan in varying concentrations (from 0.01 to 0.5% w/w) were characterized for *in vitro* antimicrobial activity against *P. acnes* (ATCC 6919), adhesivity and in vitro skin permeation. The antimicrobial activity of triclosan hydrogel patches was evident when the triclosan content was 0.05% w/w and it improved with the escalation in the amount of triclosan. *In vitro* permeation studies carried out on triclosan hydrogel patches using hairless mouse skin clearly indicated the significant increase in the amount of triclosan transported into the skin as compared to the amount transported across the skin [45].

4.9. Solid Lipid Nanoparticles

Solid lipid nanoparticles (SLN TM, Lipoearls TM) are advanced drug administration systems that are introduced for combining the advantages but avoiding the disadvantages of conventional colloidal drug carrier systems like polymeric nanoparticles, liposomes and microparticles and emulsions. They have been proved to be promising delivery strategy for efficient administration of many active constituents by numerous application pathways. SLNs have revealed a great ability to efficiently deliver various topical agents and even cosmeceuticals and their applications are continuously being unraveled. It was reported the successful fabrication of SLNs for improved dermal delivery of tretinoin using the novel solvent emulsification diffusion method. Interestingly, SLN-based tretinoin gels were greatly able to improve the tolerability of tretinoin as compared to commercialized products when valued by the Draize patch test in rabbits [14, 45].

4.10. Aerosol Foams

They have become an exceedingly common kind of topical preparation for a diversity of skin disorders like acne. The vehicle base of the foam could possess a liquid or semi-solid consistency that contains the same physicochemical properties of conventional vehicles like creams, lotions and gels, but it balances desirable characterstics such as moisturizing/fast-drying effects, or higher drug bioavailability. The aerosol base is dispensed through a gas-pressurized can that discharges the foam. The product features are determined by the type of formulation and the dispensing container that are selected to suit the specific therapy needs. In acne, foams may be preferred for application on large hairy surfaces or on the face as cleansers, because they are easier to spread [22].

Table **3** shows the summary of novel drug delivery systems for antiacne agents.

Table 3. Novel drug delivery systems for antiacne agents [14, 16, 22, 28, 45, 46].

Drug delivery systems	Drug enclosed	Limitations with conventional therapy	Merits
Nanoparticles	Minocycline	Lack of drug loading and entrapment efficiency due to hydrophilicity of the drug	Enhanced drug loading and entrapment efficiency and controlled release
	Azelaic acid	Fewer side effects	Enhanced drug retention at PSU and stability
	Triclosan	Insufficient permeation and absorption *via* cutaneous route	Non-irritant to skin, enhanced stability
	CPA	Systemic antiandrogenic effects	Increased skin penetration and absorption
Niosomes	Tretinoin	Photodegradation	Increased accumulation in superficial stratum and stability, Increased drug release and entrapment efficiencies
Liposomes	Isotretinoin	Skin irritation, very low water solubility, difficulty to incorporate in topical base, photodegradation	Potential for skin targeting, prolonging drug release, reduction of photodegradation and skin irritation
	Clindamycin hydrochloride	Lesser reduction in number of lesions	Enhanced antiacne activity and sustained release of drug
	Tretinoin	Skin irritant, photo instability	Enhanced local tolerability and 5-6 times increase comedolytic activity, Reduced photo instability
	Salicylic acid	Skin irritation	Increased entrapment efficiency and stability
	BPO	Skin irritation	Improved antibacterial activity, reduced irritation
Solid lipid nanoparticles	Isotretinoin	Teratogenicity, mucocutaneous problems like cheilitis, dermatitis, conjunctivitis, blepharitis, skin fragility and xerosis, psychological disorders, erythema, dryness, itching, stinging, skin peeling	Reduced dermal irritation, increased therapeutic performance
	Retinoic acid	Sensitive to sunlight, eczematous irritation, erythema, interaction with other applied products	Comedolytic effect, reduction in RA induced irritation
	Tretinoin	Skin irritation and chemical instability	High encapsulation efficacy, physical stability and absence of cytotoxicity
	Terbinafine hydrochloride	Longer duration of treatment	Controlled release, drug targeting
Nanosuspension	Tretinoin	Poor water solubility and photostability	Improved drug permeation and UV irradiation stability
Nanoemulsion	Tretinoin, Tetracycline	Skin irritation, a burning sensation, and peeling	Enhanced drug permeation and antibacterial activity
Nano lipid carriers	Tretinoin, Tetracycline	Skin irritation, a burning sensation, and peeling	Enhanced drug permeation and antibacterial activity

(Table 3) contd.....

Drug delivery systems	Drug enclosed	Limitations with conventional therapy	Merits
Microemulsions	Azelaic acid	Large and frequent dosing	Enhanced stability
	Tretinoin	systemic side effects	Reducing frequency of administration, potentially decreasing side effects, improved patient compliance sustaining drug delivery
	Retinoic acid	Systemic side effects	Enhanced skin accumulation of retinoic acid
Microspheres	BPO	Skin irritation	Appropriate reduction in P. acnes count, reduced skin irritation
	Retinoid	Skin irritation and instability	Reduced irritation and enhanced stability
Hydrogels	Triclosan	Insufficient permeation and absorption *via* cutaneous route	Enhanced transdermal penetration

CONCLUSION

Novel drug delivery systems display a strong base for topical management of acne in order to enhance the therapeutic performance of the topical antiacne agents with improved patience compliance and a concomitant reduction in their side effects. Amongst various drug delivery systems: liposomes have been extensively explored and their ability to optimize and improve topical therapy has been proved by several clinical trials. However, the potential of various other vesicular carriers like niosomes, aspasomes, ethosomes and transferosomes still remains to be fully investigated. Microemulsions, microsponges, solid lipid nanoparticles and hydrogels also exhibit a tremendous potential for commercialization. In fact, their potential for successful topical delivery of antiacne agents has been very well reported by *in vitro* experiments.

CONFLICT OF INTEREST

The author confirms that this article content has no conflict of interest.

ACKNOWLEDGEMENTS

Declared none.

REFERENCES

[1]   Miranda W, Maja P, Joke AB. The lipid organization in SC and model systems base on ceramides. In: Enhancement in drug delivery. USA: CRS Press Taylor & Francis Group 2007; pp. 217-20.

[2]   Blank IH. Transport across the SC. Toxicol Appl Pharmacol 1969; 14(Suppl. 3): 23-9.
[http://dx.doi.org/10.1016/S0041-008X(69)80006-2]

[3]   Scheuplein RJ, Blank IH. Permeability of the skin. Physiol Rev 1971; 51(4): 702-47.
[PMID: 4940637]

[4]   Eckert RL. Structure, function, and differentiation of the keratinocyte. Physiol Rev 1989; 69(4): 1316-46.
[PMID: 2678169]

[5]   Baker H, Kligman AM. Technique for estimating turnover time of human stratum corneum. Arch Dermatol 1967; 95(4): 408-11.
[http://dx.doi.org/10.1001/archderm.1967.01600340068016] [PMID: 4164581]

[6]   Bouwstra JA, de Graaff A, Gooris GS, Nijsse J, Wiechers JW, van Aelst AC. Water distribution and related morphology in human stratum corneum at different hydration levels. J Invest Dermatol 2003; 120(5): 750-8.
[http://dx.doi.org/10.1046/j.1523-1747.2003.12128.x] [PMID: 12713576]

[7]   Elias PM. Epidermal lipids, barrier function, and desquamation. J Invest Dermatol 1983; 80: 44.
[http://dx.doi.org/10.1038/jid.1983.12] [PMID: 6184422]

[8]   Barry BW. Structure, function, diseases, and topical treatment of human skin. In: Dermatological formulations percutaneous absorption, 1. New York: Marcel Dekker 1983.

[9]   Rolland A, Wagner N, Chatelus A, Shroot B, Schaefer H. Site-specific drug delivery to pilosebaceous structures using polymeric microspheres. Pharm Res 1993; 10(12): 1738-44.
[http://dx.doi.org/10.1023/A:1018922114398] [PMID: 8302759]

[10]   Grams YY, Alaruikka S, Lashley L, Caussin J, Whitehead L, Bouwstra JA. Permeant lipophilicity and vehicle composition influence accumulation of dyes in hair follicles of human skin. Eur J Pharm Sci 2003; 18(5): 329-36.
[http://dx.doi.org/10.1016/S0928-0987(03)00035-6] [PMID: 12694885]

[11]   Cullander C, Guy RH. Visualization of iontophoretic pathways with confocal microscopy and the vibrating probe electrode. Solid State Ion 1992; 53-56: 197.
[http://dx.doi.org/10.1016/0167-2738(92)90382-Y]

[12]   Williams ML, Elias PM. The extracellular matrix of stratum corneum: role of lipids in normal and pathological function. Crit Rev Ther Drug Carrier Syst 1987; 3(2): 95-122.
[PMID: 3542246]

[13]   Fries JH. Chocolate: a review of published reports of allergic and other deleterious effects, real or presumed. Ann Allergy 1978; 41(4): 195-207.
[PMID: 152075]

[14]   Date AA, Naik B, Nagarsenker MS. Novel drug delivery systems: potential in improving topical delivery of antiacne agents. Skin Pharmacol Physiol 2006; 19(1): 2-16.
[http://dx.doi.org/10.1159/000089138] [PMID: 16247244]

[15]   Ballangera F, Baudrya P, N'Guyenb JM, Khammaria A, Dréno B. Heredity: a prognostic factor for acne. Dermatology 2005; 212(2): 145.: 9.

[16]   Dermatological Services - Acne. Available from: http://www.adultandpediatricdermatology.com/acne.shtml [Accessed on June 20, 2016].

[17]   Simpson NB, Cunliffe WJ. Disorders of the sebaceous glands. In: Burns T, Ed. Rook's textbook of dermatology. 7th ed. Malden, Mass.: Blackwell Science 2004; pp. 43-75.
[http://dx.doi.org/10.1002/9780470750520.ch43]

[18]   Adebamowo CA, Spiegelman D, Berkey CS, et al. Milk consumption and acne in adolescent girls. Dermatol Online J 2006; 12(4): 1.
[PMID: 17083856]

[19]   Arbesman H. Dairy and acnethe iodine connection. J Am Acad Dermatol 2005; 53(6): 1102.
[http://dx.doi.org/10.1016/j.jaad.2005.05.046] [PMID: 16310091]

[20]   Fulton JE Jr, Plewig G, Kligman AM. Effect of chocolate on acne vulgaris. JAMA 1969; 210(11): 2071-4.
[http://dx.doi.org/10.1001/jama.1969.03160370055011] [PMID: 4243053]

[21]   Acne Scars - The Physical Effects of Acne. Available from: http://www.proactiv.com.au/physical-effects-of- acne.aspx [Accessed Date: June 20, 2016].

[22]   Taglietti M, Hawkins CN, Rao J. Novel topical drug delivery systems and their potential use in acne vulgaris. Skin Therapy Lett 2008; 13(5): 6-8.
[PMID: 18648713]

[23]   Chiou WL. Low intrinsic drug activity and dominant vehicle (placebo) effect in the topical treatment of acne vulgaris. Int J Clin Pharmacol Ther 2012; 50(6): 434-7.
[http://dx.doi.org/10.5414/CP201694] [PMID: 22677304]

[24]   Chiou WL. Topical treatment of skin infection. US Patent US8846646 B2, 2014.

[25]   Lamel SA, Sivamani RK, Rahvar M, Maibach HI. Evaluating clinical trial design: systematic review of randomized vehicle-controlled trials for determining efficacy of benzoyl peroxide topical therapy for acne. Arch Dermatol Res 2015; 307(9): 757-66.
[http://dx.doi.org/10.1007/s00403-015-1568-9] [PMID: 26048131]

[26]   Schäfer-Korting M, Korting HC, Ponce-Pöschl E. Liposomal tretinoin for uncomplicated acne vulgaris. Clin Investig 1994; 72(12): 1086-91.
[http://dx.doi.org/10.1007/BF00577761] [PMID: 7711421]

[27]   Brisaert M, Gabriëls M, Matthijs V, Plaizier-Vercammen J. Liposomes with tretinoin: a physical and chemical evaluation. J Pharm Biomed Anal 2001; 26(5-6): 909-17.
[http://dx.doi.org/10.1016/S0731-7085(01)00502-7] [PMID: 11600303]

[28]   Elka T, Biana G. Vesicular carriers enhanced delivery through the skin. In: Enhancement in drug delivery. USA: CRS Press Taylor & Francis Group 2007; pp. 255-63.

[29]   Peter AM, Kathleen MB. Lipids of Physiologic Significance. In: Harper's Illustrated Biochemistry. 26th Edition. USA: McGraw-Hill Companies, Inc. 2003; p. 120.

[30]   Patel VB, Misra AN, Marfatia YS. Preparation and comparative clinical evaluation of liposomal gel of benzoyl peroxide for acne. Drug Dev Ind Pharm 2001; 27(8): 863-9.
[http://dx.doi.org/10.1081/DDC-100107251] [PMID: 11699839]

[31]   Gollnick H, Cunliffe W, Berson D, et al. Management of acne: a report from a global alliance to improve outcomes in acne. J Am Acad Dermatol 2003; 49(1)(Suppl.): S1-37.
[http://dx.doi.org/10.1067/mjd.2003.618] [PMID: 12833004]

[32]   Burkhart CN, Specht K, Neckers D. Synergistic activity of benzoyl peroxide and erythromycin. Skin Pharmacol Appl Skin Physiol 2000; 13(5): 292-6.
[http://dx.doi.org/10.1159/000029936] [PMID: 10940820]

[33]   Gruber DM, Sator MO, Joura EA, Kokoschka EM, Heinze G, Huber JC. Topical cyproterone acetate treatment in women with acne: a placebo-controlled trial. Arch Dermatol 1998; 134(4): 459-63.
[http://dx.doi.org/10.1001/archderm.134.4:459] [PMID: 9554298]

[34]   Eremia S. Chemical Peels and Microdermabrasion. In: Office-Based Cosmetic Procedures and Techniques. 1st ed. UK: Cambridge University Press 2010; pp. 338-42.
[http://dx.doi.org/10.1017/CBO9780511674839]

[35]   Small R, Hoang D, Linder J. Chemical Peels. In: A Practical Guide to Chemical Peels, Microdermabrasion & Topical Products. USA: Lippincott Williams & Wilkins 2013; pp. 43-5.

[36]   Namdeo A, Jain NK. Niosomes as drug carriers. Indian J Pharm Sci 1996; 58: 41-6.

[37]   Uchegbu IF, Vyas SP. Non-ionic surfactant based vesicles (niosomes) in drug delivery. Int J Pharm 1998; 172: 33-70.
        [http://dx.doi.org/10.1016/S0378-5173(98)00169-0]

[38]   Manconi M, Sinico C, Valenti D, Loy G, Fadda AM, Fadda AM. Niosomes as carriers for tretinoin. I. Preparation and properties. Int J Pharm 2002; 234(1-2): 237-48.
        [http://dx.doi.org/10.1016/S0378-5173(01)00971-1] [PMID: 11839454]

[39]   Manconi M, Valenti D, Sinico C, Lai F, Loy G, Fadda AM. Niosomes as carriers for tretinoin. II. Influence of vesicular incorporation on tretinoin photostability. Int J Pharm 2003; 260(2): 261-72.
        [http://dx.doi.org/10.1016/S0378-5173(03)00268-0] [PMID: 12842345]

[40]   Gopinath D, Ravi D, Rao BR, Apte SS, Renuka D, Rambhau D. Ascorbyl palmitate vesicles (Aspasomes): formation, characterization and applications. Int J Pharm 2004; 271(1-2): 95-113.
        [http://dx.doi.org/10.1016/j.ijpharm.2003.10.032] [PMID: 15129977]

[41]   Embil K, Nacht S. Microsponge delivery systems (MDS) a topical delivery system with reduced irritancy incorporating multiple mechanisms for triggering the release of active agents. J Microencapsul 1996; 13: 575-88.
        [http://dx.doi.org/10.3109/02652049609026042] [PMID: 8864994]

[42]   Gasco MR, Gallarate M, Pattarino F. *In vitro* permeation of azelaic acid from microemulsions. Int J Pharm 1991; 69: 193-6.
        [http://dx.doi.org/10.1016/0378-5173(91)90361-Q]

[43]   Hoffman AS. Hydrogels for biomedical applications. Adv Drug Deliv Rev 2002; 54(1): 3-12.
        [http://dx.doi.org/10.1016/S0169-409X(01)00239-3] [PMID: 11755703]

[44]   Lee TW, Kim JC, Hwang SJ. Hydrogel patches containing triclosan for acne treatment. Eur J Pharm Biopharm 2003; 56(3): 407-12.
        [http://dx.doi.org/10.1016/S0939-6411(03)00137-1] [PMID: 14602184]

[45]   Sinha P, Srivastava S, Mishra N, Yadav NP. New perspectives on antiacne plant drugs: contribution to modern therapeutics. BioMed Res Int 2014; 2014: 301304.
        [http://dx.doi.org/10.1155/2014/301304] [PMID: 25147793]

[46]   Mortazavi SA, Pishrochi S, Jafari Azar Z. Formulation and *in vitro* evaluation of tretinoin microemulsion as a potential carrier for dermal drug delivery. Iran J Pharm Res 2013; 12(4): 599-609.
        [PMID: 24523740]

6

Possible Role of Phosphatidylglycerol-Activated Protein Kinase C-βII in Keratinocyte Differentiation

Lakiea J. Bailey[2], Vivek Choudhary[1,2] and Wendy B. Bollag[*, 1,2]

[1]*Charlie Norwood VA Medical Center, One Freedom Way, Augusta, GA 30904, USA*
[2]*Department of Physiology, 1120 15th Street, Medical College of Georgia at Augusta University (formerly Georgia Regents University), Augusta, GA 30912, USA*

Abstract:

Background:

The epidermis is a continuously regenerating tissue maintained by a balance between proliferation and differentiation, with imbalances resulting in skin disease. We have previously found that in mouse keratinocytes, the lipid-metabolizing enzyme phospholipase D2 (PLD2) is associated with the aquaglyceroporin, aquaporin 3 (AQP3), an efficient transporter of glycerol. Our results also show that the functional interaction of AQP3 and PLD2 results in increased levels of phosphatidylglycerol (PG) in response to an elevated extracellular calcium level, which triggers keratinocyte differentiation. Indeed, we showed that directly applying PG can promote keratinocyte differentiation.

Objective:

We hypothesized that the differentiative effects of this PLD2/AQP3/PG signaling cascade, in which AQP3 mediates the transport of glycerol into keratinocytes followed by its PLD2-catalyzed conversion to PG, are mediated by protein kinase CβII (PKCβII), which contains a PG-binding domain in its carboxy-terminus. Method: To test this hypothesis we used quantitative RT-PCR, western blotting and immunocytochemistry.

Results:

We first verified the presence of PKCβII mRNA and protein in mouse keratinocytes. Next, we found that autophosphorylated (activated) PKCβII was redistributed upon treatment of keratinocytes with PG. In the unstimulated state phosphoPKCβII was found in the cytosol and perinuclear area; treatment with PG resulted in enhanced phosphoPKCβII localization in the perinuclear area. PG also induced translocation of phosphoPKCβII to the plasma membrane. In addition, we observed that overexpression of PKCβII enhanced calcium- and PG-induced keratinocyte differentiation without affecting calcium-inhibited keratinocyte proliferation.

Conclusion:

These results suggest that the PG produced by the PLD2/AQP3 signaling module may function by activating PKCβII.

Keywords: Aquaporin-3 (AQP3), Epidermis, Keratin-10, Phospholipase D2 (PLD2), Skin, Kinase.

1. INTRODUCTION

The epidermis forms the mechanical and water permeability barrier of the skin, allowing terrestrial existence and protecting from various environmental insults. The predominant cells comprising the epidermis are keratinocytes, which form a stratified epithelium. At the basement membrane, the basal keratinocytes continuously proliferate to replace

[*] Address correspondence to this author at the Department of Physiology, 1120 15th Street, Medical College of Georgia at Augusta University, Augusta, GA 30912, USA, E-mail: wbollag@augusta.edu

damaged cells and those sloughed to the surroundings. As they move upwards into the upper epidermal layers, the keratinocytes growth arrest and differentiate, expressing different sets of genes and proteins as they become more and more differentiated. A great deal is known about the signals that regulate proliferation and differentiation, including the fact that elevated extracellular calcium concentrations trigger keratinocyte differentiation [1]. Nevertheless, a complete understanding of these processes, and the signaling molecules that modulate them, requires further study.

We have previously shown that the lipid-metabolizing enzyme phospholipase D2 (PLD2) and the water and glycerol channel aquaporin-3 (AQP3) physically and functionally associate in keratinocytes to produce phosphatidylglycerol (PG) [2, 3]. PG levels are increased biphasically in response to increasing concentrations of calcium, with a maximal effect at approximately 125µM [3]. This dose response is similar to that reported for calcium-induced keratinocyte differentiation [4], suggesting the possibility that the PLD2/AQP3/PG signaling module might mediate keratinocyte differentiation. This idea is supported by our finding that manipulation of this module inhibited proliferation and promoted differentiation of keratinocytes [5]. In particular, treatment of keratinocytes with liposomes formed from egg-derived PG promoted the differentiation and inhibited the proliferation of rapidly growing keratinocytes [5, 6]. The mechanism by which PG exerted this effect, however, is unclear.

The protein kinase C (PKC) enzymes comprise a family of enzymes with 10 isoforms that are differentially regulated. The classical (or conventional) PKC isoforms, which include PKCα, PKCβI, PKCβII and PKCγ, require acidic phospholipids and are activated by increased diacylglycerol and calcium levels triggered upon phosphoinositide hydrolysis initiated by receptor engagement by various hormones, growth factors and other ligands. Different PKC isoforms are encoded by separate genes except for PKCβI and PKCβII, which represent splice variants of mRNA transcribed from a single gene; PKCβI and PKCβII differ in their C-terminal V5 regions. In PKCβII, this region is the location of the PG-binding domain and contains the molecular determinant necessary for nuclear translocation and enzyme activation [7, 8]. In HL60 leukemia cells, PG in the nuclear membrane selectively stimulates PKCβII activity 3-6 fold above the level achieved in the presence of optimal concentrations of calcium, diacylglycerol and phosphatidylserine [9]. In fibroblasts, entry into mitosis is dependent upon activation of PKCβII by PG [10]. Furthermore, the sequence in PKCβII responsible for binding to PG has been localized to the 13 amino acids in the C-terminus unique to PKCβII [7].

We hypothesized that PKCβII might serve as an effector enzyme for PG in keratinocytes to promote early keratinocyte differentiation. We tested this idea by examining the redistribution of phospho-PKCβII in keratinocytes treated with a moderately elevated calcium concentration (which maximally increases PG levels [3]) and PG liposomes. We also assessed the effect of overexpression of PKCβII on the calcium-induced inhibition of proliferation and stimulation of keratin 10 levels. We provide evidence for PKCβII activation in response to an elevated extracellular calcium concentration and PG liposomes as well as the ability of PKCβII to promote early keratinocyte differentiation.

2. METHODS

2.1. Culture of Primary Mouse Keratinocytes

Primary murine epidermal keratinocytes were prepared from 1 to 3 day old neonatal ICR CD-1 outbred mice as described in [11]. Treatment of mice conformed to policies in the Guide for the Care and Use of Laboratory Animals and monitored by the Institutional Animal Care and Use Committee (IACUC) of Augusta University. Harvested keratinocytes were plated at a density of 25,000 cells/cm^2 and incubated overnight at 37°C with 5% carbon dioxide in Plating Medium composed of calcium-free minimum essential medium alpha (MEMα) supplemented with 2% dialyzed fetal bovine serum, 25µM CaCl$_2$, 5ng/mL epidermal growth factor, 2mM glutamine, ITS+, 100U/mL penicillin, 100µg/mL streptomycin and 0.25µg/mL fungizone as in [12]. After approximately 24 hours, Plating Medium was replaced with either a laboratory-prepared serum-free keratinocyte medium (SFKM) or commercially purchased Keratinocyte-serum free medium (K-SFM) (Gibco, Gaithersburg, MD). Initial experiments used SFKM containing 25µM CaCl$_2$, 90µg/mL bovine pituitary extract, ITS+, 5ng/mL epidermal growth factor, 2mM glutamine, 0.05% BSA, 100U/mL penicillin, 100µg/mL streptomycin and 0.25µg/mL fungizone as described by Griner *et al.* [12]. Our laboratory subsequently switched to commercial K-SFM supplementing pre-prepared K-SFM with 50µM CaCl$_2$, 2.5µg recombinant human EGF and 25mg bovine pituitary extract per the supplier's recommendations [13]. Medium was replaced every 1-2 days.

2.2. Preparation of PG Liposomes

Liposomes were prepared from egg-derived PG (Avanti Polar Lipids, Alabaster, AL). Briefly, PG in organic solvent was distributed into amber glass vials as 1mg aliquots, the solvent evaporated with nitrogen gas and the lipid stored under nitrogen at -20°C until use. For experiments, 0.5 mL serum-free medium was added to the amber vial to hydrate the lipid film followed by bath sonication using a Branson Sonifier with a microprobe and a cup horn.

2.3. RT-PCR and Quantitative RT-PCR Analysis

Cultured primary mouse keratinocytes, epidermis or skin were collected in 0.5-1mL of Trizol and RNA was extracted according to the manufacturer's protocol. The epidermis was isolated following overnight incubation of neonatal mouse skin in 0.25% trypsin in Hank's buffered saline solution at 4°C to allow the enzyme to permeate along the dermal-epidermal junction of the skin. After a brief incubation at 37°C to promote trypsin proteolysis, the epidermis was manually separated from the dermis using forceps. Total skin was extracted immediately after harvest. Mouse brain tissue was also collected and immediately RNA-extracted. First-strand cDNA synthesis was performed using Thermoscript RT-PCR System and oligo(dT) nucleotides (Sigma-Aldrich, St. Louis, MO) according to the manufacturer's protocol. RT-PCR was performed using JumpStart RedTaq reaction mix (Sigma-Aldrich) and the primers for PKCβII and GAPDH (mPKCβ forward: 5'-GCTGACAAGGGCCCAGCCTC-3'; reverse: 5'-GTGTGGTTCCGTGCCGCAGAG-3' and mGAPDH forward: 5'-GCGGCACGTCAGATCCA-3'; reverse: 5' CATGGCCTTCCGTGTTCCCTA-3'), also according to the manufacturer's protocol. The reaction parameters consisted of heat activation at 94°C for 2 minutes followed by 35 cycles of denaturation at 94°C for 15 seconds, annealing at 50°C for 30 seconds and elongation at 72°C for 30 seconds. The amplified product was resolved on a 1% TAE agarose gel. Quantitative RT-PCR was performed using Taqman probes (ThermoFisher Scientific, Waltham, MA) and analyzed by the delta-delta Ct method as described previously [13].

2.4. Western Blot Analysis

Near-confluent cultures of keratinocytes were incubated in SFKM (25µM $CaCl_2$) or K-SFM (50µM $CaCl_2$) alone or with medium containing the desired treatment, elevated calcium (125µM $CaCl_2$) or 100µg/mL PG for 24 hours. Cells were then harvested in lysis buffer, with 30µL/cm^2 of heated buffer (containing 0.1875M Tris-HCl, pH 8.5, 3% SDS and 1.5mM EDTA) added to each well. Protein concentrations were determined using a BioRad protein assay with BSA as the standard. After protein determination, 3X sample buffer (containing 30% glycerol, 15% β-mercaptoethanol and 1% bromophenol blue) was added to each sample to constitute Laemmli buffer. Total protein was also extracted from mouse brain, homogenized epidermis and freshly isolated keratinocytes after shearing using an 18-gauge needle. Samples were stored at -20°C until analysis at which time protein samples were heated to near boiling and equal amounts were loaded onto 8% SDS polyacrylamide gels, separated by electrophoresis and transferred to Immobilon-FL transfer membranes (Millipore, Billerica, MA). After washing and blocking, the membranes were incubated overnight with primary antibody [recognizing PKCβII (Abcam, Cambridge, MA), pPKCβII (pSer^{660}, Epitomics, Burlingame, CA), 1:10,000; K10 (Covance, Denver, PA), 1:15,000; and actin (Sigma-Aldrich or Santa Cruz, Santa Cruz, CA), 1:15,000] followed by secondary AlexaFluor florescent antibodies (Invitrogen, Carlsbad, CA or Licor, Lincoln, NE, 1:10,000), all diluted in Odyssey blocking buffer containing Tween-20 (LiCor). Immunoreactive bands corresponding to the proteins of interest were visualized *via* an Odyssey®SA infrared imaging system from Li-Cor and quantified with the internal software according to the manufacturer's instructions. The data are reported as means ± SEM after normalization to actin levels.

2.5. [³H]Thymidine Incorporation into DNA

DNA proliferation assays were performed on primary mouse keratinocytes overexpressing PKCβII or empty vector incubated in SFKM containing 25µM or 125µM calcium. Briefly, cells were transfected as previously described and exposed to experimental treatments for 24 hours. The cells were then incubated with 1µCi/mL [³H]thymidine (Moravek Biochemicals, Brea, CA) for 1 hour at 37°C. Reactions were terminated and macromolecules precipitated with cold trichloroacetic acid and the cells solubilized in 0.3M sodium hydroxide. [³H] Thymidine incorporation was measured in an aliquot using Ecolite scintillant (MP Biomedicals, Santa Ana, CA) and a Beckman Coulter LS 6500 multi-purpose scintillation counter (Brea, CA).

2.6. Immunocytochemistry

For immunocytochemistry PKCβII-specific and phosphoPKCβII-specific antibodies were generously provided by Dr. Denise Cooper (University of South Florida, Tampa, FL) [14]. The antibody recognizing PKCβII was raised against residues 655 to 671 (the C-terminus specific to PKCβII), and the phospho-specific antibody recognizes PKCβII phosphorylated on serine 660 of the C-terminus (residues 657-673) [14]. Primary murine keratinocytes were plated on glass BD BioCoat fibronectin-coated slides and at near-confluence were incubated in SFKM (25μM CaCl$_2$) or SFKM containing 100μg/ml PG at 37°C. After the desired incubation period, cells were washed with PBS and fixed in 4% paraformaldehyde. After permeabilization in 0.2% Triton X-100, the slides were blocked in buffer containing 10% goat serum and 1% BSA in PBS and incubated in buffer containing either phospho-PKCβII (1:500) or keratin-10 (Abcam, 1:250) overnight. The slides were then incubated in Cy3-conjugated secondary goat anti-rabbit IgG antibody (1:150) in 10% goat serum at room temperature and mounted with ProLong Antifade with DAPI (Invitrogen). Staining was visualized by multiphoton microscopy with a Zeiss LSM 510 confocal laser scanning microscope with a Meta System equipped with a Coherent Mira 900 tunable Ti:Sapphire laser for multi-photon excitation at 488nm, 543nm and 760nm wavelengths (Carl Zeiss Microscopy, Germany).

2.7. Keratinocyte Transfection

Primary mouse keratinocytes were transfected with wild-type PKCβII plasmid in a pcDNA3 vector backbone (or the vector plasmid) *via* AMAXA nucleofection (Lonza, Cologne, Germany), using an Amaxa Nucleofector Kit for primary endothelial cells as in [15] according to the manufacturer's instructions. The authors reported 40-60% transfection efficiency with this method [15]. The PKCβII plasmid was a generous gift from Dr. Lan Ko, (Augusta University). Transfected cells were then incubated in RPMI medium containing 10% fetal bovine serum and antibiotic/antimycotic (100U/mL penicillin, 100μg/mL streptomycin and 0.25μg/mL fungizone) for 20 minutes, plated in Plating Medium (described above) and allowed to attach overnight. After 24 hours the plating medium was replaced with K-SFM (containing 50μM CaCl$_2$).

2.8. Statistics

All experiments were performed independently a minimum of three times. Values were analyzed for statistical significance by analysis of variance or repeated measures analysis of variance with a Student-Newmann-Keuls or Dunn's *post-hoc* test using Prism (GraphPad Software, San Diego, CA). All quantitative data were expressed in the form of bar graphs, with the bars representing mean ± standard error of the mean (SEM).

3. RESULTS

3.1. PKCβII is Expressed in Mouse Keratinocytes

PKCβII is known to bind to and be activated by PG to trigger cell cycle progression in human leukemia cells [8]. However, although multiple PKC isozymes have been identified in keratinocytes, there has been some debate regarding the presence of PKCβ in these cells [16 - 19], with an initial report failing to detect PKCβ in mouse keratinocytes using northern analysis [16]. Two subsequent studies found PKCβ in human skin [17], mouse keratinocytes [18] and mouse skin [19]. To resolve this issue, we first sought to determine if PKCβ could be detected by semi-quantitative RT-PCR using mouse brain as a positive control. PKCβ was found to be transcribed in primary mouse keratinocytes (Fig. **1A**). Although the mRNA was much less abundant than in brain (Fig. **1B**), quantitative RT-PCR using Taqman assays indicated that the cycle threshold was within a detectable range (approximately 30 cycles). The difference in the amount of cDNA amplified and separated also likely explains the slight apparent differences in molecular weight of the PKCβ band observed in brain and keratinocytes with semi-quantitative RT-PCR (Fig. **1A**), since greatly different amounts of nucleic acid can separate slightly differently by electrophoresis. We next sought to determine whether the PKCβII protein was expressed using a PKCβII-specific antibody obtained from Dr. Denise Cooper [14]. This antibody was raised against residues 655 to 671 (the C-terminus specific to PKCβII). Using this antibody it was shown that keratinocytes also express PKCβII protein (Fig. **1C**). To ensure that expression of the enzyme was not an artifact of culture, we also demonstrated PKCβII protein expression in freshly isolated keratinocytes and epidermis (Fig. **1D**), as well as mRNA expression in total skin (Fig. **1B**). Therefore, we hypothesized that PKCβII might be an effector enzyme for PG in keratinocytes.

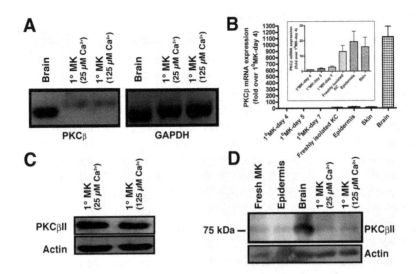

Fig. (1). PKCβII protein is expressed in primary mouse epidermal keratinocytes, freshly isolated epidermal keratinocytes and the epidermis. (A) RNA was isolated from primary mouse keratinocytes (1°MK) cultured to near confluence before incubation for 24 hours in medium containing basal (25μM) or moderately elevated (125μM) extracellular Ca^{2+} concentrations as indicated and PKCβ expression monitored by semi-quantitative RT-PCR. (B) RNA was isolated from primary mouse keratinocytes (1°MK) incubated in medium containing a basal (50μM) extracellular Ca^{2+} concentration, freshly isolated keratinocytes (before plating), isolated epidermis, total skin and brain as indicated and PKCβ expression monitored by quantitative RT-PCR using primer-probe sets from Applied Biosystems and a StepOne system as described in Methods. Results are expressed as the fold change in normalized cycle threshold relative to primary cultures of primary mouse keratinocytes (1°MK) cultured for 4 days, analyzed using the ΔΔCt method with GAPDH as the normalization control. Note that the brain expresses a significantly greater amount of PKCβ than do keratinocytes or skin tissue; therefore, in the inset the values obtained only from 1°MK cultured for the indicated number of days, freshly isolated keratinocytes (KC), isolated epidermis or total skin are plotted using a different scale. (C) Protein lysates were prepared from primary mouse keratinocytes (1°MK) cultured in medium containing basal (25μM) or moderately elevated (125μM) extracellular Ca^{2+} concentrations. (D) Protein lysates prepared from primary mouse keratinocytes (1°MK) cultured in medium containing basal (25μM) or 125μM Ca^{2+}, freshly isolated keratinocytes (fresh MK) or a homogenate of epidermis were analyzed by western blotting. Western analysis was performed using the PKCβII antibody obtained from Dr. Denise Cooper (University of South Florida, Tampa, FL). Commercially available antibodies yielded similar results. Brain was used as a positive control.

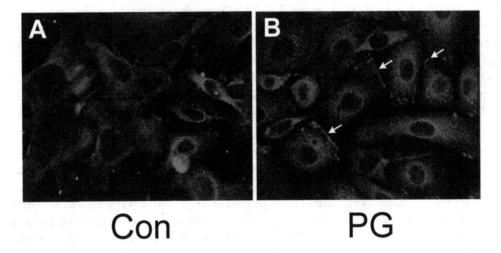

Fig. (2). PG stimulates phosphoPKCβII redistribution in keratinocytes. Keratinocytes grown on fibronectin-coated slides were stimulated for 60 minutes with medium containing a basal (25μM) calcium concentration (A) without (Con) or (B) with 100μg/mL egg PG (PG), provided in the form of liposomes. Cells were then stained with an antibody recognizing phosphorylated PKCβII, an Alexa468-conjugated secondary antibody and the nuclear stain, DAPI, and visualized using a multiphoton Zeiss microscope. The primary antibody was omitted to serve as a negative control and showed no staining for PKCβII although DAPI was visualized (data not shown).

3.2. PKCβII is Redistributed Upon Provision of PG

We have shown that PG can inhibit proliferation and promote differentiation of keratinocytes, and based on the literature demonstrating that PKCβII is a PG-activated enzyme, we hypothesized that stimulation of PKCβII activity by PG may be the mechanism by which the lipid signal exerts its effects. Phosphorylation and translocation to cell membranes are considered hallmarks of PKC activation [20]. We utilized immunocytochemical techniques to visualize the cellular localization of phosphorylated/activated PKCβII upon treatment with PG, again using an antibody provided by Dr. Cooper recognizing PKCβII phosphorylated on serine 660 of the C-terminus (residues 657-673). Primary mouse keratinocytes plated on collagen-coated slides were subjected to immunohistochemical analysis. Under basal conditions, autophosphorylated PKCβII (phosphoPKCβII) was found diffusely throughout the entire cell with increased staining around the perinuclear area (Fig. **2**, left panel). A 1h treatment with PG (100μg/mL egg-derived PG in the form of liposomes) increased staining in the perinuclear area (Fig. **2A**, right panel) compared to the control (Fig. **2B**, left panel). In addition, PG induced localization of PKCβII in the plasma membrane (Fig. **2B**, right panel, arrows). Since PKCβII requires phospholipids for its activity, translocation to the membrane is thought to mark activation of the enzyme [21, 22]. These results suggest that, as in leukemia cells [7 - 9], PG activates PKCβII. Treatment of keratinocytes with PG followed by western analysis with the antibody recognizing phosphoPKCβII also showed a trend towards enhanced autophosphorylation (activation) of PKCβII (to a value of 1.32 ± 0.13-fold over the control of 1.0; n=6), but the increase did not quite achieve statistical significance (p=0.054).

3.3. A Moderately Elevated Extracellular Calcium Concentration Induces the Autophosphorylation/ Activation of PKCβII

We have previously observed an ability of moderately elevated extracellular calcium concentrations to increase PG levels in keratinocytes [3], suggesting the possibility that PG-activated PKCβII may play a role in calcium-induced differentiation. To explore this possibility we over-expressed PKCβII and first assessed the effect of calcium on the autophosphorylation/activation of this enzyme. Primary mouse keratinocytes were transfected with either an empty vector or PKCβII plasmid vector, as described in the Materials and Methods section, and then cultured in the presence or absence of an elevated extracellular calcium concentrations. Total and autophosphorylated PKCβII levels were increased in mouse keratinocytes transfected with PKCβII plasma vector, and autophosphorylation of this overexpressed PKCβII was stimulated in response to elevated extracellular calcium (125μM) (Figs. **3A-C**).

3.4. Over-Expression of PKCβII has no Effect on Calcium-Induced Inhibition of Proliferation but Increases the Levels of Keratin-10, a Marker of Early Keratinocyte Differentiation, in Primary Mouse Keratinocytes

To determine whether this over-expression of PKCβII affected the ability of elevated calcium levels to inhibit keratinocyte proliferation, we treated vector- and PKCβII-transfected cells with medium containing basal calcium levels or a moderately elevated calcium concentration. Proliferation was assessed by measuring the incorporation of [^{3}H]thymidine into the DNA of dividing cells. In cells expressing basal, physiological levels of PKCβII, that is, transfected with empty vector plasmid, stimulation with elevated extracellular calcium resulted in calcium-induced inhibition of proliferation (Fig. **3D**), as described elsewhere [23]. A similar inhibition was observed in the PKCβII-transfected cells, although this effect did not achieve statistical significance, suggesting that this enzyme likely does not mediate the anti-proliferative effect of an elevated calcium concentration.

Expression levels of keratin-10, a marker of keratinocyte differentiation, were also examined in cells over-expressing PKCβII. There was no change in the keratin-10 expression of keratinocytes over-expressing PKCβII and cultured under basal conditions. PKCβII over-expression in combination with an elevated extracellular calcium concentration, however, resulted in a substantial up-regulation in keratin-10 expression, with p<0.01 versus all other conditions (Fig. **4**). These results suggest that PKCβII alone is not sufficient to induce an increase in keratin-10 expression, but instead works in concert with calcium to promote early differentiation, but not growth arrest, in primary mouse keratinocytes.

3.5. Over-Expression of PKCβII Affects the Pattern of Keratin-10 Distribution and Results in an Altered Morphology of Cells Grown in the Presence of Phosphatidylglycerol

Our previous findings suggested that PG stimulates keratinocyte differentiation and inhibits proliferation [5, 6]; therefore, we next examined the morphological effect of PG on keratinocytes over-expressing PKCβII. Mouse keratinocytes were again transfected with either PKCβII or empty vector and were then cultured on collagen-coated slides in medium containing basal calcium with or without 100µg/ml egg PG. The cells were then fixed, permeabilized and stained with an antibody specific for keratin-10 (Fig. **5**). Interestingly, treatment with PG led to morphological changes consistent with later differentiation in cells transfected with PKCβII (Fig. **5A-D**), as well as the formation of keratin-10 filaments, changes that were not seen in cells transfected with empty vector and stimulated with PG (Fig. **5D**). Thus, PG in PKCβII-overexpressing cells induced enlargement and flattening reminiscent of the alterations observed with later keratinocyte differentiation; these changes also were not seen in keratinocytes overexpressing PKCβII in the absence of PG (Fig. **5A**). These data suggest that keratinocyte differentiation in response to elevated calcium concentrations may be mediated through the activation of PKCβII induced by increased production of PG. This hypothesis is consistent with the observed ability of PKCβII overexpression to increase keratin-10 levels in the presence of a moderately elevated calcium concentration and of PG to promote differentiative changes in PKCβII-overexpressing keratinocytes.

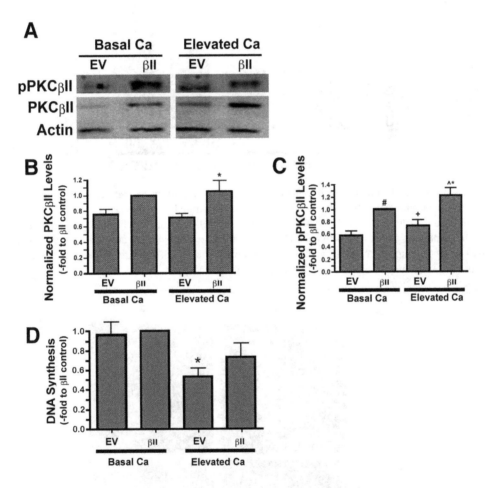

Fig. **(3)**. **Overexpressed PKCβII is autophosphorylated/activated in response to an elevation of extracellular calcium concentration in mouse keratinocytes but has no effect on calcium-inhibited proliferation.** Mouse keratinocytes were nucleofected with wild-type PKCβII (βII) or empty vector (EV) and then cultured in the presence of basal (25µM) or a moderately elevated extracellular calcium level (Ca; 125µM) for 24h. Cells were harvested and lysates were resolved on 8% SDS gels, transferred to PVDF membranes and probed with antibodies recognizing total PKCβII, autophosphorylated PKCβII and actin. **(A)** A representative experiment is illustrated. **(B)** Total PKCβII and **(C)** pPKCβII levels were quantified, normalized to actin and expressed relative to the PKCβII-transfected cells under basal conditions. Data represent the means ± SEM from at least 3 separate experiments. For total PKCβII, *$p < 0.05$ vs EV or EV+Ca and for autophosphorylated PKCβII, #$p < 0.01$ vs EV, *$p < 0.01$ vs EV+Ca, ^$p < 0.001$ vs EV, +$p < 0.05$ vs βII. **(D)**Keratinocytes nucleofected with wild-type PKCβII (βII) or empty vector (EV) were cultured in the presence of basal (25µM) or a moderately elevated extracellular calcium level (Ca; 125µM) for 24h. [³H]Thymidine was added to the medium for 1 hour and DNA synthesis measured as described in Materials and Methods. [³H]Thymidine incorporation into DNA is expressed as the percentage of the control value and shown as the mean ± SEM (n=4; *$p < 0.01$ vs EV or βII).

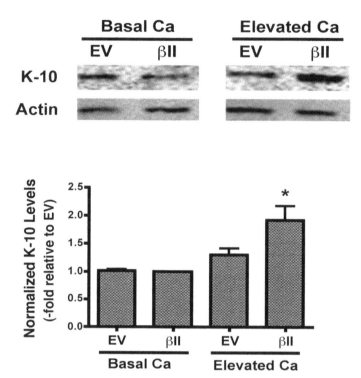

Fig. (4). Overexpressed PKCβII enhances calcium-induced keratin-10 protein expression (differentiation). Keratinocytes nucleofected with wild-type PKCβII (βII) or empty vector (EV) were cultured in the presence of basal (25μM) or a moderately elevated extracellular calcium level (Ca; 125μM) for 24h. Following cell harvest total lysates were resolved on 8% SDS gels, transferred to PVDF membranes and probed with antibodies recognizing keratin-10 (K10) and actin. A representative experiment is shown. Keratin-10 levels (normalized to actin and expressed relative to the PKCβII-transfected cells under basal conditions) were quantified and expressed as the mean ± SEM (n=4; *p<0.01 vs EV, βII or EV+Ca).

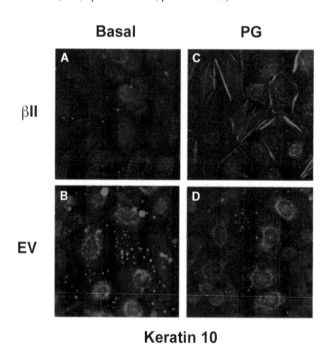

Fig. (5). PKCβII overexpression increases the PG-induced formation of keratin-10-containing intermediate filaments. Mouse keratinocytes were nucleofected with wild-type **(A and C)** PKCβII (βII) or **(B and D)** empty vector (EV) and then cultured on coated glass slides in the **(C and D)** presence or **(A and B)** absence of 100μg/mL PG in 25μM calcium-containing medium for 24h. Cells were fixed, permeabilized, probed with an antibody recognizing keratin-10 and visualized with an Alexa468-conjugated secondary antibody. Immunofluorescence was examined by confocal microscopy.

4. DISCUSSION

Disruption in the normal form and function of skin can result in a significant amount of human suffering. Several human skin diseases, such as psoriasis, a hyperproliferative disorder of the epidermis, and the non-melanoma skin cancers (basal and squamous cell carcinoma) are the result of a breakdown in the carefully controlled program regulating the proliferation and differentiation of keratinocytes. Approximately 7 million Americans and as much as 3 percent of the world population suffer from the devastating effects of psoriasis (www.healthline.com/health /psoriasis/facts-statistics-infographic). Although usually not a fatal condition, the physical and emotional impact of psoriasis has been reported to be comparable with that of other serious medical conditions, including heart and lung disease, depression and cancer ([24, 25] and www.aad.org/media/stats/conditions/psoriasis). Basal and squamous cell carcinomas are the two most common skin cancers in the world, with more than 3.5 million new diagnoses each year in the United States (http://www.cancer.org). Our results contribute to the body of knowledge regarding the pathways regulating the normal growth and differentiation of epidermal keratinocytes that are dysregulated in these diseases. Our study provides insight into a possible role of PKCβII in keratinocyte differentiation. On the other hand, an inhibitor of PKC has been proposed as therapeutic option for psoriasis, based on its ability to reduce cytokine production in psoriatic patients [26]. Our results suggest that targeting a PKC inhibitor more towards PKCθ and PKCα, and less towards PKCβ, might improve the efficacy of such a therapy (although PKCα has also been demonstrated to play a role in keratinocyte differentiation [27]).

Although the precise mechanisms regulating the progression of keratinocytes through the multilayered stratified structure of the epidermis remain unknown, our laboratory has proposed a potential signaling module involving PG generation by a signaling module composed of AQP3 and PLD2. We have previously shown a functional and physical interaction between PLD2 and the glycerol channel AQP3 [2, 3]. Notably, the PLD2/AQP3 signaling module was observed to be abnormal in psoriasis and non-melanoma skin cancers [28], suggesting a possible involvement of dysregulation of this module in such hyperproliferative skin diseases. Our laboratory has further shown that: (1) PLD2 can utilize AQP3-transported glycerol to generate PG, (2) elevated calcium concentrations increase PG levels and (3) this increase is likely mediated by PLD [3]. Maximal stimulation of calcium-induced PG formation was observed at a calcium concentration optimal for stimulation of markers of early differentiation (*e.g.*, keratin-10) [3, 4]. These findings, combined with the observation that the C-terminal PKCβII V5 region binds PG and contains the molecular determinant necessary for translocation and activation of the enzyme [7, 8], led us to suspect that PKCβII may be the mediator of PG's ability to promote keratinocyte maturation. Here, we present evidence that PKCβII is present in mouse keratinocytes (Fig. 1), consistent with previous reports [18, 19]. Although the brain expresses significantly more PKCβ than do keratinocytes, keratinocytes express PKCβ mRNA, although the band migrated slightly differently than the amplicon from brain, likely because of the difference in amounts in the two tissues, since abundance can alter electrophoretic separation. Nevertheless, PKCβ mRNA was also demonstrated by quantitative RT-PCR using Taqman assays. Since the Taqman probe only binds to the specific amplicon of interest, artifactual amplification of incorrect sequences will not be detected. In addition, we noted that mRNA levels tended to increase under conditions when keratinocytes would be expected to show less stem cell character and greater differentiation. This idea likely explains why PKCβ expression tends to rise with increasing time in culture as the cells reach confluence and begin to undergo contact-induced differentiation [29] and also to be higher in freshly isolated keratinocytes, which contain differentiated cells that do not attach to the tissue culture plastic upon seeding for culture. Expression tends to be higher also in epidermis and skin, as these tissues also contain large numbers of differentiated keratinocytes. The presence of PKCβ has also been detected in human skin [17]; nevertheless, a dearth of PKCβ isoform-specific antibodies with reactivity in formalin-fixed, paraffin-embedded tissue samples has hampered a complete characterization of PKCβII protein expression in human skin.

We also found that PKCβII is translocated/activated in response to PG treatment (Fig. 2). In addition, PKCβII over-expression induces an up-regulation of keratin-10 upon calcium-induced stimulation of differentiation (Fig. 4), but has no effect on calcium-induced inhibition of proliferation (Fig. 3). Finally, overexpression of PKCβII in keratinocytes promotes keratin-10 filament formation and results in morphology consistent with later differentiation upon treatment with PG (Fig. 5). On the other hand, it could be argued that a toxic effect of the liposomal matrix is responsible for the reorganization of keratin filaments observed in (Fig. 5), since the concentration of egg PG used, 100 μg/mL, translates to approximately 120-130 μM, near the threshold for toxicity observed by Mayhew *et al.* [30]. Nevertheless, overall cell morphology was not markedly affected by PG as seen in (Fig. 2), suggesting that toxicity is likely not an issue.

Calcium functions as a precise regulator of keratinocyte maturation and is essential for normal differentiation [4, 31 - 33], such that an increase in extracellular calcium concentration can initiate this process. Thus, keratinocytes grown in a low-calcium medium proliferate and maintain an immature state *in vitro*, but will transition to a more differentiated state when exposed to elevated extracellular calcium levels [34, 35]. Consistent with this effect, a calcium gradient has been observed in the epidermis *in situ*, with the lowest concentration observed in the basal layer where keratinocytes are actively proliferating and gradually increasing outward towards the more differentiated granular layer [33]. The observation that extracellular calcium is able to increase PG levels led us to test whether PKCβII plays a role in calcium-induced differentiation. Thus, we experimentally altered the expression of PKCβII and recorded the effect of this manipulation on keratinocyte proliferation and differentiation. Proliferation was assessed by measuring the incorporation of [^{3}H]thymidine into DNA in cells transfected with vector or PKCβII. In cells expressing basal, physiological levels of PKCβII (*i.e.*, vector-transfected cells), stimulation with elevated extracellular calcium resulted in calcium-induced inhibition of proliferation (Fig. **3**), as described by Bikle and colleagues [23]. However, overexpression of PKCβII did not substantially alter this calcium-elicited inhibition, suggesting that PKCβII is not involved in the initial growth arrest triggered by calcium.

In an effort to determine if PKCβII plays a role in keratinocyte differentiation we next evaluated the effect of PKCβII overexpression on the levels of keratin-10, a marker of early differentiation, in the presence and absence of elevated extracellular calcium. Although we did not detect a statistically significant change in the levels of keratin-10 under basal conditions, PKCβII overexpression in combination with elevated extracellular calcium resulted in a substantial up-regulation of keratin-10 levels (Fig. **4**). These results suggest that PKCβII alone is not sufficient to induce an increase in keratin-10 expression, but instead works in concert with calcium to promote early differentiation in primary mouse keratinocytes.

These results suggest that PKCβII can be activated not only by PG, but also by agents, such as extracellular calcium, that stimulate keratinocyte differentiation. This result, as well as our previous data indicating that PG can induce keratinocyte differentiation [5], prompted us to test the morphological effect of PG on keratinocytes overexpressing PKCβII. Interestingly, treatment with PG led to morphological changes consistent with entry into later differentiation in cells transfected with PKCβII. This morphological change was not detected in keratinocytes that were expressing basal levels of PKCβII (Fig. **5**), suggesting that overexpressed PKCβII must be activated (by PG or the PG produced upon elevation of extracellular calcium levels) in order to exert its prodifferentiative effect.

CONCLUSION

In summary, we show that PKCβII is present in mouse keratinocytes and is translocated and/or activated upon stimulation of the AQP3/PLD2/PG signaling module by a moderate elevation of extracellular calcium levels (which increases PG levels [3]) or direct provision of PG. We provide further evidence suggesting that PKCβII, activated in response to an elevated calcium level or provision of PG, can promote keratinocyte differentiation. This result suggests a potential mechanism by which PG affects keratinocyte function.

LIST OF ABBREVIATIONS

AQP3	=	Aquaporin-3
K10	=	Keratin-10
K-SFM	=	Keratinocyte serum-free medium
PG	=	Phosphatidylglycerol
PKC	=	Protein kinase C
PKCβII	=	Protein kinase C-betaII
PLD2	=	Phospholipase D2
SFKM	=	Serum-free keratinocyte medium

HUMAN AND ANIMAL RIGHTS

All experiments were performed using protocols approved by the institutional animal care and use committee as described in Methods (section 2.1). No human subjects were used for these studies.

CONFLICT OF INTEREST

The authors declare no conflict of interest, financial or otherwise.

ACKNOWLEDGEMENTS

This work was submitted in partial fulfillment for the requirements of a doctoral degree to LJB. This work was supported in part by award #AR045212 from the National Institutes of Health/National Institute of Arthritis, Musculoskeletal and Skin Diseases to WBB; LJB was supported in part by a minority supplement to this award. VC was supported by start-up funds from the Department of Physiology at Augusta University. WBB was also supported by a VA Research Career Scientist Award. The contents of this article do not represent the views of the Department of Veterans Affairs or the United States Government.

REFERENCES

[1]   Qin H, Zheng X, Zhong X, Shetty AK, Elias PM, Bollag WB. Aquaporin-3 in keratinocytes and skin: its role and interaction with phospholipase D2. Arch Biochem Biophys 2011; 508(2): 138-43.
[http://dx.doi.org/10.1016/j.abb.2011.01.014] [PMID: 21276418]

[2]   Zheng X, Bollinger W. Aquaporin 3 colocates with phospholipase d2 in caveolin-rich membrane microdomains and is downregulated upon keratinocyte differentiation. J Invest Dermatol 2003; 121(6): 1487-95.
[http://dx.doi.org/10.1111/j.1523-1747.2003.12614.x] [PMID: 14675200]

[3]   Zheng X, Ray S, Bollag WB. Modulation of phospholipase D-mediated phosphatidylglycerol formation by differentiating agents in primary mouse epidermal keratinocytes. Biochim Biophys Acta 2003; 1643(1-3): 25-36.
[http://dx.doi.org/10.1016/j.bbamcr.2003.08.006] [PMID: 14654225]

[4]   Yuspa SH, Kilkenny AE, Steinert PM, Roop DR. Expression of murine epidermal differentiation markers is tightly regulated by restricted extracellular calcium concentrations in vitro. J Cell Biol 1989; 109(3): 1207-17.
[http://dx.doi.org/10.1083/jcb.109.3.1207] [PMID: 2475508]

[5]   Bollag WB, Xie D, Zhong X, Zheng X. A potential role for the phospholipase D2-aquaporin-3 signaling module in early keratinocyte differentiation: Production of a novel phosphatidylglycerol lipid signal. J Invest Dermatol 2007; 127: 2823-31.
[http://dx.doi.org/10.1038/sj.jid.5700921] [PMID: 17597824]

[6]   Xie D, Seremwe M, Edwards JG, Podolsky R, Bollag WB. Distinct effects of different phosphatidylglycerol species on mouse keratinocyte proliferation. PLoS One 2014; 9(9): e107119.
[http://dx.doi.org/10.1371/journal.pone.0107119] [PMID: 25233484]

[7]   Gökmen-Polar Y, Fields AP. Mapping of a molecular determinant for protein kinase C betaII isozyme function. J Biol Chem 1998; 273(32): 20261-6.
[http://dx.doi.org/10.1074/jbc.273.32.20261] [PMID: 9685375]

[8]   Murray NR, Fields AP. Phosphatidylglycerol is a physiologic activator of nuclear protein kinase C. J Biol Chem 1998; 273(19): 11514-20.
[http://dx.doi.org/10.1074/jbc.273.19.11514] [PMID: 9565565]

[9]   Murray NR, Burns DJ, Fields AP. Presence of a beta II protein kinase C-selective nuclear membrane activation factor in human leukemia cells. J Biol Chem 1994; 269(33): 21385-90.
[PMID: 8063766]

[10]   Parekh DB, Ziegler W, Parker PJ. Multiple pathways control protein kinase C phosphorylation. EMBO J 2000; 19(4): 496-503.
[http://dx.doi.org/10.1093/emboj/19.4.496] [PMID: 10675318]

[11]   Bailey LJ, Choudhary V, Merai P, Bollag WB. Preparation of primary cultures of mouse epidermal keratinocytes and the measurement of phospholipase D activity. Methods Mol Biol 2014; 1195: 111-31.
[http://dx.doi.org/10.1007/7651_2014_80] [PMID: 24840936]

[12]   Griner RD, Qin F, Jung E, et al. 1,25-dihydroxyvitamin D3 induces phospholipase D-1 expression in primary mouse epidermal keratinocytes. J Biol Chem 1999; 274(8): 4663-70.
[http://dx.doi.org/10.1074/jbc.274.8.4663] [PMID: 9988703]

[13]   Choudhary V, Olala LO, Qin H, *et al.* Aquaporin-3 re-expression induces differentiation in a phospholipase D2-dependent manner in aquaporin-3-knockout mouse keratinocytes. J Invest Dermatol 2015; 135(2): 499-507.
        [http://dx.doi.org/10.1038/jid.2014.412] [PMID: 25233074]

[14]   Chappell DS, Patel NA, Jiang K, *et al.* Functional involvement of protein kinase C-betaII and its substrate, myristoylated alanine-rich C-kinase substrate (MARCKS), in insulin-stimulated glucose transport in L6 rat skeletal muscle cells. Diabetologia 2009; 52(5): 901-11.

[15]   Helfrich I, Schmitz A, Zigrino P, *et al.* Role of aPKC isoforms and their binding partners Par3 and Par6 in epidermal barrier formation. J Invest Dermatol 2007; 127(4): 782-91.
        [http://dx.doi.org/10.1038/sj.jid.5700621] [PMID: 17110935]

[16]   Dlugosz AA, Mischak H, Mushinski JF, Yuspa SH. Transcripts encoding protein kinase C-alpha, -delta, -epsilon, -zeta, and -eta are expressed in basal and differentiating mouse keratinocytes *in vitro* and exhibit quantitative changes in neoplastic cells. Mol Carcinog 1992; 5(4): 286-92.
        [http://dx.doi.org/10.1002/mc.2940050409] [PMID: 1379814]

[17]   Fisher GJ, Tavakkol A, Leach K, *et al.* Differential expression of protein kinase C isoenzymes in normal and psoriatic adult human skin: reduced expression of protein kinase C-beta II in psoriasis. J Invest Dermatol 1993; 101(4): 553-9.
        [http://dx.doi.org/10.1111/1523-1747.ep12365967] [PMID: 8409523]

[18]   Fischer SM, Lee ML, Maldve RE, *et al.* Association of protein kinase C activation with induction of ornithine decarboxylase in murine but not human keratinocyte cultures. Mol Carcinog 1993; 7(4): 228-37. [eng.].
        [http://dx.doi.org/10.1002/mc.2940070405] [PMID: 8352882]

[19]   Hara T, Saito Y, Hirai T, *et al.* Deficiency of protein kinase Calpha in mice results in impairment of epidermal hyperplasia and enhancement of tumor formation in two-stage skin carcinogenesis. Cancer Res 2005; 65(16): 7356-62.
        [http://dx.doi.org/10.1158/0008-5472.CAN-04-4241] [PMID: 16103087]

[20]   Mochly-Rosen D, Das K, Grimes KV. Protein kinase C, an elusive therapeutic target? Nat Rev Drug Discov 2012; 11(12): 937-57.
        [http://dx.doi.org/10.1038/nrd3871] [PMID: 23197040]

[21]   Shirai Y, Saito N. Activation mechanisms of protein kinase C: maturation, catalytic activation, and targeting. J Biochem 2002; 132(5): 663-8.
        [http://dx.doi.org/10.1093/oxfordjournals.jbchem.a003271] [PMID: 12417013]

[22]   Corbalán-García S, Gómez-Fernández JC. Classical protein kinases C are regulated by concerted interaction with lipids: the importance of phosphatidylinositol-4,5-bisphosphate. Biophys Rev 2014; 6(1): 3-14.
        [http://dx.doi.org/10.1007/s12551-013-0125-z] [PMID: 28509956]

[23]   Tu C-L, Chang W, Bikle DD. The extracellular calcium-sensing receptor is required for calcium-induced differentiation in human keratinocytes. J Biol Chem 2001; 276(44): 41079-85.
        [http://dx.doi.org/10.1074/jbc.M107122200] [PMID: 11500521]

[24]   Rapp SR, Feldman SR, Exum ML, Fleischer AB Jr, Reboussin DM. Psoriasis causes as much disability as other major medical diseases. J Am Acad Dermatol 1999; 41(3 Pt 1): 401-7.
        [http://dx.doi.org/10.1016/S0190-9622(99)70112-X] [PMID: 10459113]

[25]   de Arruda LH, De Moraes AP. The impact of psoriasis on quality of life. Br J Dermatol 2001; 144(Suppl. 58): 33-6.
        [http://dx.doi.org/10.1046/j.1365-2133.2001.144s58033.x] [PMID: 11501512]

[26]   Skvara H, Dawid M, Kleyn E, *et al.* The PKC inhibitor AEB071 may be a therapeutic option for psoriasis. J Clin Invest 2008; 118(9): 3151-9.
        [http://dx.doi.org/10.1172/JCI35636] [PMID: 18688284]

[27]   Jerome-Morais A, Rahn HR, Tibudan SS, Denning MF. Role for protein kinase C-alpha in keratinocyte growth arrest. J Invest Dermatol 2009; 129(10): 2365-75.
        [http://dx.doi.org/10.1038/jid.2009.74] [PMID: 19340015]

[28]   Voss KE, Bollag RJ, Fussell N, By C, Sheehan DJ, Bollag WB. Abnormal aquaporin-3 protein expression in hyperproliferative skin disorders. Arch Dermatol Res 2011; 303(8): 591-600.
        [http://dx.doi.org/10.1007/s00403-011-1136-x] [PMID: 21400035]

[29]   Lee Y-S, Yuspa SH, Dlugosz AA. Differentiation of cultured human epidermal keratinocytes at high cell densities is mediated by endogenous activation of the protein kinase C signaling pathway. J Invest Dermatol 1998; 111(5): 762-6.
        [http://dx.doi.org/10.1046/j.1523-1747.1998.00365.x] [PMID: 9804335]

[30]   Mayhew E, Ito M, Lazo R. Toxicity of non-drug-containing liposomes for cultured human cells. Exp Cell Res 1987; 171(1): 195-202.
        [http://dx.doi.org/10.1016/0014-4827(87)90262-X] [PMID: 3622630]

[31]   Bikle DD, Pillai S. Vitamin D, calcium, and epidermal differentiation. Endocr Rev 1993; 14(1): 3-19.
        [PMID: 8491153]

[32]   Menon GK, Elias PM, Lee SH, Feingold KR. Localization of calcium in murine epidermis following disruption and repair of the permeability barrier. Cell Tissue Res 1992; 270(3): 503-12.
        [http://dx.doi.org/10.1007/BF00645052] [PMID: 1486603]

[33]   Menon GK, Grayson S, Elias PM. Ionic calcium reservoirs in mammalian epidermis: ultrastructural localization by ion-capture cytochemistry. J Invest Dermatol 1985; 84(6): 508-12.
        [http://dx.doi.org/10.1111/1523-1747.ep12273485] [PMID: 3998499]

[34]   Ng DC, Su MJ, Kim R, Bikle DD. Regulation of involucrin gene expression by calcium in normal human keratinocytes. Front Biosci 1996; 1: a16-24.
[http://dx.doi.org/10.2741/A101] [PMID: 9159190]

[35]   Bikle DD, Oda Y, Xie Z. Calcium and 1,25(OH)2D: interacting drivers of epidermal differentiation. J Steroid Biochem Mol Biol 2004; 89-90(1-5): 355-60.
[http://dx.doi.org/10.1016/j.jsbmb.2004.03.020] [PMID: 15225800]

7

Pyoderma Gangrenosum of the Face: A Rare Presentation and a Rapid Resolution

Julia Shah[*], Lorie Gottwald, Ashley Sheskey and Craig Burkhart

Department of Dermatology, University of Toledo College of Medicine, Toledo, USA

Abstract:

Background:

Pyoderma Gangrenosum (PG) is a disorder of neutrophil chemotaxis that often affects the lower extremities of patients with concurrent autoimmune disorders.

Result and Discussion:

Resolution of lesions typically requires a minimum of six weeks of treatment with systemic steroids. We present a unique case of multifocal PG involving the hand and face that healed after ten days of treatment with oral prednisone.

Keywords: Pyoderma Gangrenosum, Neutrophil chemotaxis, Seronegative Arthritis, MCPJ, Prednisone theraphy, IgG.

1. INTRODUCTION

A 51-year-old female with a history of Seronegative Arthritis presented with lesions on multiple parts of her body that had erupted over the past eighteen months. She described the lesions as large, painful papules which she would "pop" for relief. The distribution involved a new, active lesion on the right knuckle and lesions in various stages of healing on the left nostril and left cheek. She reported previous lesions on the jaw, genital mucosa, and toe. She believed the lesions were precipitated by small cuts or injuries and noted flares when she was stressed.

Physical examination revealed two erythematous, eroded papules on the left jawline (Fig. **1**), a vesicle with surrounding erythema on the rim of the left nostril (Fig. **2**), and a hemorrhagic, necrotic plaque on the right fifth metacarpal phalangeal joint (MCPJ) (Fig. **3**).

A punch biopsy of the active lesion over the right fifth MCPJ was conducted. The patient was given mupirocin 2% topical ointment and instructed to apply it to the lesions three times daily.

The radial side of the right fifth MCPJ biopsy was submitted for immunofluorescence and stained negative for IgG, IgA, C3, fibrinogen, and albumin. The ulnar side of the biopsy sample was fixed with H&E staining. The sample spanned from the epidermis to the subcutaneous fat. There was marked irregular epidermal hyperplasia bordering an ulcer with underlying dense neutrophilic infiltrate and an undermining edge within the dermis. There were interstitial neutrophils and crushed lymphocytes in between the collagen bundles, but there was no definite evidence of vasculitis. There was no evidence of viral inclusions, interface dermatitis, or malignancy.

The findings of an undermined edge and neutrophilic dermatosis were consistent with a diagnosis of Pyoderma Gangrenosum (PG). The patient was started on a 10 day course of 60 mg oral Prednisone therapy.

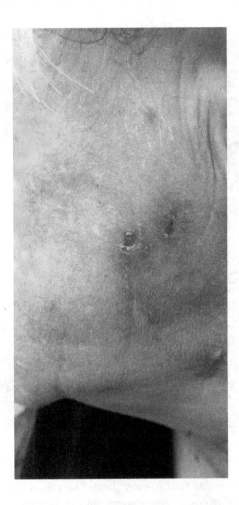

Fig. (1). left jaw.

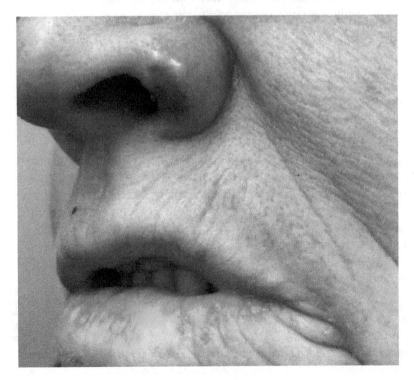

Fig. (2). left nostril.

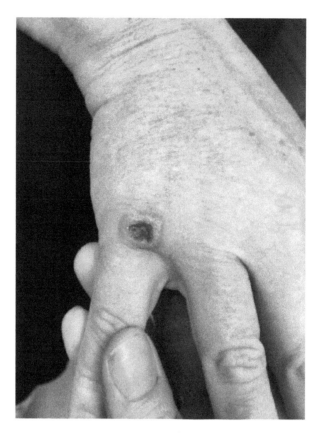

Fig. (3). Right fifth metacarpal phalangeal joint.

She was briefly lost to follow up and was seen 6 weeks later. The patient reported compliance with corticosteroid therapy and resolution of the lesions after course completion. On examination, resolution of the lesions on her hands and face was noted, with some mild scarring on her hand. She reported no new lesions at this time. She was instructed to follow up as needed and if any new ulcerations developed.

2. DISCUSSION

PG is characterized as a disorder of neutrophil chemotaxis [1]. The neutrophilic infiltration seen in PG is thought to be driven by the elevated levels of inflammatory mediators, such as IL-8 (neutrophil chemotactic factor), which are observed in the tissues [2]. The dense neutrophilic infiltrate present in our patient's lesion with a lack of infectious or malignant cause made PG the most likely diagnosis.

The *Journal of the American Medical Association Dermatology* recently published this consensus for the diagnostic criteria for PG: the presence of major criterion (a biopsy of an ulcer edge demonstrating a neutrophilic infiltrate) and the presence of at least four of the eight minor criteria (Fig. **4**)[1]. Minor criteria include: (1) exclusion of infection; (2) pathergy; (3) history of inflammatory bowel disease or inflammatory arthritis; (4) history of papule, pustule, or vesicle ulcerating within 4 days of appearing; (5) peripheral erythema, undermining border, and tenderness at ulceration site; (6) multiple ulcerations, at least 1 on an anterior lower leg; (7) cribriform or "wrinkled paper" scar(s) at healed ulcer sites; and (8) decreased ulcer size within 1 month of initiating immunosuppressive medication(s) [1]. Our patient's case is consistent with the major criterion, and the first, second, third, fourth, fifth, and eighth aforementioned minor criteria.

The exact cause of PG is unknown, but patients tend to be between the age of 20-50 and males and females are equally affected [3]. Ulcerative PG, the most common variant, is typically found on the lower extremities [2]. The multi-focal ulcerative presentation above the waist is relatively rare but was shown in our patient. PG has also a tendency to cause pathergy, a phenomenon where minor trauma contributes to significant, non-healing skin damage [4, 5]. This is consistent with our patient's history of injuries preceding the formation of new PG lesions.

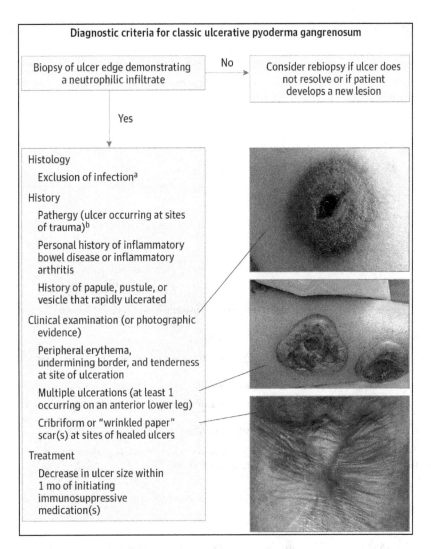

Fig. (4). JAMA Diagnostic Criteria of Ulcerative Pyoderma Gangrenosum A Delphi Consensus of International Experts[1].

PG has a well-known association with other neutrophilic and inflammatory disorders, including Inflammatory Bowel Disease (IBD), Rheumatoid Arthritis (RA), seronegative arthritis, autoimmune hepatitis [2, 6]. IBD is by far the most commonly observed. Some even classify seronegative arthritis and PG as extra-cutaneous manifestations of IBD. Our patient's history of seronegative arthritis may be associated with her skin disease. Affected patients exemplify a triad of IBD, PG, and seronegative arthritis concurrently [7]. PG has rarely been documented to occur with seronegative arthritis but without IBD – however, our patient is one such case [6].

PG has also been documented to occur as an adverse drug reaction. Paradoxically, these reactions are to the immunosuppressive drugs used to treat autoimmune conditions (*e.g.* IBD or RA) that occur with PG. A case report from the *European Journal of Dermatology* describes extensive ulcerative PG that developed in a psoriasis patient after 4 years of infliximab therapy [8]. Infliximab, an immunosuppressive agent, has also been reported to cause PG in at least two patients with ulcerative colitis, and one patient with RA [8].

Due to the rarity of PG, very few large-scale studies have been conducted comparing treatment options. First line treatment for limited PG, defined as involving <5% of the body, is systemic or topical corticosteroids [2]. In a study conducted by the University of Nottingham, 47% of patients receiving .75mg/kg/day of prednisolone experienced resolution of PG at the end of a 6-month treatment period [9, 10]. Patients in this study first began seeing improvement in symptoms after 6 weeks of oral prednisolone [10].

CONCLUSION

On average, most studies involving systemic steroid treatment for PG yield results after 6 weeks of treatment [9 - 11]. By contrast, our patient reported complete resolution of symptoms after a ten day treatment period with prednisone.

The only other record of an abridged interval for steroid treatment is a case report of malignant pyoderma gangrenosum of the parotid gland with dexamethasone pulse therapy (100 mg dexamethasone in 500 ml 5% dextrose infused over 3-4 hours each day). The steroid treatment infusion occurred over three consecutive days and, even then, complete healing did not occur for 6 weeks [11]. By comparison, our patient's resolution of symptoms after just a 10-day treatment with oral prednisone is remarkable.

CONFLICT OF INTEREST

The authors declare no conflict of interest, financial or otherwise.

ACKNOWLEDGEMENTS

Declared none.

REFERENCES

[1]   Maverakis E, Ma C, Shinkai K, *et al.* Diagnostic criteria of ulcerative pyoderma gangrenosum: A delphi consensus of international experts. JAMA Dermatol 2018; 154(4): 461-6.
        [http://dx.doi.org/10.1001/jamadermatol.2017.5980] [PMID: 29450466]

[2]   Alavi A, French LE, Davis MD, Brassard A, Kirsner RS. Pyoderma gangrenosum: An update on pathophysiology, diagnosis and treatment. Am J Clin Dermatol 2017; 18(3): 355-72.
        [http://dx.doi.org/10.1007/s40257-017-0251-7] [PMID: 28224502]

[3]   Ahronowitz I, Harp J, Shinkai K. Etiology and management of pyoderma gangrenosum: A comprehensive review. Am J Clin Dermatol 2012; 13(3): 191-211.
        [http://dx.doi.org/10.2165/11595240-000000000-00000] [PMID: 22356259]

[4]   Zuo KJ, Fung E, Tredget EE, Lin AN. A systematic review of post-surgical pyoderma gangrenosum: Identification of risk factors and proposed management strategy. J Plast Reconstr Aesthet Surg 2015; 68(3): 295-303.
        [http://dx.doi.org/10.1016/j.bjps.2014.12.036] [PMID: 25589459]

[5]   Patel DK, Locke M, Jarrett P. Pyoderma gangrenosum with pathergy: A potentially significant complication following breast reconstruction. J Plast Reconstr Aesthet Surg 2017; 70(7): 884-92.
        [http://dx.doi.org/10.1016/j.bjps.2017.03.013] [PMID: 28476284]

[6]   Olivieri I, Costa AM, Cantini F, Niccoli L, Marini R, Ferri S. Pyoderma gangrenosum in association with undifferentiated seronegative spondylarthropathy. Arthritis Rheum 1996; 39(6): 1062-5.
        [http://dx.doi.org/10.1002/art.1780390627] [PMID: 8651972]

[7]   Card TR, Langan SM, Chu TP. Extra-Gastrointestinal manifestations of inflammatory bowel disease may be less common than previously reported. Dig Dis Sci 2016; 61(9): 2619-26.
        [http://dx.doi.org/10.1007/s10620-016-4195-1] [PMID: 27193564]

[8]   Vestita M, Guida S, Mazzoccoli S, Loconsole F, Foti C. Late paradoxical development of pyoderma gangrenosum in a psoriasis patient treated with infliximab. Eur J Dermatol 2015; 25(3): 272-3.
        [PMID: 25786592]

[9]   Quist SR, Kraas L. Treatment options for pyoderma gangrenosum. *Journal der Deutschen Dermatologischen Gesellschaft = Journal of the German Society of Dermatology.* JDDG 2017; 15(1): 34-40.

[10]   Ormerod AD, Thomas KS, Craig FE, *et al.* Comparison of the two most commonly used treatments for pyoderma gangrenosum: Results of the STOP GAP randomised controlled trial. BMJ 2015; 350: h2958.
        [http://dx.doi.org/10.1136/bmj.h2958] [PMID: 26071094]

[11]   Ambooken B, Khader A, Muhammed K, Rajan U, Snigdha O. Malignant pyoderma gangrenosum eroding the parotid gland successfully treated with dexamethasone pulse therapy. Int J Dermatol 2014; 53(12): 1536-8.
        [http://dx.doi.org/10.1111/ijd.12519] [PMID: 25312614]

8

Assessment of the Degree of Skin Hypopigmentation in Patients with Vitiligo by using Mexametry

N.V. Deeva[*], Yu.M. Krinitsyna, S.V. Mustafina, O.D. Rymar and I.G. Sergeeva

Novosibirsk State University, Institute of Molecular Pathology and Pathomorphology, Research Institute of Internal and Preventive Medicine – Branch of the Institute of Cytology and Genetics, Novosibirsk, Russia

Abstract:

This study is an assessment of the degree of skin hypopigmentation in patients with vitiligo.

Material and Methods:

The study followed 47 patients with vitiligo (33 female and 14 male patients; the average age was 38.0 ± 18.0 years). The mean disease duration was 15.5 ± 14.1 years. We determined the melanin levels in the patches of vitiligo and on the healthy skin of the face, trunk, and extremities by using mexametry.

Results:

High melanin levels were found in patches on and around the mouth. Melanin levels did not differ in vitiligo patches and on healthy skin of chins and buttocks. All patients had no melanin in the patches on their cheeks. Having vitiligo for a long time reduces melanin levels in the skin of the forehead. High melanin levels in healthy skin are associated with stored melanin in vitiligo patches in axillary areas, on the back, brachiums, and femurs.

Conclusions:

There are significant differences in the melanin levels in the vitiligo patches and healthy skin, which have specific features depending on the localization. Analysis of melanin levels may be useful in choosing a method and evaluating the effectiveness of the planned therapy.

Keywords: Vitiligo, Melanin, Mexametry, Melanin levels, Hypopigmentation, Skin.

1. INTRODUCTION

Vitiligo is a disease characterised by patches of skin hypopigmentation tending to peripheral growth and develops because of the disappearance of melanocytes or disruption of their functional activity [1].

Because the pathogenesis of vitiligo is still not fully understood, the methods of treating this disease are often ineffective, despite the application of evidence-based medicine. Therefore, in addition to conventional methods of diagnosis, instrumental analyses are important for studies of human skin *in vivo*, because these analytical tools are standardised and objectively reflect the distribution of pigment in the lesions. One such analytical method is mexametry. It allows researchers to quantify the distribution of the pigment in the skin of patients with vitiligo, to determine the characteristics of the disease in patients, and to monitor changes in the pigment content in the patches during the process of therapy.

* Address correspondence to this author at the Novosibirsk State University, 2 Pirogova Str., Novosibirsk, Russia, 630090;
  E-mail: pikelgaupt1991@gmail.com

2. MATERIAL AND METHODS

We studied 47 patients with vitiligo, 33 (70.2%) women and 14 (29.8%) men aged from 8 to 77 years with a mean age of 38.0 ± 18.0 years. The mean duration of the disease was 15.5 ± 14.1 years. This study was approved by Local ethics committee of Research Institute of Internal and Preventive Medicine – Branch of the Institute of Cytology and Genetics. The subjects in this study were recruited after obtaining written informed consent.

Twelve (25.5%) vitiligo patients had diffused telogen hair loss and 12 (25.5%) had onychodystrophy (which encompasses a wide spectrum of nail disorders). Thirteen (27.7%) patients had autoimmune thyroiditis, 4 (8.5%) had halo naevus, and 1 (2.1%) had psoriasis. Family history of the patients with the disease revealed that 14 (29.8%) had relatives with vitiligo, 3 (6.4%) had a family history of rheumatoid arthritis, and 1 (2.1%) had a family history of psoriasis.

Vitiligo was evaluated according to the Vitiligo Global Issues Consensus Conference (2012) Vitiligo Disease Activity score (VIDA) disease activity classification scale [2 - 4]. The generalised form of vitiligo was observed in 26 patients (55.3%), mixed in 9 (19.1), acrofacial in 4 (8.5%), focal and universal in 3 (6.4%) each, and segmental in 2 (4.3%). The progressing type of vitiligo was noted in 39 patients (83.0%), while stable and unstable forms were noted in 4 (8.5%) patients each.

We determined melanin levels by mexametry. The measurement of melanin distribution in the skin was based on the definition of light absorption. The range of values was denoted by 1-100 conventional units (c.u.). The error of this method does not exceed 0.1%.

We determined melanin levels in the patches of vitiligo and healthy skin at 19 locations: forehead, eyelids, cheeks, lips, chin, neck, breast, axillary areas, back, buttocks, inguinal folds, brachiums, elbows, forearms, the back of brushes, femurs, knees, shins, and the back of the feet. A total of 346 measurements were performed in the patches of vitiligo and 474 measurements on healthy skin.

We defined skin type using the Fitzpatrick skin type scale classification. The majority of patients with vitiligo had phototype 2 in 24 (51.1%) patients and phototype 3 in 16 (34.0%) patients; phototype 4 occurred in 3 (6.4%) and phototypes 1 and 5 occurred in 2 (4.3%) patients.

Statistical data processing was performed using the program Statistica 10.0 (StatSoft, Tulsa, OK, USA). The results are presented as the mean value of the indicator and its standard deviation (M ± SD) or percentage incidence. To assess group differences, Student's t-test was calculated and Spearman's rank correlation coefficient (r) was used for the characterisation of the binding forces between the parameters. Test results that produced P values < 0.05 were regarded as statistically significant.

3. RESULTS

The patches of vitiligo were diagnosed on the back of brushes in 32 (68.1%) patients; on the eyelids in 29 (61.7%); on the axillary areas in 27 (57.5%); on the breast and on the back of the feet in 25 (53.2%); on the forearms, shins, and back in 23 (49.0%); on the knees and elbows in 20 (42.6%); on the inguinal folds in 18 (38.3%); on the femurs in 15 (31.9%); on the neck, chin, and lips in 12 (25.5%); and on the brachiums in 10 (21.3%). Hypopigmented patches were seen less often on the buttocks in 9 (19.2%), on the cheeks in 6 (12.8%), and on the forehead in 5 (10.6%).

The melanin levels in healthy skin of patients with vitiligo were approximately 6-13 c.u. on the eyelids, cheeks, lips, chin, neck, back, buttocks, axillary areas, and inguinal folds, but the melanin levels in the vitiligo patches in these areas differed significantly Fig. (1). The melanin levels in the vitiligo patches and healthy skin did not differ significantly on the chin and buttocks ($P > 0.05$) Table (1). Melanin was almost absent in vitiligo patches on the cheeks (1 c.u.) in all patients.

Table 1. The average melanin levels in the healthy skin and patches of vitiligo in patients, c.u. (M ± SD).

Localisation	Melanin levels, c.u.	
	healthy skin	vitiligo patches
Forehead	15.8 ± 4.5	2.4 ± 2.2***
Eyelids	9.2 ± 8.0	1.1 ± 0.6***
Cheeks	11.3 ± 5.6	1.0 ± 0.0***
Lips	12.1 ± 4.6	8.1 ± 5.0*

(Table 1) contd.....

Localisation	Melanin levels, c.u.	
Neck	12.5 ± 7.7	1.3 ± 0.6***
Breast	5.0 ± 5.4	1.5 ± 2.2**
Axillary areas	13.1 ± 9.0	2.8 ± 4.1***
Back	12.7 ± 11.1	2.4 ± 2.7***
Inguinal folds	13.8 ± 7.8	3.7 ± 4.8***
Brachiums	16.5 ± 12.3	2.0 ± 1.8**
Elbows	17.7 ± 11.2	2.2 ± 2.3***
Forearms	19.0 ± 10.9	3.0 ± 5.1***
The back of brushes	16.7 ± 11.5	1.5 ± 1.3***
Femurs	14.1 ± 10.7	4.8 ± 3.6**
Knees	19.2 ± 7.6	5.5 ± 5.6***
Shins	16.4 ± 10.4	3.3 ± 3.1***
The back of feet	21.7 ± 9.8	3.2 ± 4.0***
Chin	13.7 ± 6.0	10.8 ± 6.9
Buttocks	6.6 ± 7.4	2.7 ± 2.8

Note: * – $P < 0.05$, ** – $P < 0.01$, *** – $P < 0.001$

Table (2) shows the correlation between melanin levels in vitiligo patches and the duration of the disease. We found a negative correlation ($r = -0.89$; $P < 0.05$) between the melanin levels in vitiligo patches of the forehead and the disease duration. Thus, a longer duration of disease affects the decrease in the melanin level in the skin of only the forehead. We also found a positive correlation, but not a significant one, between the duration of vitiligo and the melanin levels in the patches on the chin, neck, buttocks, femurs, axillary areas, and inguinal folds. This implies that a high melanin level is preserved better in these areas compared to that at other locations over the course of time.

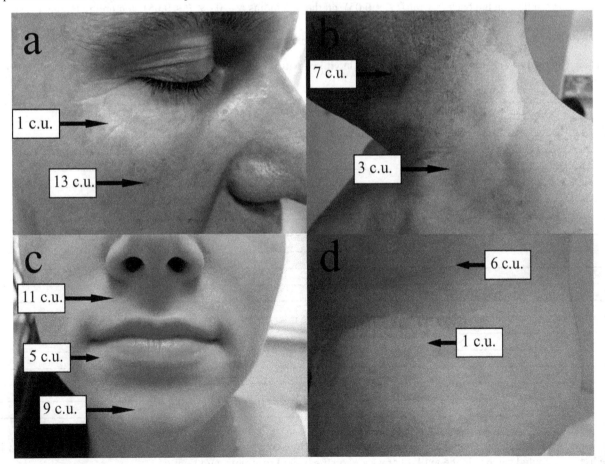

Fig. (1). The melanin levels was determined in patients with vitiligo: a) in vitiligo patches (1 c.u.) and healthy skin (13 c.u.) on the eyelids; b) in vitiligo patches (3 c.u.) and healthy skin (7 c.u.) on the neck; c) in vitiligo patches on the lips (5 c.u.), shin (9 c.u.) and healthy skin (11 c.u.); d) in vitiligo patches (1 c.u.) and healthy skin (6 c.u.) on the buttocks.

Table 2. Correlation (r) between melanin levels in vitiligo patches and duration of disease in patients.

Localisation	The correlation coefficient (r) with a duration of disease
Forehead	-0.89*
Eyelids	-0.14
Lips	-0.07
Chin	0.14
Neck	0.15
Breast	-0.08
Axillary areas	0.08
Back	-0.33
Buttocks	0.05
Inguinal folds	0.02
Brachiums	-0.32
Elbows	-0.35
Forearms	-0.06
The back of brushes	-0.13
Femurs	0.12
Knees	-0.21
Shins	-0.16
The back of feet	-0.02

Note: * – $P < 0.05$

Table (**3**) show the correlation between melanin levels in vitiligo patches and healthy skin in the corresponding locations. We found a positive correlation between vitiligo patches and the following body locations: the axillary areas ($r = 0.55$; $P < 0.05$), on the back ($r = 0.61$; $P < 0.05$), on the brachiums ($r = 0.68$; $P < 0.05$), and on the femurs ($r = 0.63$; $P < 0.05$).

Table 3. Correlation (r) between the melanin levels in vitiligo patches and healthy skin in the corresponding localisation in patients.

Localisation in vitiligo patches and healthy skin	The correlation coefficient (r)
Forehead	0.87
Eyelids	0.04
Lips	0.27
Chin	0.29
Neck	-0.21
Breast	0.37
Axillary areas	0.55*
Back	0.61*
Buttocks	0.74
Inguinal folds	0.28
Brachiums	0.68*
Elbows	0.09
Forearms	-0.04
The back of brushes	0.09
Femurs	0.63*
Knees	0.44
Shins	-0.04
The back of feet	-0.28

Note: * – $P < 0.05$

Thus, we found that high melanin levels relative to healthy skin is associated with a high preservation of melanin in the hypopigmented patches in the axillary areas and on the back, brachiums, and femurs.

4. DISCUSSION

Vitiligo is a common skin disorder of depigmentation that can occur in any location of the body. The localisation of vitiligo on the trunk is an independent risk factor for patients with nonsegmental vitiligo developing thyroid dysimmunity, although very few researchers have studied this association using multivariate logistic regression [5]. In our study, 13 (27.7%) patients had autoimmune thyroiditis, 4 (8.5%) had halo naevus, and 1 (2.1%) had psoriasis. In our study, the progressing type of vitiligo was noted in 39 patients (83.0%), while stable and unstable forms were noted in 4 (8.5%) patients each. Among our patients, most of them had a nonsegmental vitiligo with varying degrees of prevalence and a progressive process of the disease, probably explaining one of the reasons for patients' admission to the method with this disease.

There are conflicting and insufficient data on the location in the vitiligo patches. Thus, in a study of 21 patients whose mean age was 44.3 years, the assessment of vitiligo patches was carried out only in 7 locations: on the trunk (28.6%), legs (19.1%), feet (14.3%), hands (14.3%), the back of brushes (9.5%), wrists (9.5%) and face (4.8%) [6]. We determined melanin levels in the patches of vitiligo and healthy skin at 19 locations. The patches of vitiligo were most often diagnosed on the back of brushes, on the eyelids, on the axillary areas, on the breast and on the back of the feet in our study.

The presence of periorbital vitiligo was significantly related to the ocular findings, revealing concordances between periorbital and genitalial localisations of vitiligo [7].

We found that the highest average melanin levels in vitiligo patches on the chin were 10.8 ± 6.9 c.u. and around the mouth (lips) were 8.1 ± 5.0 c.u. The melanin levels in vitiligo patches and healthy skin were not significantly different ($P > 0.05$) on the chin and buttocks. The melanin levels in vitiligo patches on the cheeks were absent in all patients.

We found that a longer duration of disease affects the decrease in the melanin level in the skin of only the forehead ($r = -0.89$; P <0.05). We also found that high melanin levels in healthy skin are associated with a high preservation of melanin in the hypopigmented patches in the axillary regions ($r = 0.55$; P <0.05) and on the back ($r = 0.61$; P <0.05), brachiums ($r = 0.68$; P <0.05), and femurs ($r = 0.63$; P <0.05).

The evaluation of the effectiveness of the planned therapy is important for determining the predictions. However, there is currently no standardized method for measuring vitiligo damage. Objective and non-invasive methods for measuring and controlling the degree of pigmentation compared to the surrounding normal skin can be useful for assessing the effectiveness and monitoring of treatment [7]. Reflectance spectrophotometers have been used for many years to measure the level of skin pigmentation. Diffuse reflection spectroscopy (DRS) can be a suitable method for measuring skin color and melanin content of human skin in out [8].

A rather large number of studies on instrumental methods for studying human skin *in vivo* have been carried out, which are more standardized and therefore more objective. The method of mexametry was used to quantify the allergic or inflammatory reaction caused by UV damage, as well as to confirm the diagnosis of hemangioma, also used to determine the degree of skin tanning, phototype, evaluation of the effectiveness of bleaching procedures, to confirm the diagnosis of melanoma, individual studies to assess the effectiveness of treatment vitiligo after the procedures. However, data on the amount of melanin in all locations in vitiligo patches and on healthy skin, correlation between melanin levels in vitiligo patches and duration of disease, correlation between the melanin levels in vitiligo patches and healthy skin in the corresponding localisation, together with the clinical features of the disease, are obtained for the first time.

We found that the visual assessment of depigmentation in some cases does not correspond to the melanin levels in the patches of vitiligo. With an equal indirect visual assessment of depigmentation in the patches of vitiligo, melanin levels may be equal to 1 c.u. (absence of melanin), 3 c.u. and even 10 c.u. This requires further study regarding the choice of therapy in these areas of the skin.

CONCLUSION

There are significant differences in the melanin levels in the vitiligo patches and healthy skin, which have specific features depending on the localization. Analysis of melanin levels may be useful in choosing a method and evaluating the effectiveness of the planned therapy.

HUMAN AND ANIMAL RIGHTS

No Animals/Humans were used for studies that are base of this research.

CONFLICT OF INTEREST

The authors declare no conflict of interest, financial or otherwise.

ACKNOWLEDGEMENTS

Declared none.

REFERENCES

[1]   Taieb A, Picardo M. Epidemiology, definitions and classification. In: Picardo M, Taieb A, Eds. Vitiligo. Heidelberg: Springer Verlag 2010; pp. 13-24.
[http://dx.doi.org/10.1007/978-3-540-69361-1_2]

[2]   Ezzedine K, Lim HW, Suzuki T, et al. Revised classification/nomenclature of vitiligo and related issues: the Vitiligo Global Issues Consensus Conference. Pigment Cell Melanoma Res 2012; 25(3): E1-E13.
[http://dx.doi.org/10.1111/j.1755-148X.2012.00997.x] [PMID: 22417114]

[3]   Njoo MD, Westerhof W, Bos JD, Bossuyt PM. The development of guidelines for the treatment of vitiligo. Arch Dermatol 1999; 135(12): 1514-21. [https://doi.org/10.1001/archderm.135.12.1514]. [PMID: 10606057].
[http://dx.doi.org/10.1001/archderm.135.12.1514] [PMID: 10606057]

[4]   Taïeb A, Picardo M. Clinical practice. Vitiligo. N Engl J Med 2009; 360(2): 160-9.
[PMID: 19129529]

[5]   Gey A, Diallo A, Seneschal J, et al. Autoimmune thyroid disease in vitiligo: multivariate analysis indicates intricate pathomechanisms. Br J Dermatol 2013; 168(4): 756-61. [https://doi.org/10.1111/bjd.12166]. [PMID: 23253044].
[http://dx.doi.org/10.1111/bjd.12166] [PMID: 23253044]

[6]   Linthorst Homan MW, Wolkerstorfer A, Sprangers MA, van der Veen JP. Digital image analysis vs. clinical assessment to evaluate repigmentation after punch grafting in vitiligo. J Eur Acad Dermatol Venereol 2013; 27(2): e235-8. [https://doi.org/10.1111/j.1468-3083.2012.04568.x]. [PMID: 22621363].
[http://dx.doi.org/10.1111/j.1468-3083.2012.04568.x] [PMID: 22621363]

[7]   Bulbul Baskan E, Baykara M, Ercan I, Tunali S, Yucel A. Vitiligo and ocular findings: a study on possible associations. J Eur Acad Dermatol Venereol 2006; 20(7): 829-33. [https://doi.org/10.1111/j.1468-3083.2006.01655.x]. [PMID: 16898906].
[PMID: 16898906]

[8]   Hegyi V, Petrovajová M, Novotný M. An objective assessment of melanin in vitiligo skin treated with Balneo PUVA therapy. Skin Res Technol 2014; 20(1): 108-15. [https://doi.org/10.1111/srt.12092]. [PMID: 23800185].
[http://dx.doi.org/10.1111/srt.12092] [PMID: 23800185]

9

Two-phase Surgery using a Dermal Regeneration Material for Nail Unit Melanoma

Shiro Iino[1,*], Suguru Sato[1], Natsuki Baba[1], Naoki Maruta[1], Wataru Takashima[1], Noritaka Oyama[1], Takahiro Kiyohara[2], Masato Yasuda[3] and Minoru Hasegawa[1]

[1]Department of Dermatology, Division of Medicine, Faculty of Medical Sciences, University of Fukui, Fukui, Japan
[2]Department of Dermatology, Kansai Medical University, Osaka, Japan
[3]Department of Plastic Surgery, University of Saga, Saga, Japan

Abstract:

Background:

Nail unit melanoma (NUM) poses a considerable treatment challenge, particularly in cases with in situ or early invasive lesions, and wide excision with phalanx amputation. For post-excisional skin defects, stump plasty and/or split-thickness skin grafting may cause persisted irritation and ulceration as a post-operative complication, because of the insufficient underlying tissue volume, vascularity, and stability.

Objective:

To seek out other superior management avoiding disadvantages associated with the conventional NUM surgery.

Method:

Three consecutive cases with NUM were treated by a novel two-phase surgical procedure using a commercially available dermal regeneration template; as the first phase, the lesional nail unit was excised and subsequently covered by a dermal regeneration template onto the phalangeal bone surface, allowing development of robust granulation with extracellular matrix and vascular network. Thereafter, the second phase employed a full-thickness skin grafting.

Results:

All three cases accomplished complete removal of the NUM lesion, and achieved a good cosmetic and functional outcome, maintaining physiological firmness, contour, and less contraction and atrophy of the overlying skin. They did not complain of major post-operative complications.

Conclusion:

Our two-phase approach using a dermal regeneration material is a satisfactory and straightforward technique, achieving a substantial benefit functionally and cosmetically in the post-operative period. We propose that the additional use of a tissue regeneration material can provide superior results for the reconstruction step of excised NUM.

Keywords: Nail unit melanoma, Dermal regeneration template, Preserved subcutaneous, Vascular network, Skin grafting, Surgery.

1. INTRODUCTION

Nail unit melanoma (NUM) is a relatively rare clinical form of malignant melanoma. The prevalence of NUM

---

* Address correspondence to this author at the Department of Dermatology, Faculty of Medical Sciences, University of Fukui, 23-3 Matsuoka-Shimoaizuki, Eiheiji, Fukui 910-1193, Japan; E-mail: shiro@u-fukui.ac.jp

represents <2% of Caucasian [1] and 15-35% of dark-skinned ethnic origin [2, 3] of overall patients with melanomas. Invasive NUM is often reconstructed using stump plasty combined with wide skin excision and bone amputation, whereas non-invasive disease may undergo full-thickness skin grafting on the exposed phalangeal bone. The excision and reconstruction procedures are usually managed in tandem at the same time. Most NUM is non-invasive to the bone layer, and only limited cases require amputation of the underlying bone to avoid the potential local recurrence [4]. Because of the unique properties and portion of the nail unit, the conventional procedures for the nail unit surgery may bring an intense operative stress and inevitable post-operative complication, such as shortening, contour irregularity, lesser volume, and persisted irritation and ulceration of the affected fingers [5, 6], causing a cosmetic and functional morbidity. Considering the balance between surgical invasiveness and site specificity in the digits, therefore, adequate reconstruction procedures concerning segmental arrangement need to be warranted for the NUM surgery. Here, we present three cases of NUM that were successfully treated by a two-phase surgical operation using a commercially available dermal regeneration template INTEGRA® (Ethicon, Inc, Plainsboro, NJ) and later reconstructed by using preserved subcutaneous vascular network skin grafting (PSVNSG) [7]. All the cases achieved good clinical and cosmetic outcomes during the long term of follow-up, accomplishing complete removal of the NUM.

2. CASE REPORTS

2.1. Case 1

A 60-year-old Japanese man was presented with longitudinal melanonychia suspicious for NUM in situ on his left thumb (Fig. **1a**). We performed a wide skin excision extending vertically to the subperiosteal layer (Fig. **1b**), and then placed a dermal regeneration template, INTEGRA®, directly onto the phalangeal bone surface with anchoring suture (Fig. **1c**). Pathological examination of the excised subungual skin revealed atypical melanocytes scattered along the basement membrane (Fig. **1d**), compatible with NUM in situ. The lateral and vertical margins were free of tumor. A month after placing the INTERA® template, the surgical defect was fully covered by abundant granulation bed (Fig. **1e**), followed by a PSVNSG donated from his subclavicular skin (Fig. **1f**). Subsequently, a local injection of IFN-β was done as an adjuvant therapy. One year after the skin grafting, the patient's affected thumb has almost recovered to the original length and volume, and maintained its contour and texture (Fig. **1g**). He has had no recurrence of NUM and no post-operative complication, such as irritation and fragility of the overlying skin, for 4 years after surgery.

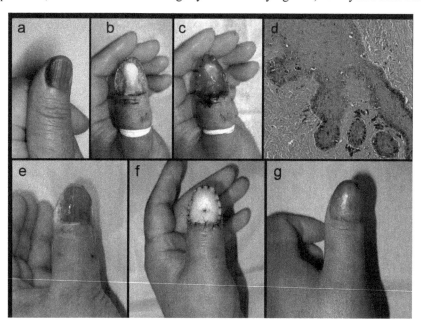

Fig. (1). Clinical course and histopathological features of case 1.
(a) Left thumb NUM in situ. **(b)** Wide skin excision extending vertically to the subperiosteal layer. **(c)** INTEGRA® was directly placed onto the exposed bone and tissue. **(d)** Histologically, numerous atypical melanocytes were scattered along the basement membrane. **(e)** The regenerated dermal tissue induced by INTEGRA® fully covered the defect within one month after the lesional excision as the first phase operation. **(f)** Reconstruction with a PSVNSG technique using a graft from the patient's clavicular skin. **(g)** Postoperative appearance one year after the skin grafting.

2.2. Case 2

A 62-year-old Japanese man presented to our hospital for evaluation of possible NUM on his left great toe (Fig. **2a**). At the first examination, however, the pigmented nail unit was fully covered with the dirty marks and crusts. Therefore, we first biopsied the lesional skin for the confirmative diagnosis of melanoma, performed a wide skin excision including the periosteal layer tissue, and then scraped the minimum amount of neighboring bone that was subsequently covered by the INTEGRA® template (Figs. **2b**, **2c**). Pathologically, the tumor mass consisted of atypical melanocytic nests at the hyponychium and intraepidermal spreading of individual melanoma cells along the basement membrane (Fig. **2d**), without lateral and vertical margin involvements. A month later, the regenerated dermal tissue covered the entire surgical defect (Fig. **2e**), and a PSVNSG was performed using the patient's abdominal skin (Fig. **2f**), with local injection of IFN-β for adjuvant therapy. Six months after the skin grafting, his great toe retained substantial volume and firmness with smooth texture of the overlying skin, although it was slightly shortened compared to the contralateral great toe (Fig. **2g**). He remains free from the local recurrence of melanoma during 1-year of follow-up, as well as incidence of post-operative complication in the grafted skin.

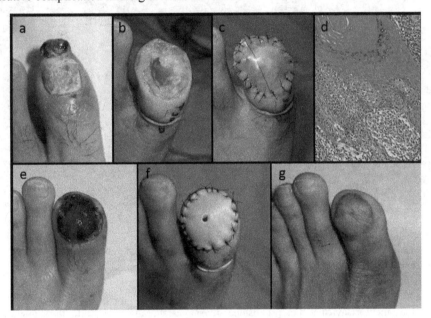

Fig. (2). Clinical course and histopathological features of case 2.
(a) NUM with a nodule on the hyponychium on the left great toe. **(b)** Wide skin excision extending vertically to the subperiosteal layer, with minimized amputation of the neighboring bone. **(c)** Placement of INTEGRA® directly onto the surgical defect. **(d)** Presentation of atypical melanocytes scattered along the basement membrane of the nail matrix with nodular invasion at the hyponychium. **(e)** INTEGRA* developed the regenerated dermal tissue entirely covering the defect within one month after the first phase operation. **(f)** Reconstruction with PSVNSG using a graft harvested from the patient's abdominal skin. **(g)** Postoperative outcome six months after the skin grafting

2.3. Case 3

A 78-year-old Japanese man with NUM experienced nail destruction on his right thumb prior to his first admission (Fig. **3a**). We performed a wide skin excision, as was in our two cases described above, and disconnected the protuberant distal phalanx (Fig. **3b**). Subsequently, the INTEGRA® template was sutured briefly onto the defected tissue (Fig. **3c**). Pathological examination revealed atypical melanocytes scattering along the basement membrane and nodular invasion to the nail bed (Fig. **3d**), all of which were completely resected. One month later, the regenerated dermal tissue completely covered the surgical defect (Fig. **3e**). A PSVNSG was then performed using a graft harvested from the patients' subclavicular skin (Fig. **3f**). After the operation, he was followed by a local injection of IFN-β. One year after the skin grafting, the affected thumb had maintained the substantial volume with only minimal shortening from its original length (Fig. **3g**). There is no recurrence of melanoma.

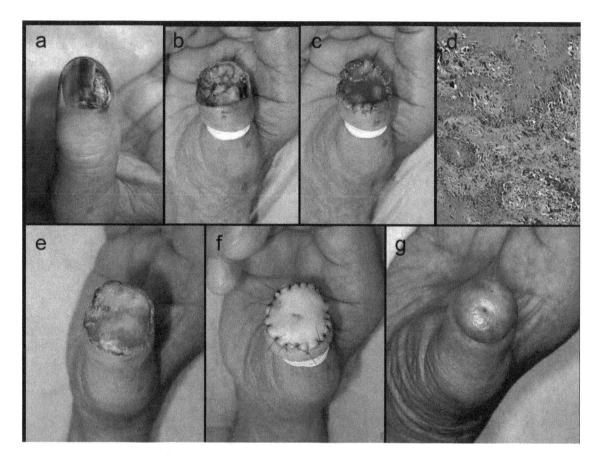

Fig. (3). Clinical course and histopathological features of case 3.
(a) NUM with nail destruction on the right thumb. **(b)** Wide skin excision extending vertically to the subperiosteal layer and amputation of the distal phalanx. **(c)** INTEGRA® was sutured directly onto the surgical defect without debriding the bone. **(d)** Atypical melanocytes were seen along the basement membrane with nodular invasion at the nail bed. **(e)** Regenerated dermal tissue induced by INTEGRA® fully covered the defect within one month after the first phase operation. **(f)** Reconstruction with PSVNSG utilizing a graft from the patient's clavicular skin. **(g)** Postoperative appearance at one year after the skin grafting.

3. DISCUSSION

We treated three cases of NUM by a two-phase surgical procedure designed to maintain, as much as possible, their original length, contour, and volume of the affected fingers, and obtained a favorable outcome in terms of cosmetic and functional reconstruction. This approach utilized a dermal regeneration template INTEGRA®, attributing to shift towards a later reconstruction step with PSVNSG.

INTEGRA® is a bilaminar membrane system consisting of porous bovine tendon collagen and shark glycosaminoglycan (chondroitin-6-sulfate), covered with the superficial silicone layer as a temporary epidermal substitute. The structure and regeneration process of this dermal template have been well described by Burke *et al.* [8]; the spongy bovine collagen layer acts as a scaffolding matrix to support the ingrowth of host fibroblasts and endothelial cells, known as a tri-dimensional neo-dermis, and is gradually saturated with integration of host (endogenous) collagens and extracellular matrices. After vascularization in the regenerated dermis, the superficial silicone layer is easily removed and replaced with an epidermal autograft onto the surface. The regenerated dermal tissue induced by INTEGRA® is applicable for covering any type of small tissue defects with capillary beds, like exposed bone or tendon [9]. In our present case series and initial trial [10], the INTEGRA® template may thus provide a safety and satisfactory regeneration result within at least one month after invasive excision to the subperiosteal tissue layer of the nail unit.

PSVNSG, first reported in 1980, is a method for full-thickness skin grafting that preserves the vascular network within the areolar tissue between the dermis and fat layer [7]. It is considered to organize superior results in the overall reconstruction outcomes compared to other skin graft methods. However, PSVNSG requires preparation of the sufficient post-excisional wound bed to ensure the proper skin engraftment [11]. On this basis, the combined use of the INTEGRA® template and PSVNSG can be a preferable approach for the NUM surgery, although the template would also provide a potential benefit with split-/full-thickness skin graft procedure.

Another advantage of our two-phase reconstruction method is that we can confirm a conclusive diagnosis of the excised skin lesion histologically between the two phases, achieving a curative skin grafting at the second reconstruction step. This enables us to keep the opportunity for further excision in the case of an incomplete excision, without compromising our repair. In such a case, we would simply remove and then reput the INTEGRA® following further excision.

CONCLUSION

Based on the several post-operative performance, we propose that the two-phase method using a dermal regeneration material is an advanced and reliable option for the treatment of NUM.

HUMAN AND ANIMAL RIGHTS

Not applicable.

CONFLICT OF INTEREST

The authors declare no conflict of interest, financial or otherwise.

ACKNOWLEDGEMENTS

Declared none.

REFERENCES

[1]   Haneke E. Textbook of Dermatologic Surgery. 1st ed. Padova, Italy: Piccin, Co. 2008.

[2]   Eedy DJ. Surgical treatment of melanoma. Br J Dermatol 2003; 149(1): 2-12.
        [http://dx.doi.org/10.1046/j.1365-2133.149.s64.8_65.x] [PMID: 12890188]

[3]   Phan A, Touzet S, Dalle S, Ronger-Savlé S, Balme B, Thomas L. Acral lentiginous melanoma: A clinicoprognostic study of 126 cases. Br J Dermatol 2006; 155(3): 561-9.
        [http://dx.doi.org/10.1111/j.1365-2133.2006.07368.x] [PMID: 16911282]

[4]   Izumi M, Ohara K, Hoashi T, et al. Subungual melanoma: Histological examination of 50 cases from early stage to bone invasion. J Dermatol 2008; 35(11): 695-703.
        [http://dx.doi.org/10.1111/j.1346-8138.2008.00551.x] [PMID: 19120763]

[5]   Duarte AF, Correia O, Barros AM, Azevedo R, Haneke E. Nail matrix melanoma in situ: Conservative surgical management. Dermatology (Basel) 2010; 220(2): 173-5.
        [http://dx.doi.org/10.1159/000266038] [PMID: 20016126]

[6]   Duarte AF, Correia O, Barros AM, Ventura F, Haneke E. Nail melanoma in situ: clinical, dermoscopic, pathologic clues, and steps for minimally invasive treatment. Dermatol Surg 2015; 41(1): 59-68.
        [http://dx.doi.org/10.1097/DSS.0000000000000243] [PMID: 25521106]

[7]   Tsukada S. Transfer of free skin grafts with a preserved subcutaneous vascular network. Ann Plast Surg 1980; 4(6): 500-6.
        [http://dx.doi.org/10.1097/00000637-198006000-00009] [PMID: 7002007]

[8]   Burke JF, Yannas IV, Quinby WC Jr, Bondoc CC, Jung WK. Successful use of a physiologically acceptable artificial skin in the treatment of extensive burn injury. Ann Surg 1981; 194(4): 413-28.
        [http://dx.doi.org/10.1097/00000658-198110000-00005] [PMID: 6792993]

[9]   Chou TD, Chen SL, Lee TW, *et al.* Reconstruction of burn scar of the upper extremities with artificial skin. Plast Reconstr Surg 2001; 108(2): 378-84.
        [http://dx.doi.org/10.1097/00006534-200108000-00015] [PMID: 11496178]

[10]   Iino S, Kiyohara T, Hasegawa M, *et al.* Proceedings of the 29th Annual Meeting of the Japanese Association of Dermatologic Surgery. 1994 Sep 13-14; Wakayama, Japan: Wakayama Medical University 1995.

[11]   Shimada K, Aoki Y, Ide Y, Ishikura N, Kawakami S. Burn due to misuse of an acetylene gas burner: A case report. Burns 1999; 25(7): 666-8.
        [http://dx.doi.org/10.1016/S0305-4179(99)00044-3] [PMID: 10563697]

10

Detection of TGF-β1, HGF, IGF-1 and IGF-1R in Cleft Affected Mucosa of the Lip

Elga Sidhom[*] and Mara Pilmane

Institute of Anatomy and Anthropology, Riga Stradins University, Riga, Latvia

Abstract:

Background:

Orofacial clefts are one of the most common birth defects with multifactorial and only partly understood morphopathogenesis.

Objective:

The aim of this study was to evaluate the presence of TGF-β1, HGF, IGF-1 and IGF-1R in cleft affected mucosa of the lip.

Methods:

Lip mucosa tissue samples were obtained during surgical cleft correction from seven 2 to 6 months old children. Prepared tissue sections were stained by immunohistochemistry for TGF-β1, HGF, IGF-1 and IGF-1R. The intensity of staining was graded semiquantitatively.

Results:

We found numerous TGF-β1 and HGF-containing epithelial and connective tissue cells, moderate number of IGF-1 immunoreactive cells and even less pronounced presence of IGF-1R-positive cells.

Conclusion:

TGF-β1 and HGF are present in defective epithelia and soft tissue in cleft affected lip. Expressions of IGF-1 and IGF-1R show significant differences, and both factors play a role in the morphopathogenesis of clefts.

Keywords: TGF-β1, HGF, IGF-1, IGF-1R, Cleft, Orofacial defects, Lip mucosa.

1. INTRODUCTION

Orofacial clefts - cleft lips, alveolar ridges and palates are one of the most common birth defects with multifactorial and only partly understood morphopathogenesis. Over 500 different complex genetic disorders include cleft formation [1].

TGF-β1 (Transforming growth factor beta 1) belongs to the TGF-β superfamily of approximately 40 cytokines and takes part in controlling proliferation, differentiation and survival in various cell types [2]. TGF-β1 is secreted by myofibroblasts, inflammatory cells, endothelial cells and epithelial cells and takes part in burn scar contracture formation [3]. Similarly, TGF-β1 also modulates wound inflammation and granulation tissue formation [4]. To date, the role of TGF in the formation of clefts has been evaluated in several studies. TGF-β3 is found to be decreasingly expressed in glands and epithelium of unaffected cleft of lip, alveolus with or without cleft palate compared to healthy

* Address correspondence to this author at the Institute of Anatomy and Anthropology, Riga Stradins University, Kronvalda blvd. 9, Riga, LV-1010, Latvia; E-mail: Elga.Sidhoma@rsu.lv

tissue [5]. Simultaneously, TGF-alpha has been studied in nonsyndromic clefts and healthy control tissue samples; it has been shown to have low protein expression in glands of cleft of the lip or palate tissue, as well as unaffected control tissue obtained from the lip and alveolus [6].

HGF (Hepatocyte growth factor) is secreted by tumor stromal cells; and cancer-associated fibroblasts promote growth, survival and migration of cancer cells in an HGF-dependent manner [7]. HGF is thought to be responsible for cancer cell migration, as well as their invasion *via* cytoskeletal assembly, reorganization and dynamics. HGF contributes to cytoskeleton remodeling, interactions and distribution [8].

IGF-1 (Insulin like growth factor 1) is phylogenetically ancient neurotrophic hormone with essential role in central nervous system development and maturation. It is especially important in cellular neuroplasticity and signals through its glycoprotein receptor IGF-1R (Insulin like growth factor 1 receptor) [9]. IGF-1 regulates survival and differentiation of many types of cells, including stem cells and placental cells, and stimulates prenatal and postnatal growth. In prenatal life, the synthesis of IGF-1 itself is regulated by various paracrine and endocrine factors and is synthesized as required. IGF-1R is a transmembrane tetramer receptor and its downregulation is associated with the inhibition of differentiation and induction of apoptosis [10]. IGF-1 and IGF-1R also play an initial role in cancerogenesis and their activity leads to increased mitogenesis, cell cycle progression and protection against apoptosis [11].

The aim of this study was to evaluate the presence of TGF-β1, HGF, IGF-1 and IGF-1R in cleft affected mucosa of the lip.

2. MATERIALS AND METHODS

Lip mucosa tissue samples were obtained during surgical lip correction from seven 2 to 6 months old children (five boys and two girls) in the Cleft Lip and Palate Centre at the Institute of Stomatology of Riga Stradins University. Six were patients with unilateral cleft lip and palate and one patient was with bilateral cleft lip and palate.

The study was performed in accordance with the 1964 Declaration of Helsinki. All tissue samples were obtained after receiving written informed consent from the parents of the patients. The study was approved by the Ethical Committee at Riga Stradins University, permit issued in 2003.

Lip mucosa tissue was fixed in Stefanini's solution [12]. Stefanini's solution was made of 20 g paraformaldehyde, 150 ml picric acid, 425 ml Sorensen's phosphate buffer (pH 7.2) and 425 ml distilled water, and stored in fridge. Further tissue samples were dehydrated and embedded in paraffin. Four micrometers thick sections were prepared and further stained routinely with hematoxylin and eosin [13].

TGF-β1 (code orb7087, obtained from rabbit, dilution 1:100, Biorbyt Limited, Cambridge, UK), HGF (catalog number AF-294-NA, Lot number ALP01, obtained from goat, dilution 1:300, R&D Systems, USA), IGF-1 (catalog number MAB291, Lot number 56408, obtained from mouse, dilution 1:50, R&D Systems, USA) and IGF-1R (catalog number AF-305-NA, Lot number VL03, obtained from goat, dilution 1:100, R&D Systems, USA) primary antibodies were used by biotin – streptavidin immunohistochemistry (IMH) [14].

Lip mucosa tissue samples were deparaffinized and washed in alcohol and water, then washed for 10 minutes in wash buffer (Tris-buffered saline) and placed for 5 minutes in EDTA boiling buffer in microwave; then cooled down and washed twice for 5 minutes in wash buffer. To decrease background staining, we used normal blocking serum for 20 minutes. All tissue samples were incubated with primary antibodies for 1 hour. Further, washing for 10 minutes in wash buffer and incubation for 30 minutes with LSAB+LINK with biotin related secondary antibodies (code K1015, DakoCytomation, Denmark) was performed. Afterwards we performed another washing for 5 minutes in wash buffer. Lip mucosa samples were incubated for 25 minutes with LSAB+LINK with enzyme peroxidase labeled streptavidine (code K0690, DakoCytomation, Denmark), which was followed by 5 minutes washing in wash buffer and 10 minutes processing with liquid DAB substrate-chromogen system (code K3468, DakoCytomation, Denmark) to obtain positive structure staining in brown color. Samples were then rinsed in running water and counterstained with hematoxylin to stain the nuclei blue.

All antibodies used in the study were tested for positive and negative control.

Image processing and analysis was performed using Image Pro Plus 6.0 software (Media Cybernetics, Silver Spring, Maryland, USA).

The intensity of immunostaining was graded semiquantitatively and labeled as follows: no positive structures in the visual field were labeled as 0, few positive structures in the visual field were labeled with +, moderate number of positive structures in the visual field were labeled with ++, numerous positive structures in the visual field were labeled with +++, abundance of positive structures in the visual field was marked with ++++ [15].

3. RESULTS

Mostly numerous (+++) TGF-β1-containing structures were detected in all lip tissue samples (Fig. **1**). TGF-β1 is found to be expressed in epitheliocytes, as well as fibroblasts and macrophages in subepithelial tissue. In one patient's tissue sample, we observed factor positive salivary glands, while another tissue sample showed patchy immunoreactivity. Occasional endothelial cells of the capillary walls were also immunopositive for TGF-β1.

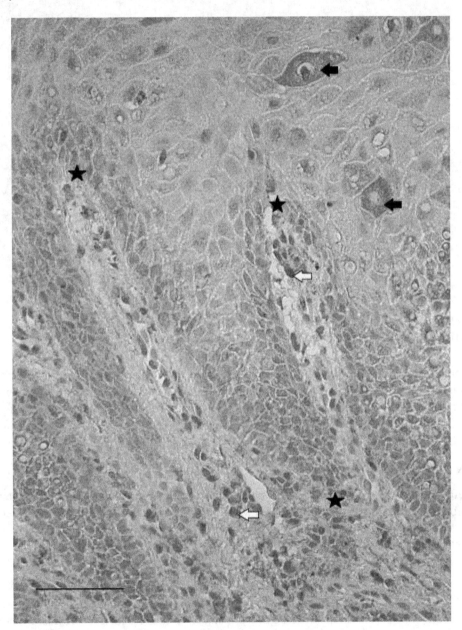

Fig. (1). Numerous TGF-β1-positive fibroblasts and macrophages in subepithelial tissue (white arrows), as well as TGF-β1-containing epithelial cells (black arrows). Occasional endothelial cells of the capillary walls are immunopositive for TGF-β1. Epithelium-connective tissue junction is marked with stars. TGF-β1 IMH, x250, scale bar: 4.1 μm.

HGF-positive epitheliocytes, macrophages, as well as fibroblasts were found in all patients' tissue samples. In epithelia, we detected mostly numerous (+++) HGF-positive cells, meanwhile HGF-positive fibroblasts and macrophages observed in subepithelial tissue varied from few (+) to abundance (++++) in the visual field (Fig. **2**).

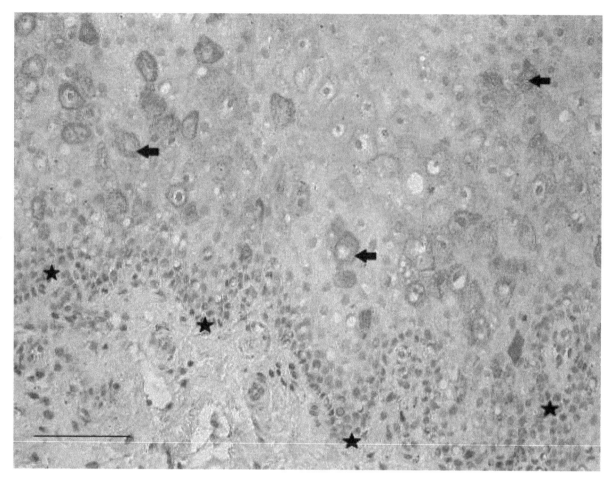

Fig. (2). Numerous HGF-positive epithelial cells (black arrows) in cleft affected lip mucosa. Epithelium-connective tissue junction is marked with stars. HGF IMH, x200, scale bar: 7.25 µm.

Mostly moderate (++) number of IGF-1-containing epithelial cells and connective tissue cells (fibroblasts, macrophages) (Fig. **3**), as well as IGF-1R-containing epithelial cells were found in most of our lip mucosa tissue samples. The expression of both factors was often with patchy distribution and the immunoreactive cells were observed in scattered regions. Simultaneously the immunoreactivity of IGF-1R in subepithelial tissue was weak and only some of the tissue samples contained few IGF-1R-positive fibroblasts and macrophages.

4. DISCUSSION

Orofacial clefts are constituted of cleft lip, cleft palate, and cleft lip and palate. Clefts are the largest group of craniofacial malformations. As there is strong familial association, major etiology factor is the genetic component. While cleft palate or cleft clip and palate require surgical correction due to difficulty in breastfeeding, untreated cleft lip or cleft lip and palate leads to social discrimination [16]. Orofacial clefting is associated with delayed facial growth or fusion. Various signaling pathways have been suggested as the culprit for the development of the facial malformations while one detailed mechanism is not known yet [17]. In the current study, we evaluated lip mucosa tissue samples obtained from seven children with cleft lip and palate.

TGF-β1 contributes to the formation of collagenous connective tissue and is expressed by large amount of fibroblasts and chronic inflammatory cells in reactive gingival overgrowths [18]. Compared with typical wounds there is a higher ratio of TGF-β1 in fetal wounds. Fetal wounds are known to heal rapidly and without scar formation early in gestation [19]. Various studies using animal models have looked at the role of TGF in the formation of clefts. It has been found that the loss of TGF-β signaling in the palatal epithelium leads to soft palate muscle cell proliferation and differentiation defects [20]. We found numerous TGF-β1-containing epithelial cells, fibroblasts and macrophages. Some of the endothelial cells in capillaries of our tissue samples were also immunopositive for TGF-β1 and in certain conditions endothelial cells can contain growth factors. We suggest that TGF-β1 takes part in the formation of both defective epithelia and soft tissue in cleft affected lip.

Our tissue samples showed prominent immunoreactivity also for HGF with overall numerous HGF-positive epithelial and subepithelial cells. HGF is associated with head and neck squamous cell carcinoma and contributes to proliferation, metastasis, angiogenesis, the tumor microenvironment and the immune system [21]. Apart from tumorogenesis, it has been shown that HGF is responsible for the development of *stria vascularis* and nonsensory structures of the cochlea. Lack of HGF signaling in the inner ear leads to hearing loss [22]. HGF is a mitogen and motility factor and primarily regulates epithelial cell function. HGF actively augments the proliferation of corneal epithelial cells in normal and inflammatory conditions [23]. Thus, HGF also takes part in the development of the defective epithelia and soft tissue in cleft affected lip mucosa.

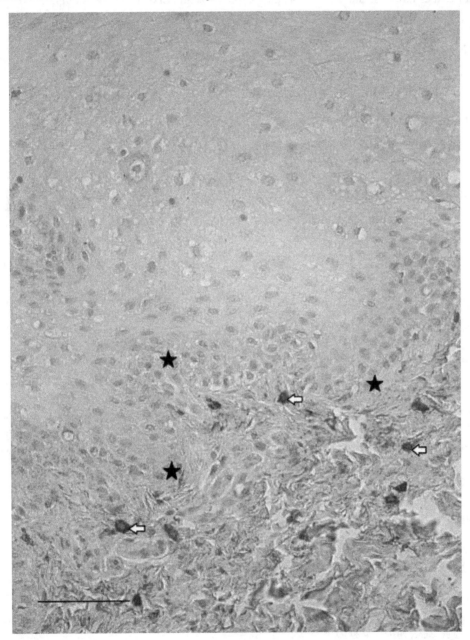

Fig. (3). IGF-1-immunoreactive cells (white arrows) in subepithelial tissue of cleft affected lip tissue. Epithelium-connective tissue junction is marked with stars. IGF-1 IMH, x250, scale bar: 4.1 μm.

IGF-1 is known to take part in the postnatal facial development as it regulates vertical face growth [24]. IGF-1 also stimulates proliferation, wound healing and differentiation processes of periodontal ligament cells under inflammatory conditions [25]. Furthermore, IGF-1 and IGF-1R are expressed early during embryogenesis and have shown antagonizing effects. Overexpression of IGF-1 leads to anterior expansion of head neural tissue and ectopic eyes, while IGF-1R depletion greatly reduces head structures [26]. We found moderate number of IGF-1-containing epithelial cells and connective tissue cells, as well as IGF-1R-containing epithelial cells. Simultaneously only few IGF-1R-positive connective tissue cells were found in some of the studied tissue samples. Therefore, we suggest that expressions of IGF-1 and IGF-1R show significant differences, and both factors play a role in the morphopathogenesis of clefts.

CONCLUSION

TGF-β1 and HGF are present in defective epithelia and soft tissue in cleft affected lip. Expressions of IGF-1 and IGF-1R show significant differences, and both factors play a role in the morphopathogenesis of clefts.

HUMAN AND ANIMAL RIGHTS

No Animals/Humans were used for studies that are base of this research.

CONFLICT OF INTEREST

The authors declare no conflict of interest, financial or otherwise.

ACKNOWLEDGEMENTS

Riga Stradins University project "Longitudinal research on cleft morphopathogenesis".

REFERENCES

[1]   Wójcicki P, Koźlik MJ, Wójcicka K. Genetic factors in selected complex congenital malformations with cleft defect. Adv Clin Exp Med 2016; 25(5): 977-87.
[http://dx.doi.org/10.17219/acem/61911] [PMID: 28028964]

[2]   Rider CC, Mulloy B. Heparin, Heparan sulphate and the TGF-β Cytokine superfamily. Molecules 2017; 22(5): E713.
[http://dx.doi.org/10.3390/molecules22050713] [PMID: 28468283]

[3]   Tan J, Wu J. Current progress in understanding the molecular pathogenesis of burn scar contracture. Burns Trauma 2017; 5: 14.
[http://dx.doi.org/10.1186/s41038-017-0080-1] [PMID: 28546987]

[4]   Koivisto L, Heino J, Häkkinen L, Larjava H. Integrins in wound healing. Adv Wound Care (New Rochelle) 2014; 3(12): 762-83.
[http://dx.doi.org/10.1089/wound.2013.0436] [PMID: 25493210]

[5]   Rullo R, Gombos F, Ferraraccio F, et al. TGFbeta3 expression in non-syndromic orofacial clefts. Int J Pediatr Otorhinolaryngol 2006; 70(10): 1759-64.
[http://dx.doi.org/10.1016/j.ijporl.2006.05.019] [PMID: 16837067]

[6]   Rullo R, Gombos F, Ferraraccio F, et al. TGF alpha has low protein expression in nonsyndromic clefts. J Craniofac Surg 2007; 18(6): 1276-80.
[http://dx.doi.org/10.1097/scs.0b013e3180de6506] [PMID: 17993868]

[7]   Owusu BY, Galemmo R, Janetka J, Klampfer L. Hepatocyte growth factor: A key tumor-promoting factor in the tumor microenvironment. Cancers (Basel) 2017; 9(4): E35.
[http://dx.doi.org/10.3390/cancers9040035] [PMID: 28420162]

[8]   Xiang C, Chen J, Fu P. HGF/Met Signaling in Cancer Invasion: The impact on cytoskeleton remodeling. Cancers (Basel) 2017; 9(5): E44.
[http://dx.doi.org/10.3390/cancers9050044] [PMID: 28475121]

[9]   Dyer AH, Vahdatpour C, Sanfeliu A, Tropea D. The role of Insulin-Like growth factor 1 (IGF-1) in brain development, maturation and neuroplasticity. Neuroscience 2016; 325: 89-99.
[http://dx.doi.org/10.1016/j.neuroscience.2016.03.056] [PMID: 27038749]

[10]   Youssef A, Aboalola D, Han VK. The roles of Insulin-Like growth factors in mesenchymal stem cell niche. Stem Cells Int 2017.
[http://dx.doi.org/10.1155/2017/9453108]

[11]   Kasprzak A, Kwasniewski W, Adamek A, Gozdzicka-Jozefiak A. Insulin-like growth factor (IGF) axis in cancerogenesis. Mutat Res Rev Mutat Res 2017; 772: 78-104.
[http://dx.doi.org/10.1016/j.mrrev.2016.08.007] [PMID: 28528692]

[12]   Stefanini M, De Martino C, Zamboni L. Fixation of ejaculated spermatozoa for electron microscopy. Nature 1967; 216(5111): 173-4.
[http://dx.doi.org/10.1038/216173a0] [PMID: 4862079]

[13]   Fischer AH, Jacobson KA, Rose J, Zeller R. Hematoxylin and eosin staining of tissue and cell sections. CSH Protoc 2008.
       [http://dx.doi.org/10.1101/pdb.prot4986]

[14]   Hsu SM, Raine L, Fanger H. The use of antiavidin antibody and avidin-biotin-peroxidase complex in immunoperoxidase technics. Am J Clin
       Pathol 1981; 75(6): 816-21.
       [http://dx.doi.org/10.1093/ajcp/75.6.816] [PMID: 6167159]

[15]   Pilmane M, Luts A, Sundler F. Changes in neuroendocrine elements in bronchial mucosa in chronic lung disease in adults. Thorax 1995;
       50(5): 551-4.
       [http://dx.doi.org/10.1136/thx.50.5.551] [PMID: 7541167]

[16]   Beaty TH, Marazita ML, Leslie EJ. Genetic factors influencing risk to orofacial clefts: today's challenges and tomorrow's opportunities.
       F1000 Res 2016; 5: 2800.
       [http://dx.doi.org/10.12688/f1000research.9503.1] [PMID: 27990279]

[17]   Kurosaka H. The roles of hedgehog signaling in upper lip formation. Biomed Res Int 2015; 6.
       [http://dx.doi.org/10.1155/2015/901041]

[18]   Epivatianos A, Andreadis D, Iordanidis S. Myofibroblasts and transforming growth factor-beta1 in reactive gingival overgrowths. J Oral
       Maxillofac Res 2013; 4(1): e3.
       [http://dx.doi.org/10.5037/jomr.2013.4103] [PMID: 24422026]

[19]   Namazi MR, Fallahzadeh MK, Schwartz RA. Strategies for prevention of scars: what can we learn from fetal skin? Int J Dermatol 2011;
       50(1): 85-93.
       [http://dx.doi.org/10.1111/j.1365-4632.2010.04678.x] [PMID: 21039435]

[20]   Iwata J, Suzuki A, Yokota T, et al. TGFβ regulates epithelial-mesenchymal interactions through WNT signaling activity to control muscle
       development in the soft palate. Development 2014; 141(4): 909-17.
       [http://dx.doi.org/10.1242/dev.103093] [PMID: 24496627]

[21]   Hartmann S, Bhola NE, Grandis JR. HGF/Met signaling in head and neck cancer: impact on the tumor microenvironment. Clin Cancer Res
       2016; 22(16): 4005-13.
       [http://dx.doi.org/10.1158/1078-0432.CCR-16-0951] [PMID: 27370607]

[22]   Shibata S, Miwa T, Wu HH, Levitt P, Ohyama T. Hepatocyte growth factor-c-MET signaling mediates the development of nonsensory
       structures of the mammalian cochlea and hearing. J Neurosci 2016; 36(31): 8200-9.
       [http://dx.doi.org/10.1523/JNEUROSCI.4410-15.2016] [PMID: 27488639]

[23]   Omoto M, Suri K, Amouzegar A, et al. Hepatocyte growth factor suppresses inflammation and promotes epithelium repair in corneal injury.
       Mol Ther 2017.
       [http://dx.doi.org/10.1016/j.ymthe.2017.04.020]

[24]   Masoud MI, Marghalani HY, Alamoudi NM, El Derw D, Masoud IM, Gowharji NF. Longitudinal relationship between insulin-like growth
       factor-1 levels and vertical facial growth. J Orofac Orthop 2015; 76(5): 440-50.
       [http://dx.doi.org/10.1007/s00056-015-0305-5] [PMID: 26272169]

[25]   Reckenbeil J, Kraus D, Stark H, et al. Insulin-like growth factor 1 (IGF1) affects proliferation and differentiation and wound healing
       processes in an inflammatory environment with p38 controlling early osteoblast differentiation in periodontal ligament cells. Arch Oral Biol
       2017; 73: 142-50.
       [http://dx.doi.org/10.1016/j.archoralbio.2016.10.010] [PMID: 27769028]

[26]   Richard-Parpaillon L, Héligon C, Chesnel F, Boujard D, Philpott A. The IGF pathway regulates head formation by inhibiting Wnt signaling in
       Xenopus. Dev Biol 2002; 244(2): 407-17.
       [http://dx.doi.org/10.1006/dbio.2002.0605] [PMID: 11944947]

11

Prospective Pilot Evaluation of the Efficacy and Safety of Topical Ingenol Mebutate Gel for Localized Patch/Plaque Stage Mycosis Fungoides

Eve Lebas[1], Charlotte Castronovo[1], Jorge E. Arrese[2], Florence Libon[1], Nazli Tassoudji[1], Laurence Seidel[3] and Arjen F. Nikkels[1,*]

[1]*Dermatology (Dermato-oncology unit), University Hospital Centre, CHU du Sart Tilman, Liège, Belgium*
[2]*Dermatopathology, University Hospital Centre, CHU du Sart Tilman, Liège, Belgium*
[3]*Biostatistics University Hospital Centre, CHU du Sart Tilman, Liège, Belgium*

Abstract:

Background:

Mycosis Fungoides (MF) is the most frequent type of the primary cutaneous NK/T-cell lymphomas. Ingenol mebutate (IM) displays *in vitro* pro-apoptotic properties on neoplastic lymphocytes.

Objectives:

To evaluate the efficacy and safety of IM gel as topical treatment for MF.

Materials and Methods:

Ten male patients with longstanding classic type MF (n=9) and follicular MF (FMF; n=1), T2bN0M0B0, stage Ib, resistant to systemic methotrexate or acitretin therapies for at least 3 months, were included in this pilot study. In these patients, 11 target patch/plaque stage lesions with an area ≤ 25 cm^2 were selected for IM therapy (0,05%, 2 weekly applications). The primary endpoint was the improvement of the CAILS scores. Biopsies were performed before and after treatment from 10 target lesions. Relapse rates were evaluated at 6 months.

Results:

The mean CAILS score of treated target lesions was reduced by 58.2%. The mean erythema, scaling and plaque elevation scores were improved by 73.6%, 93.9% and 97.9% ($p<0.0001$), respectively, while the lesion size remained unchanged ($p=0.34$). A complete or partial clearance of histological and immunohistochemical features was observed in 6/10 (60%) and 4/10 (40%) of the MF or FMF target lesions, respectively. Monoclonal TCR rearrangement was evidenced in 100% (7/7) of the patients and in 3/7 (43%) after treatment. The relapse rate at 6 months was 18%. All the patients experienced burning sensations, oozing and crusting.

Conclusion:

IM gel warrants further investigation and development as a potential topical treatment for localized patch/plaque stage MF and FMF.

Keywords: Ingenol Mebutate, Mycosis Fungoides, PCNKTCL, Alternative Topical Treatment Option.

* Address correspondence to this author at the Department of Dermatology, CHU of Sart Tilman, University of Liège, B-4000, Liège, Belgium; E-mail: af.nikkels@chu.ulg.ac.be

1. INTRODUCTION

Ingenol Mebutate (IM) is a macrocyclic diterpene ester and originates from the plant *Euphorbia peplus* (PEP005, 0,015%, 0,05%, Picato° gel, Leo Pharma) [1, 2]. For decades the sap from *E. peplus* has been used as traditional medicine for various types of skin cancer [1, 2]. Both the EMA and the FDA recognize IM gel as a field-directed treatment for Actinic Keratosis (AK) [1, 2]. IM also revealed to be an efficacious topical treatment for other cutaneous (Fig. 3) epithelial cancers, including superficial basal cell carcinoma [3 - 5], Bowen's disease [6, 7] and murine cutaneous squamous cell carcinoma [8]. IM has also demonstrated activity against melanoma cell lines *in vitro* [9, 10] and, *in vivo*, for Dubreuilh's melanoma of the face [11].

IM and other ingenol derivatives activate multiple signaling pathways in cancer cells, including the intracellular pro-apoptotic Protein Kinase C (PKC) δ, α and ε, NF-κB1, ERK, JNK and Akt pathways [10, 12]. The activation of these PKC's leads to a rapid cancer cell apoptosis and a neutrophil-mediated immunostimulation of antibody-dependent cellular cytotoxic response [13]. The IM-induced pro-inflammatory and pro-apoptotic storm could potentially be of therapeutic benefit for atypical lymphocytes. Ingenol 3-angelate has previously been demonstrated to be effective against murine B-lymphoma cells [12]. IM induced apoptosis in acute myeloid leukemia cells by activating the PKC isoform PKCδ [14].

The classic type of Mycosis Fungoides (MF) is the most frequent form of the primary Cutaneous T/NK Cell Lymphomas (pCTNKCL). MF follows typically an indolent cutaneous disease course and is an ideal candidate for skin-directed therapies. Its folliculotropic variant (FMF) is a more rare and late-stage FMF may present a more aggressive disease course [15 - 18].

In the view of the action mechanisms of IM, we were interested to evaluate whether IM gel 0,05% had a potential effect on patch/plaque stage lesions in MF and FMF patients that were previously resistant to systemic methotrexate or acitretin.

This prospective pilot study assessed the improvement of the CAILS (Composite Assessment of Index Lesion Severity) score [19] and the histological cure rate 2 months after using IM gel on 11 target lesions in 10 patients with histologically confirmed, longstanding patch/plaque stage MF and FMF.

2. MATERIALS AND METHODS:

2.1. Institutional Ethics

This prospective pilot study was performed in accordance with the ethical standard of the University Hospital Committee on institutional human experimentation and with the Helsinki Declaration of 1975, and amended in 2013. The aims of the study and all the procedures were explained to all the patients and all signed an informed consent.

2.2. Patient Selection

At baseline, the patients had to present patch/plaque stage lesions that were not responding to at least 3 months of oral methotrexate or acitretin treatments. Patients were selected between Feb and May 2017. The individual patient demographics, including age, gender, type of underlying MF, TNMB staging and disease stage, mSWAT (modified Severity-Weighted Assessment Tool) score of the underlying MF at baseline, as well as the site of the selected target lesion are summarized in Table **1**. All the patients had longstanding patch/plaque type classic type MF (n=9) or FMF (n=1). The diagnosis of classic type MF or FMF was made histologically at least 4 years before inclusion in the study and sustained by an immunohistochemical CD3+, CD4+, CD45R0+ and CD8- expression profile of the MF infiltrate and by the presence of a monoclonal T-Cell Receptor (TCR) rearrangement (10/10 cases).

Table 1. Patient Demographics.

Patient	Gender, Age	Type, TNMB, Stage, mSWAT	Target Lesion Site(s)	Duration of MF (years)
1	M, 64 years	FMF, T2bN0M0B0, Ib, 30	Perineal	> 7
2	M, 52 years	MF, classic type T2bN0M0B0, Ib, 82	Left arm	> 5
3	M, 70 years	MF, classic type T2bN0M0B0, Ib, 56	Left arm	> 8
4	M, 62 years	MF, classic type T2bN0M0B0, Ib, 84	Right arm	> 5
5	M, 73 years	MF, classic type T2bN0M0B0, Ib, 74	Chest	> 4
6	M, 76 years	MF, classic type T2bN0M0B0, Ib, 88	Knee	> 5

(Table 1) contd.....

Patient	Gender, Age	Type, TNMB, Stage, mSWAT	Target Lesion Site(s)	Duration of MF (years)
7	M, 79 years	MF, classic type T2bN0M0B0, Ib, 48	Knee	> 8
8	M, 80 years	MF, classic type T2bN0M0B0, Ib, 42	Axillar	> 4
9	M, 65 years	MF, classic type T2bN0M0B0, Ib, 78	Buttock	> 5
10	M, 72 years	MF, classic type T2bN0M0B0, Ib, 44	Inguinal Abdominal	> 6
	Mean age: 69 years	Mean mSWAT score: 59.6		Mean duration of MF: 5.7 years

2.3. Target Site Selection

Per patient, one or two target patch/plaque type lesion(s) of 3 to 7 cm in diameter were selected. Target lesions had to be present without any clinical changes since at least 3 months. Target lesions exceeding 25 cm^2 were excluded, as manufacturer instructions say to treat an area of not more than 25 cm^2.

2.4. Control Site Selection

One or more control lesions in the immediate vicinity of the target lesion were selected. The size of the control lesions was up to 25 cm^2. The control lesions had to present a clinical highly similar aspect as the target lesion.

2.5. Photographic Recording

Photographic recordings were made of every target lesion and control lesion(s) under standard conditions at baseline (T0) and at 2 months after therapy (T2).

2.6. Treatment Application

One tube of IM gel (0,05%, 235 µg of IM in 0,47 g of gel, Leo Pharma°) was applied to the target lesion at day 1 and day 7. The 0,05% formulation was selected, as none of the target lesions was located on the face. Patients were informed concerning potential adverse effects and how to manage them. The one-week interval between IM applications was selected to avoid too severe cutaneous adverse reactions as sometimes observed in AK patients with the 2 consecutive days IM application regimen, and furthermore, to be able to judge the severity of the cutaneous reactions after one single application and to reduce the severity the IM-treatment-related adverse effects. The control lesions did not receive any topical treatment. No other topical treatments were allowed for the target and control lesions during the entire study. The previous oral treatments were interrupted three months before inclusion.

2.7. Histology, Immunohistology and TCR

A 4-mm cutaneous punch biopsy of the target lesion was obtained under local anesthesia, fixed in neutralized formalin 4% and embedded in paraffin before and 2 months after treatment. Histopathological examination for MF criteria was performed. The histologic scoring system was the following: no change compared to baseline, a partial improvement (at least 75%) of the MF infiltrate or a total resolution (with or without persistence of post-inflammatory lymphohistiocytic infiltrate and/or post-inflammatory hyperpigmentation). Immunohistochemistry searched for CD3, CD4, CD45R0 and CD8 expressions. Immunohistological scoring was as follows: no change compared to baseline, partial resolution (at least 75% improvement) and total healing in terms of CD3, CD4, CD45R0 and CD8 expression. TCR monoclonal rearrangements were evaluated as present or absent at baseline and 2 months after treatment from 7 target lesions. No histology was performed for the control lesions.

2.8. CAILS Score

The primary endpoint in this pilot setting was the mean CAILS (Composite Assessment of Index Lesion Severity) score improvement, expressed in percentage (T0-T2), evaluating the erythema, scaling, plaque elevation and hyper/hypopigmentation scores (all: ranging from 0 (none) to 8 (very severe)) as well as the lesion size (1: up to 4 cm^2 up to maximum 4: 16-25 cm^2), as used for individual lesion evaluation, before (T0) and 2 months (T2) after treatment of the target and control lesions [19].

2.9. Local Adverse Effects

Cutaneous local adverse effects assessment was performed 5 days after the first and second IM application. The scoring of burning sensations, oozing, and crusting used the following scale: 0: none, 1: mild, 2: moderate and 3:

severe. No evaluation of eventual systemic adverse effects was included in this pilot study as no such effects were previously reported in AK studies [1 - 5].

2.10. Recurrence Rate

The clinical relapse rate of the target lesion was assessed 6 months after the initiation of the IM treatment. Relapse was defined as the re-appearance of the patch/plaque infiltration and/or erythema and/or scaling.

2.11. Statistical Analysis

A comparison of the mean relative differences (T0 and T2) between target and control was made using the Student test for the individual CAILS parameters, erythema, scaling, plaque elevation, hyper/hypopigmentation and lesion size (L. Seidel).

3. RESULTS

3.1. Histology, Immunohistology and TCR

Punch biopsies were obtained from 10 target lesions before IM treatment (T0) and at 2 months after treatment (T2). Histopathological examination revealed a complete or partial absence of histological signs and immunohistochemical features of MF or FMF in 6/11 (55%) and 4/11 (36%) target lesions, respectively (Figs. 1 and 2). Monoclonal TCR rearrangement of the target lesions before treatment was positive in 7/7 (100%) cases and in 3/7 (43%) at 2 months post-treatment.

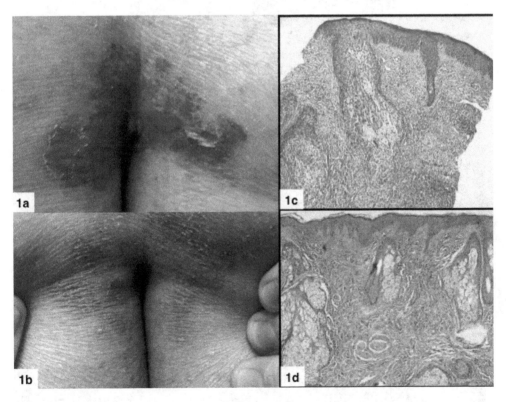

Fig. (1). a. Target lesion of a folliculotropic pCTNKCL on the buttocks. **1b.** Complete clinical cure after 2 months. **1c.** Histology illustrating folliculotropic pCTNKCL before treatment (H/E histochemical stain, 40x). **1d.** Histological clearing of atypical lymphocytes two months after IM treatment (H/E histochemical stain, 10x).

3.2. CAILS Scores

The study results are listed in Tables **2** and **3**. The mean overall CAILS score (T0-T2) was reduced by 58.2%. The erythema, scaling and plaque elevation mean scores (T0-T2) were improved by 73.6%, 93.9% and 97.7% respectively, all statistically significant (p<0.0001). No hyper or hypopigmentation was observed at baseline. Mild to moderate hyperpigmentation appeared in 8/11 (73%) of the target lesions. No reduction in lesion size was observed in any of the target and control lesions (Figs. **1-4**).

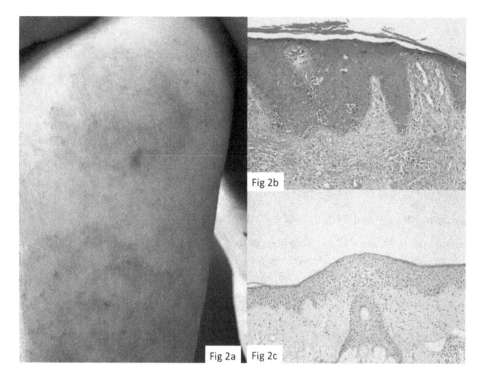

Fig. (2). a. Hyperpigmented postinflammatory target MF lesion (yellow arrow) and erythemato-squamous control MF lesion (red arrow) 2 months after treatment. **2b**. Histology illustrating patch/plaque stage MF before and **2c**. Histological clearing 2 months after treatment (H/E histochemical stain, x10).

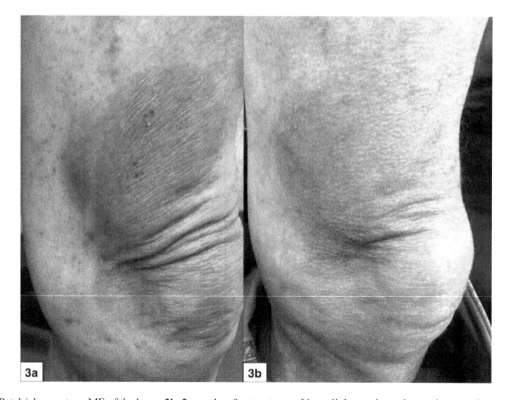

Fig. (3). a. Patch/plaque stage MF of the knee, **3b**, 2 months after treatment. Note slight persistent hyperpigmentation.

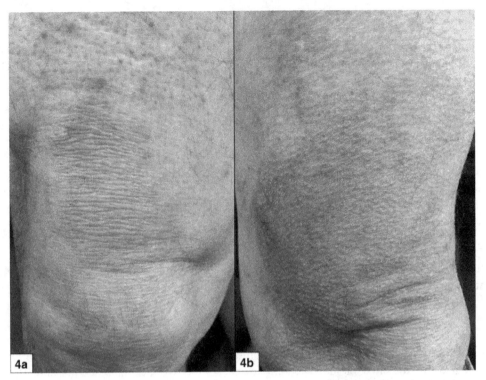

Fig. (4). a. Patch/plaque stage MF of the knee, **4b.** 2 months after treatment. Note slight persistent hyperpigmentation.

Table 2. Mean absolute differences between T0 and T2 and significance of the difference.

Variable	N	Mean	SD	SE	Min	Q1	Median	Q3	Max	Student p-value
ErythdT0T2	11	3.818	1.401	0.42	2.0	3.0	4.00	5.0	6.0	<.0001
ScalingdT0T2	11	3.273	1.421	0.43	1.0	2.0	4.00	4.0	6.0	<.0001
PlaquedT0T2	11	3.909	1.221	0.37	2.0	3.0	4.00	4.0	6.0	<.0001
HyppigmdT0T2	11	-1.636	1.433	0.43	-4.0	-2.0	-2.00	0.0	0.0	0.0036
SizedT0T2	11	0.000	0.000	0.00	0.0	0.0	0.00	0.0	0.0	
TotaldT0T2	11	9.364	2.580	0.78	6.0	7.0	9.00	12.0	14.0	<.0001

Table 3. Comparison of the relative differences (%) between Target and Control (PT0T2 et PC0C2).

Variable	N	Mean	SD	SE	Min	Q1	Median	Q3	Max	Student p-value
dErythpT0T2C	11	73.636	18.148	5.47	50.0	50.0	75.00	83.3	100.0	<.0001
dScalingpT0T	11	93.939	10.601	3.20	75.0	83.3	100.00	100.0	100.0	<.0001
dPlaquepT0T2	11	97.727	7.538	2.27	75.0	100.0	100.00	100.0	100.0	<.0001
dHyppigmpT0T	0	.	.	.	.	.	.	.	.	
dSizepT0T2C0	11	3.030	10.050	3.03	0.0	0.0	0.00	0.0	33.3	0.34
dTotalpT0T2C	11	58.235	12.910	3.89	37.5	46.2	60.00	68.3	75.0	<.0001

3.3. Recurrence

After a follow-up of 6 months after treatment, 2 out of 11 target lesions (18%) presented de novo erythema, slight infiltration and scaling, suggestive of MF recurrence. The hyperpigmentation observed at the evaluation at 2 months was significantly attenuated in 10 out of 11 cases at 6 months.

No beneficial or detrimental effects were noted for the surrounding control lesions.

3.4. Adverse Effects

Five days after the first and second application of IM, all the patients experienced treatment-related adverse effects. The scores for burning sensations, oozing and crusting were 1.6, 0.7, 1, and 1.2, 0.3, 0.5, respectively. All the patients accepted well the IM-inherent adverse effects and were never a reason to interrupt the trial.

4. DISCUSSION

Although the precise action mechanisms of IM on neoplastic lymphocytes should be further investigated, the IM-induced pro-inflammatory and pro-apoptotic storm [12] through activation of the PKC isoform PKCδ is likely to be involved in the anti-neoplastic action on MF lymphocytes [14].

As the control lesions in the direct vicinity of the target lesions were unaltered one may suggest that IM only acts locally at the site of application and does not generate a more expanded immune effect. This is in contrast to topical agents such as resiquimod, inducing not only a loco-regional immune effect, but also a systemic immune stimulation by enhancing circulating dendritic cells [20]. On the other hand, other authors described an adjuvant effect of IM by showing that its action on subcutaneous tumors simultaneously generated anti-cancer CD8+ T-cells, able to regress metastases and distant metastases by upregulating CD80 and CD86 expression on dendritic cells and by stimulating CD8+ T-cell induction when co-delivered with a protein antigen [21].

This pilot study supports the hypothesis that the action spectrum of IM is not only limited to neoplastic keratinocytes and melanocytes, but also expands to neoplastic lymphocytes of MF.

Due to the relative difficulty of finding 3 highly similar test MF lesions (IM target lesion gel, placebo gel lesion and no treatment lesion) in one patient, we decided in this pilot setting not to include a placebo gel group. Previous studies with IM on AK demonstrated that IM was significantly superior to placebo gel in terms of partial and complete clearance and the median percentage reduction in baseline AK lesions for patients treated with IM gel ranged from 75% to 100% compared with 0% for vehicle gel (P < .0001 vs vehicle) [2]. Furthermore, the 13.3% placebo effect in the AK studies could also be attributed to the natural evolution of "coming and going" of AK's. In addition, the vehicle gel could have had a keratolytic effect on the hyperkeratotic part of the AK's, explaining a placebo effect, a phenomenon that does not exist in MF lesions.

Even if only 11 target lesions of 10 T2b MF patients were included in this pilot study, the results remain interesting, in particular in comparison to other available topical treatments. In fact, for T2 MF, the topical retinoids group, including bexarotene 1% gel, tazarotene 0,1% gel and alitretinoine 0,1% gel, presented a complete cure of 21%, 33% and 100% (one single patient), respectively [22 - 24]. The potent to very strong corticosteroids achieved a complete response in 25% in T2 MF patients [25, 26]. The topical immunomodulators such as imiquimod 5% cream presented a 50% cure rate [27] and resiquimod 0.03% and 0.06% gel presented a 30% cure rate in 12 IA-IIA MF patients [20]. Topical chemotherapies using mechlorethamine or carmustine in T2 MF patients achieved about a 50% complete response [28 - 31].

IM already achieved a good clinical response after 2 months versus 10-19 months with mechlorethamine or carmustine [28 - 32] or versus 20.1 months for bexaroten gel [22]. Hence, IM gel seems to act more rapidly compared to other topical agents.

That TCR monoclonality was still present in 3 of 7 target lesions at T2 is probably related to the high sensitivity of the PCR technique, whereas the histological and immunohistological analysis do not favor anymore a diagnosis of MF. Despite this fact, there was only an 18% recurrence rate after 6 months. This may suggest that the histological and immunohistological assessment of treatment results are better predictors of a persisting favorable treatment response than TCR rearrangement analysis.

The number of cases is too small to determine whether the intensity of adverse reactions and/or the post inflammatory hyperpigmentation after application are predictive of a favorable treatment outcome or not.

The adverse effects of IM were identical to those experienced using IM gel as AK therapy [1, 2]. In general, the adverse effects were less severe following the second IM application, probably linked to an already partial remission of the target lesion after the first IM application. Hyperpigmentation of the target lesion was frequent (8 out of 11 target lesions) but faded over time.

Final dosing regimens and the place of IM among the armamentarium of topical treatments against MF should be evaluated on larger series. Whether other ingenol derivatives are also effective as anti-MF topical agent remains to be determined [33]. One major drawback of IM is that it is only approved for a body surface limited to 25 cm^2. Currently ingenol disoxate is being developed for use on larger surfaces, up to 250 cm^2, as has been recently published for field AK [34].

CONCLUSION

In conclusion, this pilot study suggests that IM gel merits further evaluation as a topical alternative treatment for patients with localized patch/plaque stage MF skin lesions not exceeding 25 cm^2, in a placebo-controlled study design. This study provides an initial proof of concept that IM also acts against neoplastic MF lymphocytes.

FINANCIAL-DISCLOSURE

Leo Pharma provided the IM gel but the authors perceived no financial compensation in what so ever form. Leo Pharma did not intervene in the design and interpretation of the study results.

HUMAN AND ANIMAL RIGHTS

No Animals were used in this research. All human research procedures followed were in accordance with the ethical standards of the committee responsible for human experimentation (institutional and national), and with the Helsinki Declaration of 1975, as revised in 2008.

CONFLICT OF INTEREST

The authors declare no conflict of interest, financial or otherwise.

ACKNOWLEDGEMENTS

Declared none.

REFERENCES

[1]   Lebwohl M, Shumack S, Stein Gold L, Melgaard A, Larsson T, Tyring SK. Long-term follow-up study of ingenol mebutate gel for the treatment of actinic keratoses. JAMA Dermatol 2013; 149: 666-70.
[http://dx.doi.org/10.1001/jamadermatol.2013.2766] [PMID: 23553119]

[2]   Keating GM. Ingenol mebutate gel 0.015% and 0.05%: in actinic keratosis. Drugs 2012; 72: 2397-405.
[http://dx.doi.org/10.2165/11470090-000000000-00000] [PMID: 23231025]

[3]   Sligh JE Jr. New therapeutic options for actinic keratosis and basal cell carcinoma. Semin Cutan Med Surg 2014; 33(4)(Suppl 76): S76-80.
[http://dx.doi.org/10.12788/j.sder.0100] [PMID: 25268601]

[4]   Cantisani C, Paolino G, Cantoresi F, Faina V, Richetta AG, Calvieri S. Superficial basal cell carcinoma successfully treated with ingenol mebutate gel 0.05%. Dermatol Ther (Heidelb) 2014; 27: 352-4.
[http://dx.doi.org/10.1111/dth.12148] [PMID: 25052730]

[5]   Siller G, Rosen R, Freeman M, Welburn P, Katsamas J, Ogbourne SM. PEP005 (ingenol mebutate) gel for the topical treatment of superficial basal cell carcinoma: results of a randomized phase IIa trial. Australas J Dermatol 2010; 51: 99-105.
[http://dx.doi.org/10.1111/j.1440-0960.2010.00626.x] [PMID: 20546215]

[6]   Micali G, Lacarrubba F, Nasca MR, Ferraro S, Schwartz RA. Topical pharmacotherapy for skin cancer: part II. Clinical applications. J Am Acad Dermatol 2014; 70: e1-e12.
[http://dx.doi.org/10.1016/j.jaad.2013.12.037] [PMID: 24831325]

[7]   Braun SA, Homey B, Gerber PA. Successful treatment of Bowen disease with ingenol mebutate. Hautarzt 2014; 65(10): 848-50.
[http://dx.doi.org/10.1007/s00105-014-3509-5] [PMID: 25217087]

[8]   Cozzi SJ, Le TT, Ogbourne SM, James C, Suhrbier A. Effective treatment of squamous cell carcinomas with ingenol mebutate gel in immunologically intact SKH1 mice. Arch Dermatol Res 2013; 305: 79-83.
[http://dx.doi.org/10.1007/s00403-012-1270-0] [PMID: 22871992]

[9]   Ogbourne SM, Suhrbier A, Jones B, et al. Antitumor activity of 3-ingenyl angelate: Plasma membrane and mitochondrial disruption and necrotic cell death. Cancer Res 2004; 64: 2833-9.
[http://dx.doi.org/10.1158/0008-5472.CAN-03-2837] [PMID: 15087400]

[10] Ersvaer E, Kittang AO, Hampson P, *et al.* The protein kinase C agonist PEP005 (ingenol 3-angelate) in the treatment of human cancer: A balance between efficacy and toxicity. Toxins (Basel) 2010; 2: 174-94.
[http://dx.doi.org/10.3390/toxins2010174] [PMID: 22069553]

[11] Mansuy M, Nikkels-Tassoudji N, Arrese JE, Rorive A, Nikkels AF. Recurrent in situ melanoma successfully treated with ingenol mebutate. Dermatol Ther (Heidelb) 2014; 4: 131-5.
[http://dx.doi.org/10.1007/s13555-014-0051-4] [PMID: 24691652]

[12] Edwards SK, Moore CR, Liu Y, Grewal S, Covey LR, Xie P. N-benzyladriamycin-14-valerate (AD 198) exhibits potent anti-tumor activity on TRAF3-deficient mouse B lymphoma and human multiple myeloma. BMC Cancer 2013; 13: 481.
[http://dx.doi.org/10.1186/1471-2407-13-481] [PMID: 24131623]

[13] Alchin DR. Ingenol mebutate: A succinct review of a succinct therapy. Dermatol Ther (Heidelb) 2014; 4: 157-64.
[http://dx.doi.org/10.1007/s13555-014-0061-2] [PMID: 25159813]

[14] Lee WY, Hampson P, Coulthard L, *et al.* Novel antileukemic compound ingenol 3-angelate inhibits T cell apoptosis by activating protein kinase Ctheta. J Biol Chem 2010; 285: 23889-98.
[http://dx.doi.org/10.1074/jbc.M109.041962] [PMID: 20472553]

[15] Jawed SI, Myskowski PL, Horwitz S, Moskowitz A, Querfeld C. Primary cutaneous T-cell lymphoma (mycosis fungoides and Sézary syndrome): Part I. Diagnosis: clinical and histopathologic features and new molecular and biologic markers. J Am Acad Dermatol 2014; 70(205): e1-e16.
[http://dx.doi.org/10.1016/j.jaad.2013.07.049] [PMID: 24438969]

[16] Jawed SI, Myskowski PL, Horwitz S, Moskowitz A, Querfeld C. Primary cutaneous T-cell lymphoma (mycosis fungoides and Sézary syndrome): Part II. Prognosis, management, and future directions. J Am Acad Dermatol 2014; 70(223): e1-e17.
[http://dx.doi.org/10.1016/j.jaad.2013.08.033] [PMID: 24438970]

[17] Demirkesen C, Esirgen G, Engin B, Songur A, Oğuz O. The clinical features and histopathologic patterns of folliculotropic mycosis fungoides in a series of 38 cases. J Cutan Pathol 2015; 42: 22-31.
[http://dx.doi.org/10.1111/cup.12423] [PMID: 25376535]

[18] Marschalkó M, Erős N, Kontár O, *et al.* Folliculotropic mycosis fungoides: clinicopathological analysis of 17 patients. J Eur Acad Dermatol Venereol 2015; 29: 964-72.
[http://dx.doi.org/10.1111/jdv.12743] [PMID: 25406034]

[19] Olsen EA, Whittaker S, Kim YH, *et al.* Clinical end points and response criteria in mycosis fungoides and Sézary syndrome: A consensus statement of the International Society for Cutaneous Lymphomas, the United States Cutaneous Lymphoma Consortium, and the Cutaneous Lymphoma Task Force of the European Organisation for Research and Treatment of Cancer. J Clin Oncol 2011; 29: 2598-607.
[http://dx.doi.org/10.1200/JCO.2010.32.0630] [PMID: 21576639]

[20] Rook AH, Gelfand JC, Wysocka M, *et al.* Topical resiquimod can induce disease regression, eradicate malignant T cells and enhance T cell effector functions in cutaneous T cell lymphoma 2015. blood-2015-02-630335.

[21] Le TT, Gardner J, Hoang-Le D, *et al.* Immunostimulatory cancer chemotherapy using local ingenol-3-angelate and synergy with immunotherapies. Vaccine 2009; 27: 3053-62.
[http://dx.doi.org/10.1016/j.vaccine.2009.03.025] [PMID: 19428919]

[22] Breneman D, Duvic M, Kuzel T, Yocum R, Truglia J, Stevens VJ. Phase 1 and 2 trial of bexarotene gel for skin-directed treatment of patients with cutaneous T-cell lymphoma. Arch Dermatol 2002; 138: 325-32.
[http://dx.doi.org/10.1001/archderm.138.3.325] [PMID: 11902983]

[23] Apisarnthanarax N, Talpur R, Ward S, Ni X, Kim HW, Duvic M. Tazarotene 0.1% gel for refractory mycosis fungoides lesions: An open-label pilot study. J Am Acad Dermatol 2004; 50: 600-7.
[http://dx.doi.org/10.1016/j.jaad.2003.09.005] [PMID: 15034511]

[24] Bassiri-Tehrani S, Ba BA, Cohen DE. Treatment of cutaneous T-cell lymphoma with alitretinoin gel. Int J Dermatol 2002; 41: 104-6.
[http://dx.doi.org/10.1046/j.1365-4362.2002.01363.x] [PMID: 11982647]

[25] Zackheim HS, Kashani-Sabet M, Amin S. Topical corticosteroids for mycosis fungoides. Experience in 79 patients. Arch Dermatol 1998; 134: 949-54.
[http://dx.doi.org/10.1001/archderm.134.8.949] [PMID: 9722724]

[26] Zackheim HS. Treatment of patch-stage mycosis fungoides with topical corticosteroids. Dermatol Ther (Heidelb) 2003; 16: 283-7.
[http://dx.doi.org/10.1111/j.1396-0296.2003.01639.x] [PMID: 14686970]

[27] Deeths MJ, Chapman JT, Dellavalle RP, Zeng C, Aeling JL. Treatment of patch and plaque stage mycosis fungoides with imiquimod 5% cream. J Am Acad Dermatol 2005; 52: 275-80.
[http://dx.doi.org/10.1016/j.jaad.2004.04.049] [PMID: 15692473]

[28] Kim YH. Management with topical nitrogen mustard in mycosis fungoides. Dermatol Ther (Heidelb) 2003; 16: 288-98.
[http://dx.doi.org/10.1111/j.1396-0296.2003.01640.x] [PMID: 14686971]

[29] Kim YH, Martinez G, Varghese A, Hoppe RT. Topical nitrogen mustard in the management of mycosis fungoides: Update of the Stanford experience. Arch Dermatol 2003; 139: 165-73.
[http://dx.doi.org/10.1001/archderm.139.2.165] [PMID: 12588222]

[30]   Talpur R, Venkatarajan S, Duvic M. Mechlorethamine gel for the topical treatment of stage IA and IB mycosis fungoides-type cutaneous T-cell lymphoma. Expert Rev Clin Pharmacol 2014; 7: 591-7.
        [http://dx.doi.org/10.1586/17512433.2014.944500] [PMID: 25068889]

[31]   Apisarnthanarax N, Wood GS, Stevens SR, *et al.* Phase I clinical trial of O6-benzylguanine and topical carmustine in the treatment of cutaneous T-cell lymphoma, mycosis fungoides type. Arch Dermatol 2012; 148: 613-20.
        [http://dx.doi.org/10.1001/archdermatol.2011.2797] [PMID: 22250189]

[32]   Zackheim HS, Epstein EH Jr, Crain WR. Topical carmustine (BCNU) for cutaneous T cell lymphoma: A 15-year experience in 143 patients. J Am Acad Dermatol 1990; 22: 802-10.
        [http://dx.doi.org/10.1016/0190-9622(90)70112-U] [PMID: 2347966]

[33]   Liang X, Grue-Sørensen G, Månsson K, *et al.* Syntheses, biological evaluation and SAR of ingenol mebutate analogues for treatment of actinic keratosis and non-melanoma skin cancer. Bioorg Med Chem Lett 2013; 23: 5624-9.
        [http://dx.doi.org/10.1016/j.bmcl.2013.08.038] [PMID: 23993332]

[34]   Bourcier M, Stein Gold L, Guenther L, Andreassen CM, Selmer J, Goldenberg G. A dose-finding trial with a novel ingenol derivative (ingenol disoxate: LEO 43204) for field treatment of actinic keratosis on full face or 250 cm2 on the chest. J Dermatolog Treat 2017; 28: 652-8.
        [http://dx.doi.org/10.1080/09546634.2017.1303568] [PMID: 28264612]

12

Wart Immunotherapies: A Short Review

Ryan S. Sefcik[1] and Craig G. Burkhart[2]

[1]*University of Toledo, College of Medicine, Toledo, Ohio, OH, USA*
[2]*Department of Medicine, University of Toledo College of Medicine, Toledo; Department of Medicine, Ohio University of Osteopathic Medicine, Athens, Ohio, OH, USA*

Abstract:

Objective:

To review the efficacy and costs of various contact immunotherapies, contact allergens, intralesional immunotherapies, and intralesional cytotoxic agents for the treatment of recalcitrant warts.

Background:

Cutaneous warts are common viral skin lesions caused by human papillomavirus that can be challenging to treat and frustrating for physicians and patients. Although several treatment options exist, there is no single treatment that can ensure a complete response with lack of lesion recurrence. Immunotherapies for recalcitrant warts present as a cost-effective, efficient therapy option for patients. Intralesional approaches have the added benefit of affecting warts at locations distant to the target location by inducing a systemic T-cell mediated response in the body.

Results:

Various contact immunotherapies, contact allergens, intralesional immunotherapies, and intralesional cytotoxic agents have shown to be effective in treating warts. The costs of each treatment varies drastically from around $10 US to over $1000 US to achieve a complete response. Several antigens were found to be both efficacious and cost effective.

Conclusion:

Although efficacy of several antigens has been confirmed by randomized studies, more randomized comparative studies will need to be performed in order to determine the best antigen and correct standardized doses for the treatment of warts in individual patients. It is important to note that individual response to antigen type and dose may vary among patients. Therefore, further studies may play an important role in the use of immunotherapies in a clinical setting.

Keywords: Warts, Immunotherapy, Immunodermatology, Cutaneous lesions, Intralesional, HPV.

1. INTRODUCTION

Cutaneous warts are common viral skin lesions caused by the infection of the human papillomavirus (HPV). Recalcitrant or recurrent warts may be disfiguring and a source of embarrassment and frustration for patients [1]. Children and immunocompromised persons tend to be most commonly affected by difficult to treat recalcitrant warts [2 - 4] Some lesions may spontaneously disappear but others may persist or even increase in number and size [2, 4, 5]. Although several potential treatment options exist for warts, there is no single treatment that ensures a complete response and lack of recurrence. Treatments may initially be effective but recurrences after treatments are common [4, 5]. Current treatment options include: topical treatments (commonly salicylic acid), cryotherapy, LASER therapy,

* Address correspondence to this author at the University of Toledo, College of Medicine, 5662 Aspen Dr, Toledo, Ohio, OH, 43615; Tel: (330)760-5154; E-mail: rsefcik16@gmail.com

photodynamic therapy, surgical excision, immunotherapies, and home remedies such as duct tape or tea tree oil [6 - 8]. Many of these options are scarring due to their destructive nature while other less invasive options may result in a lack of complete response or an increased chance of recurrence. Some may be painful or cause discomfort for the patient. Additionally, local treatments may be ineffective at treating patients with large lesions or multiple lesions. Furthermore, many of these options have unknown mechanisms of action and varying results among individuals. For this reason, treatment of warts may be challenging and frustrating for both the physician and patient [1]. Unlike the other various options, immunotherapies target specific lesions and upregulate the immune system to recognize and destroy the lesions at the target site and distant locations. This more systemic approach has shown to be an inexpensive, effective method for treatment of individuals with multiple recalcitrant warts in the literature [9]. Although the mechanism has not been completely understood, immunotherapies are believed to work by inducing a systemic T-cell mediated response at the location of contact or injection. It is also suggested that the injection itself may play a role in inducing the immune response [10]. The immunotherapies, thereby, help the body recognize the lesions and destroy them. Several specific antigens have been used for contact (topical) and intralesional immunotherapy treatments for cutaneous warts. Some contact immunotherapy antigens and contact allergens include: diphenylcyclopropenone (DPCP), Imiquimod 5% Cream, Bacillus Calmette-Guerin (BCG), dinitrochlorobenzene (DNCB), tuberculin jelly, and squaric acid dibutylester (SADBE). The most commonly studied intralesional immunotherapy antigens include: Candida albicans, measles-mumps-rubella (MMR) vaccine, tuberculin PPD, killed Myobacterium w, recombinant alpha-2 interferon, and Trichophyton. Bleomycin, an intralesional cytotoxic agent, is also commonly studied. Both intralesional immunotherapy approaches and contact immunotherapy approaches have been shown to be effective in the treatment of warts.

1.1. Efficacy of Contact Immunotherapies and Contact Allergens

Each contact immunotherapy antigen has shown to have varying, but promising, efficacies in the treatment of recalcitrant warts. Suh et al. performed an uncontrolled, open-label study which showed DPCP to have a clearance rate as high as 82.9% [11]. Imiquimod was shown to have a success rate of 44%, ranging from 27% to 89% in an evidence-based review performed by Ahn and Huang [12]. In a study on children performed by Salem et al., BCG was shown to have a complete response on 65% of children with common warts and 45% of children with plantar warts [13]. One study exploring the efficacy and safety of SADBE for the treatment of recalcitrant warts in children found that 83% of patients experienced complete clearance. However, only 60% reported no adverse side effects [14]. SADBE is limited because it can cause irritation when treating warts in the genital region [15]. There are some reports of contact dermatitis and blistering as well, especially when treated with higher concentrations [15, 16]. DNCB, although shown to be effective in the treatment of warts, is a known mutagenic and relatively expensive in comparison to other antigens. For this reason, DNCB although effective, is not often chosen because of the vast other antigens available for use immunotherapy. It has since been largely replaced by DPCP and SADBE, which are considered much safer options [17]. Tuberculin Jelly, no longer largely studied as a potential wart therapy, had shown variable efficacy in the literature. Tuberculin PPD intralesional immunotherapy appears to have replaced tuberculin jelly because of its shorter treatment response and strength [17, 18]. Contact immunotherapies present as an effective treatment for recalcitrant therapy for the treatment of recalcitrant warts. Of the contact immunotherapies, DPCP and SADBE are two of the most commonly used therapies because of their high success rates in achieving a complete response to treatment.

1.1.1. Efficacy of Intralesional Immunotherapies and Intralesional Cytotoxic Agents

Intralesional immunotherapies have been the focus of several studies found in the literature. The interest in intralesional approaches may be the result of shorter treatment times, strength, and lesser adverse side effects with promising results. Additionally, intralesional immunotherapies elicit a response of warts at locations distant to the injection site. The injection itself may also help to induce an immune response at the target site. Several antigens have presented as effective options for use in intralesional immunotherapy approaches to treat warts. In a two year study at Mayo Clinic, 80% of patients had a response to Candida antigen with 39% having a complete response to treatment. It was also found that 7 of 8 immuno-compromised patients showed a partial or complete response to the antigen [19]. Another study, which used higher doses of Candida antigen, reported complete response rates as high as 82% [20]. MMR vaccine has shown complete response rates as high as 75% in one study and 81% in another study. Both studies showed low recurrence among patients, but some patients (<30%) experienced flu-like symptoms during treatment [21 - 29]. In a study performed by Saoji et al., tuberculin PPD showed a complete response rate of 76% in four treatments with very minimal adverse reactions to the antigen [22]. Myobacterium w vaccine showed complete response rates as high as 89% in a study performed by Gupta *et al.* and 93% in a study performed by Garg and Baveja [23, 30]. Another antigen, Alpha 2- interferon, has shown 50-70% complete response rates in genital warts, specifically. One major downside to interferon is that it has a much higher costs than other potential antigens for intralesional immunotherapies [24]. As a result, other antigens are preferred over interferon. Bleomycin, a relatively costly cytotoxic agent, has shown complete response rates ranging from 14-99% in the literature [25]. Studies using Trichophyton alone were not readily found, but Trichophyton was found to increase response rates when combined with other antigens in several studies. Trichophyton combined with other antigens MMR and Candida showed a complete response rate of 71% in a study performed Johnson and Horn [26]. As shown above, various antigens for intralesional immunotherapies have shown extremely high response rates in the literature and may provide a reliable, effective option for patients in the treatment of difficult warts in the clinical setting.

1.1.2. Comparison of Costs of Immunotherapy and Other Therapies

The low costs of many of the antigens used for contact and intralesional immunotherapies present another benefit to their use. Clemens *et al.* performed a comparative study looking at the various costs of treatment options for warts. In the study, cryotherapy, a very commonly used treatment method, costs $562, while Candida antigen only costs $190. Other treatments, such as home remedies and CO_2 laser therapy, also had very low costs at $10-30 and $157, respectively. Pulse-dyed laser therapy was found to costs $360 for complete resolution in a recent study. Bleomycin and Squaric acid costs $495 and $706, respectively. In contrast, alpha-2 interferon is very expensive and typically requires several treatments resulting in an average cost of $1227. These prices represent total costs charged to patient with physician fees included.[27] DPCP costs approximately $30/session and Imiquimod costs as much as $100/session. SADBE has varying costs but is more unstable and costly than DPCP [28]. DPCP, Imiquimod, and SADBE all may require multiple sessions for a complete response. Much like candida, the MMR antigen is also relatively inexpensive at about $26 [29]. Tuberculin agents, such as PPD and BCG, are found for less than $10 [30, 31]. Killed Myobacterium w was found to be another cost-effective option at 450 rupees or approximately $7 in a study performed in India by Garg and Baveja [31]. As seen above, several of the intralesional immunotherapy antigens present as very cost-effective options in comparison to other options the patient may have for treatments. Along with being inexpensive, these immunotherapies are more beneficial because of their potential to treat warts distant to the treatment site. This phenomenon furthers the potential cost-effectiveness of the more affordable intralesional immunotherapy treatment options.

DISCUSSION

Although the mechanism of action of many of the antigens is unknown, immunotherapies provide a safe and cost-effective approach for the treatment of warts. Other more traditionally used therapies such as cryotherapy and salicylic acid, although usually effective in the treatment of warts at the target location, have a tendency to cause irritation of the skin and are not effective in treating patients with multiple warts or those with warts in several locations. Additionally, immunotherapies may even serve as a cheaper option for patients than more traditionally used options depending on the antigen. Intralesional immunotherapy is preferable because of its capability to induce a systemic response in the patient and affect warts at locations distant to the injection site. If proved effective and adopted in clinical setting, intralesional immunotherapy may lessen the frustration experienced by patients and physicians when dealing with recalcitrant warts. The appropriate dosing and location based response rates will need to be explored in future studies to determine the best practices for using intralesional approaches. Presensitization to specific antigens may serve as a means of determining the best antigen for the individual patient as well as inoculating the patient with the antigen. Initial inoculation is beneficial because it can cause the host to elicit a stronger response upon presentation of the antigen through intralesional immunotherapy injection. In addition, intralesional immunotherapies can be combined with other treatment options such as cryotherapy, laser therapy, or salicylic acid to increase the chance of a complete response. Multiple antigens can also be combined to elicit a stronger response to treatment. Finding the correct doses and combinations may be difficult to determine because responses may be different among individual patients. Therefore, future randomized studies will be important for developing a standardized protocol for treating difficult to treat warts in the clinical setting.

CONCLUSION

Immunotherapies for recalcitrant, difficult to treat cutaneous warts present as a cost-effective, efficient therapy option for patients. Intralesional approaches have the added benefit of affecting warts at locations distant to the target location by inducing a systemic T-cell mediated response in the body. Although efficacy has been confirmed by randomized studies, more randomized comparative studies will need to be performed in order to determine the best antigen and correct standardized doses for the treatment of warts in individual patients. It is important to note that individual response to antigens may vary among patients and this may further complicate the development of standardized doses. Given that patient wishes may vary and no treatment is totally curable nor painless, one should discuss the various options and choose the best option for each patient on an individual basis. Likewise, there are currently too many variables at this point to have definitive treatment plan outlined. Therefore, further studies may play an important role in the use of immunotherapies in a clinical setting.

CONFLICT OF INTEREST

The authors declare no conflict of interest, financial or otherwise.

ACKNOWLEDGEMENTS

Declared none.

REFERENCES

[1]   Lipke MM. An armamentarium of wart treatments. Clin Med Res 2006; 4(4): 273-93.
        [http://dx.doi.org/10.3121/cmr.4.4.273] [PMID: 17210977]

[2]   Leman JA, Benton EC. Verrucas. Guidelines for management. Am J Clin Dermatol 2000; 1(3): 143-9.
        [http://dx.doi.org/10.2165/00128071-200001030-00001] [PMID: 11702295]

[3]   Smolinski KN, Yan AC. How and when to treat molluscum contagiosum and warts in children. Pediatr Ann 2005; 34(3): 211-21.
        [http://dx.doi.org/10.3928/0090-4481-20050301-10] [PMID: 15792113]

[4]   Sterling JC, Handfield-Jones S, Hudson PM. Guidelines for the management of cutaneous warts. Br J Dermatol 2001; 144(1): 4-11.
        [http://dx.doi.org/10.1046/j.1365-2133.2001.04066.x] [PMID: 11167676]

[5]   Jenson AB, Kurman RJ, Lancaster WD. Tissue effects of and host response to human papillomavirus infection. Dermatol Clin 1991; 9(2): 203-9.
        [PMID: 1647900]

[6]   Sterling JC, Gibbs S, Haque Hussain SS, Mohd Mustapa MF, Handfield-Jones SE. British Association of Dermatologists' guidelines for the management of cutaneous warts 2014. Br J Dermatol 2014; 171(4): 696-712.
        [http://dx.doi.org/10.1111/bjd.13310] [PMID: 25273231]

[7]   Wenner R, Askari SK, Cham PM, Kedrowski DA, Liu A, Warshaw EM. Duct tape for the treatment of common warts in adults: a double-blind randomized controlled trial. Arch Dermatol 2007; 143(3): 309-13.
        [http://dx.doi.org/10.1001/archderm.143.3.309] [PMID: 17372095]

[8]   Pazyar N, Yaghoobi R, Bagherani N, Kazerouni A. A review of applications of tea tree oil in dermatology. Int J Dermatol 2013; 52(7): 784-90.
        [http://dx.doi.org/10.1111/j.1365-4632.2012.05654.x] [PMID: 22998411]

[9]   Aldahan AS, Mlacker S, Shah VV, et al. Efficacy of intralesional immunotherapy for the treatment of warts: A review of the literature. Dermatol Ther (Heidelb) 2016; 29(3): 197-207.
        [http://dx.doi.org/10.1111/dth.12352] [PMID: 26991521]

[10]   Nofal A, Salah E, Nofal E, Yosef A. Intralesional antigen immunotherapy for the treatment of warts: current concepts and future prospects. Am J Clin Dermatol 2013; 14(4): 253-60.
        [http://dx.doi.org/10.1007/s40257-013-0018-8] [PMID: 23813361]

[11]   Suh DW, Lew BL, Sim WY. Investigations of the efficacy of diphenylcyclopropenone immunotherapy for the treatment of warts. Int J Dermatol 2014; 53(12): e567-71.
        [http://dx.doi.org/10.1111/ijd.12688] [PMID: 25427069]

[12]   Ahn CS, Huang WW. Imiquimod in the treatment of cutaneous warts: an evidence-based review. Am J Clin Dermatol 2014; 15(5): 387-99.
        [http://dx.doi.org/10.1007/s40257-014-0093-5] [PMID: 25186654]

[13]   Salem A, Nofal A, Hosny D. Treatment of common and plane warts in children with topical viable Bacillus Calmette-Guerin. Pediatr Dermatol 2013; 30(1): 60-3.
        [http://dx.doi.org/10.1111/j.1525-1470.2012.01848.x] [PMID: 22958215]

[14]   Pandey S, Wilmer EN, Morrell DS. Examining the efficacy and safety of squaric acid therapy for treatment of recalcitrant warts in children. Pediatr Dermatol 2015; 32(1): 85-90.

[http://dx.doi.org/10.1111/pde.12387] [PMID: 25040421]

[15]   Dall' Oglio F, Nasca MR, D'Agata O, Micali G. Adult and paediatric contact immunotherapy with squaric acid dibutylester (SADBE) for recurrent, multiple, resistant, mucocutaneous anogenital warts. Sex Transm Infect 2002; 78(4): 309-10.
         [http://dx.doi.org/10.1136/sti.78.4.309-a] [PMID: 12181482]

[16]   Lee AN, Mallory SB. Contact immunotherapy with squaric acid dibutylester for the treatment of recalcitrant warts. J Am Acad Dermatol 1999; 41(4): 595-9.
         [PMID: 10495383]

[17]   Singh G, Prakash B. Topical Immunotherapy: Role in Dermatology. Recent Advances in Dermatology 2014; 3: 126.

[18]   Elela IM, Elshahid AR, Mosbeh AS. Intradermal vs intralesional purified protein derivatives in treatment of warts. Golf J Deramatol Venereol 2011; 18: 21-6.

[19]   Alikhan A, Griffin JR, Newman CC. Use of Candida antigen injections for the treatment of verruca vulgaris: A two-year mayo clinic experience. J Dermatolog Treat 2016; 27(4): 355-8.
         [http://dx.doi.org/10.3109/09546634.2015.1106436] [PMID: 26558635]

[20]   Kim KH, Horn TD, Pharis J, et al. Phase 1 clinical trial of intralesional injection of Candida antigen for the treatment of warts. Arch Dermatol 2010; 146(12): 1431-3.
         [http://dx.doi.org/10.1001/archdermatol.2010.350] [PMID: 21173332]

[21]   Zamanian A, Mobasher P, Jazi GA. Efficacy of intralesional injection of mumps-measles-rubella vaccine in patients with wart. Adv Biomed Res 2014; 3: 107.
         [http://dx.doi.org/10.4103/2277-9175.129701] [PMID: 24804181]

[22]   Saoji V, Lade NR, Gadegone R, Bhat A. Immunotherapy using purified protein derivative in the treatment of warts: An open uncontrolled trial. Indian J Dermatol Venereol Leprol 2016; 82(1): 42-6.
         [http://dx.doi.org/10.4103/0378-6323.171650] [PMID: 26728809]

[23]   Gupta S, Malhotra AK, Verma KK, Sharma VK. Intralesional immunotherapy with killed Mycobacterium w vaccine for the treatment of ano-genital warts: an open label pilot study. J Eur Acad Dermatol Venereol 2008; 22(9): 1089-93.
         [http://dx.doi.org/10.1111/j.1468-3083.2008.02719.x] [PMID: 18484970]

[24]   Kirby PK, Kiviat N, Beckman A, Wells D, Sherwin S, Corey L. Tolerance and efficacy of recombinant human interferon gamma in the treatment of refractory genital warts. Am J Med 1988; 85(2): 183-8.
         [http://dx.doi.org/10.1016/S0002-9343(88)80339-5] [PMID: 2840824]

[25]   Lewis TG, Nydorf ED. Intralesional bleomycin for warts: a review. J Drugs Dermatol 2006; 5(6): 499-504.
         [PMID: 16774100]

[26]   Johnson SM, Horn TD. Intralesional immunotherapy for warts using a combination of skin test antigens: a safe and effective therapy. J Drugs Dermatol 2004; 3(3): 263-5.
         [PMID: 15176159]

[27]   Clemons RJ, Clemons-Miller A, Johnson SM, Williamson SK, Horn TD. Comparing therapy costs for physician treatment of warts. J Drugs Dermatol 2003; 2(6): 649-54.
         [PMID: 14711145]

[28]   Sinha S, Relhan V, Garg VK. Immunomodulators in warts: Unexplored or ineffective? Indian J Dermatol 2015; 60(2): 118-29.
         [http://dx.doi.org/10.4103/0019-5154.152502] [PMID: 25814698]

[29]   Nofal A, Nofal E, Yosef A, Nofal H. Treatment of recalcitrant warts with intralesional measles, mumps, and rubella vaccine: a promising approach. Int J Dermatol 2015; 54(6): 667-71.
         [http://dx.doi.org/10.1111/ijd.12480] [PMID: 25070525]

[30]   Amirnia M, Khodaeiani E, Fouladi DF, Masoudnia S. Intralesional immunotherapy with tuberculin purified protein derivative (PPD) in recalcitrant wart: A randomized, placebo-controlled, double-blind clinical trial including an extra group of candidates for cryotherapy. J Dermatolog Treat 2016; 27(2): 173-8.
         [http://dx.doi.org/10.3109/09546634.2015.1078871] [PMID: 26295565]

[31]   Garg S, Baveja S. Intralesional immunotherapy for difficult to treat warts with Mycobacterium w vaccine. J Cutan Aesthet Surg 2014; 7(4): 203-8.
         [http://dx.doi.org/10.4103/0974-2077.150740] [PMID: 25722598]

13

Sexually Transmitted Infections in the PrEP Era. Are Family Doctors Ready to Give Advice?

Carmen Rodríguez Cerdeira[1,2,*], Sánchez Blanco E[2], Sánchez Blanco B[3,4] and Carnero Gregorio M[1,5]

[1]Efficiency, quality and costs in Health Services Research Group (EFISALUD), Galicia Sur Health Research Institute (IIS Galicia Sur). SERGAS-UVIGO
[2]Dermatology Service, Hospital do Meixoeiro and University of Vigo, Vigo, Spain
[3]Postdoctoral Researcher, Conselleria de Educación, Xunta Galicia, Vigo. Spain
[4]Predoctoral Researcher, Family Physician, EOXI, Vigo. Spain
[5]Postdoctoral Researcher, University of Vigo, Vigo, Spain

Abstract:

Background:

Pre-exposure prophylaxis (PrEP) for human immunodeficiency virus (HIV) as a method of HIV prevention is not without controversy, and there has been concern that it may lead its users to think that they no longer need other preventive measures such as condoms. Thus, healthcare providers are convinced that PrEP decreases condom use and increases sexually transmitted infections (STIs). This treatment has been studied in men who have sex with men, men and women in heterosexual HIV-discordant couples, and heterosexual men and women.

Objective:

The objective of this study was to review the current state of evidence on the association of PrEP with condom use, the incidence of STIs, and the change in sexual behaviours in populations with risky practices.

Materials and Methods:

PubMed (National Center for Biotechnology Information, Bethesda, MD, USA), Science Direct (Elsevier Ltd., Oxford, UK), and Google Scholar (Google Inc., Mountain View, CA, USA) search engines were used during the study. We used the terms HIV, PrEP, sexually transmitted infections (STIs), MSM, condom, heterosexual men / women to search the databases.

Results:

Here, we present evidence that daily oral treatment is safe and effective in these populations studied, especially when medication adherence is high. STI testing should include extra-genital testing regardless of PrEP use to prevent health deficits and onward transmission.

Conclusion:

Despite this safety and efficacy, we strongly advise that patients continue to use condoms as a prophylactic measure against other sexually transmitted diseases. This update addresses the benefits and precautions that must be taken when establishing PrEP treatment, focusing mainly on family doctorswho are best positioned to provide follow-up and advice to patients and their relatives.

Keywords: VIH, Pre-exposure prophylaxis (PrEP), Sexually transmitted infections, Syphilis, Gonorrhea, Chlamydia, Vulvovaginitis, Family Doctors.

* Address correspondence to this author at the Dermatology Service Meixoeiro hospital CHUVI, Vigo, C/Meixoeiro S/N 36200, Vigo, Spain; E-mail: carmencerdeira33@gmail.com

1. INTRODUCTION

Infection with the human immunodeficiency virus (HIV) continues to be a major sanitary, social, economic, and human health problem in the world. Recently, the so-called "pre-exposure prophylaxis" (PrEP) has been developed as a preventative strategy in which uninfected individuals with a high exposure or vulnerability to HIVare administered pharmaceutical therapy intended to prevent infection [1].

The use of antiretroviral drugs to prevent HIV infection in at-risk, uninfected individuals was initially based on efficacy demonstrated in animal models. The implementation of this strategy must be based on the scientific evidence provided by controlled clinical trials. In these trials, it is essential to pay attention to both the efficacy and the safety of a preventive intervention directed at a healthy population [2].The FDA recently approved the HIV antiretroviral drug emtricitabine/tenofovirdisoproxilfumarate as PrEP therapy for adults at high risk for sexually-acquired HIV infection [2].

The use of HIV PrEP, where seronegative individuals with high-risk sexual practices are administered with anti-retroviral drugs, could also be a contributing factor to the transmission of other STIs. We believe that such practices may lead to a significant increase in the manifestation of STIs as ulcers, such as in syphilis. Thus, a STI poses a significant public health risk in all demographic groups; all physicians should maintain a high level of awareness and should avoid stereotyping patients [3].

2. MATERIAL AND METHODS

We carried out a comprehensive search of the Cochrane Central Register of Controlled Trials, MEDLINE (PubMed), and Embase databases for articles published from March 2010 to March 2016, using the following search terms: VIH, pre-exposure prophylaxis (PrEP), sexually transmitted infections, syphilis, gonorrhea, chlamydia, and vulvovaginitis. We performed an exhaustive review of the published articles and the bibliographies of the selected manuscripts.

3. RESULTS AND DISCUSSION

The PrEP dosage is a single, once-dailytablet (emtricitabine 200 mg and tenofovir- disoproxilfumarate 300 mg). The drug is taken orally, with or without food. In addition to the medication, which should not be prescribed in more than a 90-day supply, the patient should be educated about risk reduction strategies, particularly consistent use of condoms during every sexual encounter [4].

The efficacy and safety of PrEP have been demonstrated in clinical trials and confirmed in observational studies, following the implementation of specific programs in different countries. The data are obtained from studies conducted in men who have sex with men (MSM) [5], heterosexual serodiscordant couples(regardless of the infected limb), and in users of parenteral drugs. Studies have been conducted almost exclusively with the combination of emtricitabine (FTC) and tenofovirdisoproxilfumarate (TDF), administered continuously or in intermittent patterns related to contact risk. Clinical trials and observational studies have shown that PrEP with FTC/TDF has great benefitin preventing HIV transmission, though the efficacy is highly dependent on adherence to the prescribed regimen. All studies have also analyzed the following potential drawbacks of this strategy: 1) Toxicity, whereby patients receiving FTC/TDF experience more digestive intolerance than those taking the placebo. Additionally, in those receiving FTC/TDF there is significant loss of bone mineral density and decreased clearance of creatinine, although these effects are not clinically relevant during the observed period, and are reversible after the suspension of the drugs. 2) Development of resistance; has occurred at exceptionally high rates of prophylaxis who subsequently acquire HIV infection. 3) Increase in the development of STIs whose number and type are not higher than those presented before PrEP. As reflected in the manuscript published by Lal *et al.* [6] where the authors conclude that the decrease of condom use brings with it an increase in STIs, the prevention, early detection, and treatment of STIs should be a priority in the current era of HIV PrEP.

In another study published by Hoornenborg *et al.* [7], the authors assessed 375 HIV-negative MSM enrolled in Amsterdam PrEP and detected high levels of hepatitis C virus RNA from three different genotypes (1a [73%], 4d [20%], and 2b [7%]). Therefore, the authors warn of the importance of detection and prevention of hepatitis C owing to the high rate of promiscuity in these patients.

Therefore, the benefits and risks evidenced in the PrEP studies support their administration to individuals at high risk of acquiring HIV [8].

In this study from Calabrese et al., 20 healthcare providers were interviewed.The interviews were conducted by the PI in person or by telephone between September 2014 and February 2015, and the duration of each interview was between 60 and 90 minutes. The interviews were semi-structured, following an organized thematic guide that included questions about leadership and follow-up suggestions [9].

Primary topics included PrEP experience, PrEP attitudes and prescribing intentions, patient / provider communication about sex, fair PrEP provision, and training experiences and recommendations.

In this manuscript from Krakower et al. [10],during January and February 2015, all primary care clinicians at a community health center in Boston that specializes in the care of sexual and gender minorities were invited to complete surveys regarding 35 anonymous items evaluating their experiences with the provision of PrEP. The surveys evaluated provider demographics, practice characteristics, experiences and practices with PrEP provision, perceptions about feasibility, and future prescribing intentions. Half of the respondents indicated that financial barriers had prevented patients from using PrEP [10].

In this meta-analysis Fonner et al. [11] encompassed eighteen studies, which included data from 39 papers and six conference abstracts. The results show that PrEP is attractive for people in heterosexual relationships because of their lower cost, greater availability, and lower risk of drug resistance. Regarding safety, PrEP showed no evidence of an increase in the proportion of adverse events. However, two studies reported small decreases in kidney function among those taking PrEP.

As Sheth et al. [12] reported, women are very vulnerable to HIV infections, whether due to sexual, social, or biological factors. Strategies are needed to prevent the emergence of new cases, which in the United States account for 20% of HIV cases. The World Health Organisation and Centers for Disease Control and Prevention recommend PrEP with Truvada antiviral (tenofovir/emtricitabine) in combination with protective measures to prevent infection in people at high risk of infection.

Several studies have found a 70-90% reduction in the risk of acquiring HIV in women administered oral PrEP. The adhesion is between 30% and 50% (determined by tenofovir levels in plasma). The use of gels with 1% tenofovir or vaginal rings with dapivirine has not been as effective as the use of oral PrEP. In the case of gels (application before and after having sex), the risk of acquiring HIV was reduced by up to 76% in one of the studies. In the case of vaginal rings, protection was low, but increased in women over 21 years of age.

Several factors should be considered with regard to PrEP. One is that tenofovir concentrations are higher in the rectal than in the vaginal tissue, so women should take higher doses to prevent infections. Other factors are age, presence of other sexually transmitted diseases, or viral load of sexual partners. It is also important to consider kidney and bone toxicity in long-term treatments. There appears to be no interaction between contraceptive use and prophylactic treatment with tenofovir.

One of the goals of PrEP according to Haberl [13] is to increase the perception of risk among women, since in some studies, more than 50% of women perceived being at low risk or of not being at risk of contracting HIV. A communication campaign is needed as several studies have shown that a high percentage of women had not heard of PrEP or did not know what it was.

Factors such as effectiveness, cost, side effects, and whether the doctor is guiding therapy are determinants of good adherence to this type of prophylactic treatment.

Regarding pregnancy, PrEP does not appear to affect the effectiveness of hormonal contraception. As Davey et al. [14] reported, in countries where HIV acquisition during pregnancy and postpartum periods remains high despite increased access to and initiation of antiretroviral therapy in sub-Saharan Africa, a strict follow-up of adherence by these patients is required to make PrEP a success.

Bazzi et al. [15] discussed the need to extrapolate the connotations acquired in African countries to serodiscordant couples in the United States.

Nevertheless, as Callagan et al., it appears to interfere with oral contraceptives, and unwanted pregnancies were found among users of oral contraceptives who had received PrEP [16].

Outstanding studies from Silawaspan *et al.* [17], exist in the scientific literature about attitudes, intentions, and behaviors related to PrEP, as well as concerns and obstacles by primary care physicians to prescribe PrEP. In addition, one study used a clinical case to illustratethe use of PrEP. Another study by Di Biagio *et al.* [18] was conducted in Italy, a European country in which the use of PrEP based on tenofovir and emtricitabine has not yet been approved, although in Europe, it already has the approval of the European Medicine Agency. In this study, the responses to a 21-item survey conducted among physicians at Italian centres that treat HIV patients, was analysed. The survey was conducted between 1 April and 30 May 2015.

After analysing the answers, it was found that despite the majority being familiar with PrEP, almost 47% were not clear that there was sufficient evidence supporting its use. Most believed that its use could be dangerous if it was not done properly and safely. There were also limitations in terms of its use for a specific group of people. Half of the respondents asked for more research on PrEP that could better define its role.

To date in our country, we have not found any publications concerning PrEP.

As Avuvika *et al.* [19], sexually transmitted infections (STIs) represent a public health concern due to their wide distribution and potential to lead to serious health conditions. STIs are preventable, diagnosable, and treatable. STIs most commonly occur in adolescents and young adults, and are associated with various health problems and complications in this population [20]. Elderly patients [21], particularly those who do not have a partner, have been found to be a novel group of patients. Other patient groups with high-risk practices include MSM and female sex workers. Furthermore, couples that appear to be monogamous, but in fact one individual practices sex with other partners, can also acquire an STI.

Patients seeking treatment for an STI account for a large number of Family Physician (FP) visits per year. Moreover, FP patients are reported to have a high rate of asymptomatic STIs [22].Hence, most of these patients remain undiagnosed until admission by family health services to STI units at advanced stages, by which time the infection has been disseminated and contributes to the epidemiological chain. Hence, patients with suspected STIs during an FP visit should be asked if they have a new partner, multiple partners, recent contacts, or if they are involved in high-risk sexual practices. Moreover as Rajalakshmi *et al.* [23], physicians should assess the symptomatology, including that in the genital area, and check for the presence of ulcers, vesicles,and pustules, in addition to genital, rectal, or eye discharge. Furthermore, the skin should be examined for the presence of rash or scaling, and the physical exam should include assessment for lymphadenopathy, hepatosplenomegaly, and joint pain. All patients should also undergo the required tests to exclude STIs, including HIV,hepatitis B, and possible co-infections [23].Women should undergo a pelvic examination and a pregnancy test. Also, reinforcement of human papilloma virus and hepatitis B vaccination where appropriate should be performed. Thus, a trial conducted in Spain by Hidalgo-Tenorio *et al.* [24] showed significantly higher anti-high-risk human papillomavirus antibody titres in vaccinated individuals than in unvaccinated controls.

Of more than 30 viruses, bacteria, and parasites that are reportedly transmitted through sexual contact, Rahimzadeh *et al.* [25] identified 8 species linked to the highest incidence of sexually transmitted diseases (Table 1). We begin with the STIs presenting with urethritis or cervicitis. For this, it is helpful to divide patients into two groups: those presenting with complaints consistent with urethritis or cervicitis, and those with genital ulcers. The primary pathogens responsible for urethritis and cervicitis are *Chlamydia trachomatis* and *Neisseria gonorrhoeae*, though *Trichomonasvaginalis*, *Mycoplasma*, and *Ureaplamsa* havebeen implicated as well. Urethritis is more visible in male patients, and the mucus-purulent exudate is characteristically accompanied by dysuria and pollakiuria. Cervicitis presents with redness of the cervix and mucopurulent leucorrhoea [26].

Table 1. Common STI syndromes, their pathologies, and their etiological agents.

Clinical syndromes	Associated pathologies	Etiological agents
Urethral discharge	Urethritis	*Neisseria gonorrhoeae* *Chlamydia trachomatis* *Mycoplasma genitalium* *Ureaplasma urealyticum*
	Epididymitis	
Vaginal discharge	Cervicitis	*Neisseria gonorrhoeae* *Chlamydia trachomatis* *Candida albicans* *Trichomonas vaginalis*
	Vulvovaginitis	
	Bacterial vaginosis	*Gardnerella vaginalis*

(Table 1) contd.....

Clinical syndromes	Associated pathologies	Etiological agents
Low abdominal pain	Acute pelvic inflammatory disease	*Neisseria gonorrhoeae* *Chlamydia trachomatis*
Genital ulcers	Herpes	*Herpes simplex virus* type 2 (HSV-2) and herpes simplex virus type 1 (HSV-1)
	Syphilis	*Treponema pallidum*
	Chancroid	*Haemophilus ducreyi*
	Lymphogranuloma venereum	*Chlamydia L1, L2 (serovariant L2b) y L3*
Genital Warts	Condylomata acuminata	Human papillomavirus (HPV)
	Condyloma syphilitic plane	*Treponema pallidum*
STIs that do not manifest initially at the genitals	HIV/AIDS	*VIH*
	Hepatitis B	*VHB*
	Acute cytomegalovirus infection	*CMV*
	Disseminated gonorrhoeae:	*Neisseria gonorrhoeae*
	Secondary syphilis	*Treponema pallidum*
	Lymphogranuloma venereum, Extragenital	*Chlamydia L1, L2 y L3*
	Proctoenterocolitis	*Neisseria gonorrhoeae* *Chlamydia trachomatis serotypes D-L* *Treponema pallidum* *Herpes virus* HPV
	Arthritis	*Chlamydia trachomatis* *Neisseria gonorrhoeae*

The diagnosis of non-specific urethritis is established by the presence of >5 leukocytes per gram on Gram staining (×1000) and ruling out both *N. gonorrhoeae* and *C. trachomatis*as the causative agents. Although the clinical significance is unclear, culture formycoplasma detection or nucleic acid detection by polymerase chain reaction (PCR) of *M. genitalium*, *M. hominis*, and *U. urealyticum* is recommended (Tables **2** and **3**) [27].

The diagnosis of non-specific cervicitis is established by the presence of >20-30 leukoctyes per gram on Gram staining (x1000). In this scenario, in addition to the tests already mentioned in the Table **3**,it is advisable to performculturing for Mycoplasma detection or nucleic acid detection by PCR for *M. genitalium*, *M. hominis*, and *U. urealyticum*, particularly when the investigation of *N. gonorrhoeae* and *C. trachomatis* yields a negative result [26].

It is impossible to clinically distinguish infections caused by chlamydia from those caused by gonorrhea, and they often exist as coinfections. Hence, the Centers for Disease Control and Prevention recommend the use of presumptive treatment for both chlamydia and gonorrhea in men with urethritis. In women aged <25 years with cervicitis, and women with new or multiple sexual partners, the Centers for Disease Control and Prevention also recommend presumptive treatment for chlamydia and gonorrhea. This guideline should be particularly adhered to when patient follow-up cannot be ensured [27].

Organisms that can cause genital ulcers include chancroid, herpesgenitalis, syphilis, and the lymphogranulomavenereum (LGV) serotype of *C. trachomatis*.In genital herpes, the ulcer is painful and often presents with painful, bilateral inguinal adenopathies [27]. The ulcer associated with chancroid ulcer is also painful, but painful adenopathy is unilateral. Differently, the ulcer associated with primary syphilis is painless, and though the adenopathies are bilateral,they too are painless. Finally, the ulcer associated with lymphogranuloma venereum is painless, though the associated adenopathy is painful and unilateral [28]. Syphilis can be diagnosed by darkfieldmicroscopy, PCR, or direct immunofluorescence [29]. Girometti *et al.* [30] showed the importance of the diagnosis of early syphilis as it entails a high HIV seroconversion rate and its detection should be prioritised before PrEP is prescribed.

For genital herpes, chancroid, and LGV, diagnosis is by culture, or direct immunofluorescence or PCR, if available [31].

Lymphogranuloma Venereum (LGV) is caused by specific serotypes of *C. trachomatis* and occurs sporadically in the United States. A recent increase in cases was noted in Europe, with the majority of cases affecting MSMs who were also co-infected with HIV. These patients were frequently presented with severe proctitis [32].

Genital warts should be considered, as they are common and have a strong relationship with intraepithelial squamous lesions. If a lesion is suspected (possibility of dysplasia), a biopsy should be performed under local anesthesia. This biopsy can be used either for histological analysis or for the detection of human papillomavirus via nucleic acid identification,with subsequent typing [33]. In high-income countries, accurate STI diagnostic tests are widely used, and such tests are particularly useful for diagnosing asymptomatic infections [27].

Table 2. Request for tests on men.

Location of the sample	Gonorrhea	Chlamydia	Non-specific urethritis [1]	Trichomonas	Candida	Observations
Urethral [2,3]	Gram staining + Culture	Detection of nucleic acids	Gram staining + cultivation and/or detection of nucleic acids for *M. genitalium*, *M. hominis*, and *U. urealyticum*	Culture	Not recommended	If the sample is not directly seeded, the Stuart-Amies transport medium should be used, which is the universal medium for the transport of chlamydia and viruses. The processing of the samples should be conducted within 4–6 hours at room temperature, and if this is not possible, the samples should be stored in a refrigerator at 2–8°C, following which the sample will be valid for up to 24 hours after being obtained.
Rectal [4]	Culture	Culture and/or detection of nucleic acids	Not recommended	Not recommended	Not recommended	The sample should be assessed according to the patient's sexual practices, similar to the indication used for the urethral sample. This sample is not recommended for heterosexual men
Pharyngeal [5]	Culture	Culture/PCR	Not recommended	Not recommended	Not recommended	The sample should be obtained according to the patient's sexual practices. The same indications should be followed, as for the urethral sample.

[1] As a general rule, the patient should remain without urinating for 2–4 hours prior to the urethral dose. The following materials are required for the sample protocol indicated: 3 Dacron urethral swabs, including 1 with Stuart-Amies transport medium or a similar medium (for cultivation of gonococcus and other general pathogens);another for *C. trachomatis*, which is convenient to use as a swab with the UTM (Universal Transport Medium, Copan, Italy) or a similar medium (although the technique of each manufacturer in each laboratory should be followed); and another that will serve as an extension of the Gram stain, with subsequent inoculation with Roiron or Diamond medium for the culture of trichomonas. If possible, direct seeding of the shoot should be performed on a selective agar for gonococcal isolation (GC-LECT agar or similar medium). The culture plates should be maintained at 37°C in an atmosphere with 5% CO2.

[2] It is preferable to obtain a urethral sample with a swab than a urine sample due to the greater sensitivity. Instead, Its use is relegated to: 1) population screening studies; 2) locations without laboratories that can care for the samples with minimum guarantees of quality for proper processing; and 3) cases where the patient cannot tolerate the sample study due to its invasive nature. However, it should be noted that in urine samples, only the indication of infection by *N. gonorrhoeae* and *C. trachomatis* is supported by a nucleic acid detection test.

[3] The following materials are required for the sample protocol indicated: 2 Dacron swabs, slightly moistened with physiological saline, including 1with Stuart-Amies or similar medium and another with the UTM medium. If possible, direct seeding of the shoot should be performed on a selective agar for gonococcal isolation (GC-LECT agar or similar medium). The culture plates should be maintained at 37°C in an atmosphere with 5% CO2.

[4] The following materials are required for the indicated sample protocol: 2 dry Dacron swabs, including 1 with Stuart-Amies or similar medium and another with the UTM medium. In case of direct seeding of the shoot, blood agar, Saboraud-Chloramphenicol agar, and selective agar should be used for gonococcal isolation (GC-LECT agar or similar medium). The culture plates should be maintained at 37°C, and the chocolate agar and GC-LECT agar should also be maintained at 37°C in an atmosphere with 5% CO2.

Table 3. Request for tests on women.

Location of the sample	Gonorrhea	Chlamydia	Vaginosis	Trichomonas	Candida	HPV	Observations
Urethral [1]	Not recommended	Not recommended	Not recommended	Not recommended	Not recommended	Not recommended	Only recommended in women who report symptomatology compatible with urethral syndrome
Vaginal [2,3]	Not recommended	Not recommended	Gram +/- fresh	Gram +/- fresh	Gram staining+ Gram staining +/- fresh	Not recommended	Use of Stuart-Amies medium + Roiron or Diamond medium for the cultivation of *T. vaginalis*
Endocervical [4,5,6]	Gram staining + culture	Detection of nucleic acids	Not recommended	Not recommended	Not recommended	HPV cytology and detection	Use of Stuart-Amies medium + UTM medium. Processing for <4-6 hours at room temperature, if not stored in a refrigerator at 2-8°C

(Table 3) contd.....

Location of the sample	Gonorrhea	Chlamydia	Vaginosis	Trichomonas	Candida	HPV	Observations
Rectal [7]	Culture	Culture and/or detection of nucleic acids	Not recommended	Not recommended	Not recommended	Liquid cytology in HIV patients or those with cervical cancer	Include the sample according to the patient's sexual practices. Same indications as for the urethral sample
Pharyngeal	Culture	Culture /PCR	Not recommended	Not recommended	Not recommended	Not recommended	Include the sample according to the patient's sexual practices. Same indications as for the urethral sample.

[1] Follow the procedure indicated in Table **2** and add a urine sample for the urine culture.

[2] The following materials are required for the indicated sample protocol: 2 dry Dacron swabs with Stuart-Amies transport medium or similar medium. If direct seeding of the shoot is possible, blood agar, chocolate agar, Saboraud-Chloramphenicol agar, and a selective agar should be used for gonococcal isolation (GC-LECT agar or similar medium) in case ofendocervical intake. The culture plates should be maintained at 37°C, and the chocolate agar and GC-LECT agar should also be maintained at 37°C in an atmosphere with 5% CO_2. For the cultivation of trichomonas, a Roiron or Diamond medium was inoculated with one of the intakes.

[3] If endocervical sampling is not to be performed, the inclusion of a Dacron swab with the UTM medium is acceptable for the detection of *C. trachomatis* using a nucleic acid detection test.

[4] The following materials are required for the indicated sample protocol: 2 dry Dacron endocervical swabs, including Stuart-Amies medium or similar medium and another with the UTM medium. An endocervical sample should be obtained from the cervix of the remnants of vaginal discharge,after previous cleaning, with the aid of gauze and forceps. When possible, direct seeding of the shoot should be performed on selective agar for gonococcal isolation (GC-LECT agar or similar medium). The culture plates should be maintained at 37°C in an atmosphere with 5% CO_2.

[5] It is preferable to obtain a urethral sample with a swab than a urine sample due to the greater sensitivity. Instead, its use is relegated to: 1) population screening studies; 2) locations without laboratories that can care for the samples with minimum guarantees of quality for proper processing; and 3) cases where the patient cannot tolerate the sample study due to its invasive nature. However, it should be noted that in urine samples, only the indication of infection by *N. gonorrhoeae* and *C. trachomatis* is supported by a nucleic acid detection test.

For most STIs, there are effective treatment methods (Table **4**) [34] and, in some cases, prophylaxis. Drug resistance, particularly the antibiotic resistance of gonorrhea, has markedly increased in recent years and consequently limited the treatment options. Although rare, antimicrobial resistance has been noted for other STIs as well. Therefore, early prevention and treatment are crucial [34].

Table 4. Considerations and treatment of sexually transmitted infections (STI).

STI	Treatment	Alternative regimens
Nongonococcal sexual transmitted infection	Azithromycin 1 g, orally, in a single dose Doxycycline 100 mg, orally, twice a day for 7 days	Erythromycin base 500 mg, orally, 4 times a day for 7 days Erythromycin ethyl succinate 800 mg, orally, 4 times a day for 7 days Ofloxacin 300 mg, orally, twice a day for 7 days Levofloxacin 500 mg, orally, once a day for 7 days
Gonococcal sexual transmitted infection (uncomplicated)	[A]Ceftriaxone 250 mg, IM, in a single dose, plus [B] Azithromycin 1 g, orally, in a single dose	Cefixime 400 mg, orally, in a single dose, plus [B] Azithromycin 2 g, orally, in a single dose
Gonococcal sexual transmitted Infection (complicated)	Ceftriaxone 1 g, IV, every 24 hours	Ceftriaxone 1 g, IV, every 24 hours; Cefotaxime 1 g, IV, every 8 hours; Ceftriaxone 1 g, IV, every 24 hours; or Cefotaxime 1 g, IV, every 8 hours
Trichomoniasis	Metronidazole[1] 2 g, orally, in a single dose, or Tinidazole 2 g, orally, in a single dose	Metronidazole 500 mg, orally, twice a day for 7 days
[C]Bacterial vaginosis	Metronidazole[1] 500 mg, orally, twice a day for 7 days, or Metronidazole gel, 0.75%, one full applicator (5 g) intravaginally, once a day for 5 days, or Clindamycin cream, 2%, one full applicator (5 g) intravaginally	Tinidazole 2 g, orally, once daily for 2 days, or Tinidazole 1 g, orally, daily for 5 days, or [4]Clindamycin 300 mg, orally, twice a day for 7 days, or Clindamycin ovules 100 mg, intravaginally, at bedtime for 3 days

(Table 4) contd.....

STI	Treatment	Alternative regimens
[c]Vulvovaginal candidiasis	<u>Orally</u>: Fluconazole 150 mg, orally, in a single dose <u>Intravaginally</u> Butoconazole 2% cream (single dose, bioadhesive product), 5 g, intravaginally, for 1 day, or Clotrimazole 2% cream 5 g, intravaginally, daily for 3 days OR Miconazle 2% cream 5 g, intravaginally, daily for 7 days, or Miconazle 1,200 mg vaginal suppository, one suppository for 1 day [A]Terconazole 0.4% cream 5 g, intravaginally, for 7 days, or Terconazole 0.8% cream 5 g, intravaginally, for 3 days Terconazole 80 mg vaginal suppository, daily, for 3 days,	
[2]Genital herpes	Acyclovir 400 mg, orally, 3 times a day for 7–10 days OR Acyclovir 200 mg, orally, 5 times a day for 7–10 days OR Valacyclovir 1 g, orally, twice a day for 7–10 days OR Famciclovir 250 mg, orally, 3 times a day for 7–10 days	
[3]Primary syphilis infection	Benzathine penicillin G 2.4 million units, IM, as a single dose If allergic to penicillin, consider desensitization, particularly if the patient is pregnant <u>Recommended regimen for infants and children</u> Benzathine penicillin G 50,000 units/kg, IM, up to the adult dose of 2.4 million units in a single dose	Doxycycline 100 mg, orally, twice a day for 28 days Tetracycline 500 mg, orally, 4 times a day for 28 days
Chancroid	<u>First episode:</u> Azithromycin 1 g, orally, in a single dose, or Ceftriaxone 250 mg, IM, in a single dose, or Ciprofloxacin 500 mg, orally, twice a day for 3 days., or Erythromycin base 500 mg, orally, 3 times a day for 7 days	<u>Recurrence:</u> Acyclovir 800 mg, orally, twice a day for 5 days, or Acyclovir 800 mg, orally, 3 times a day for 2 days, or Valacyclovir 500 mg, orally, twice a day for 3 days, or Valacyclovir 1 g, orally, once a day for 5 days, or Famciclovir 125 mg, orally, twice daily for 5 days, or Famciclovir 1 gram, orally, twice daily for 1 day
Lymphogranuloma venereum	Doxycycline 100 mg, orally, twice a day for 21 days	[A]Erythromycin base 500 mg, orally, 4 times a day for 21 days
[4]Genital warts (external)	Imiquimod 5% cream applied to warts, once daily at bedtime, for 3 times a week up to 16 weeks Sinecatechins 15% ointment applied to warts, 3 times a day for up to 16 weeks Podophyllinresin 10%–25%, trichloroacetic acid or bichloroacetic acid 80%–90% Cryotherapy	Intralesional interferon Podofilox 0.5% solution or gel applied to visible warts twice a day for 3 days, followed by no therapy for 4 days. Repeat up to 4 cycles Laser surgery

IM: intramuscular; IV: intravenous.

[A]Recommended treatment in pregnancy.

[B]As dual therapy, ceftriaxone and azithromycin must be administered together at the same time and day, and under direct observation.

[1]Although metronidazole crosses the placenta, data suggest that it poses a low risk to pregnant women. Recently studies have demonstrated that women can be treated with 2 g metronidazole in a single dose at any stage of pregnancy.

[c] Uncomplicated VVC and bacterial vaginosis is not usually acquired through sexual intercourse; hence, data do not support the treatment of sex partners.

[2]Treatment can be extended if disease is active after 10 days of therapy.

[3]Persons with HIV infection who have primary syphilis should be treated as those without HIV infection.

[3]Pregnant women with syphilis at any stage, who report penicillin allergy should be desensitized and treated with penicillin.

[4]Podofilox (podophyllotoxin), podophyllin, and sinecatechins use is not permitted during pregnancy. Imiquimod appears to pose a low risk but further investigation of its use in pregnancy is required.

Of note, the consultation and monitoring of the sexual health for transsexual and transvestite patients should be tailored according to the proposed sex-specific indications, and both their transgender status and sexual orientation should be taken into consideration [35].

If an STI is detected, patients should be instructed to abstain from sexual activity for at least 7 days following the initiation of treatment, regardless of the duration of treatment. The patient should also communicate to their recent sexual contacts the potential for infection, and the doctor or other health professional in-charge should ensure that these steps are completed (either at the initial stage or subsequently at an agreed time). Partner notification and presumptive treatment of risk partners should also be performed if follow-up is not guaranteed [36].

CONCLUSION

In conclusion, STIs are frequently encountered in the primary care setting. Hence, FP will be primarily responsible for the outcome of such cases, and thus influence the improvement of public health. Therefore, it is vital that FP should remain alert and familiar with the signs and symptoms of STIs, as well as the different treatment options available.

One major concern regarding broad implementation of this strategy is the possible impact on high-risk sexual behaviors (risk compensation), which can result in increased transmission of STIs other than HIV. Although the data are still limited, this effect has not been observed in those taking PrEP. However, it should be kept in mind that the study conditions may not reflect usual practices. In the study environment, pharmacological therapy was accompanied by educational strategies, behavioral reinforcement, and a free supply of condoms to the patient. This reinforces the importance of a multifaceted approach to prevention, so that the implementation of a particular strategy does not result in lax adherence to other preventative strategies.

FUNDING

This research received no specific grant from any funding agency in the public, commercial, or not-for-profit sectors.

HUMAN AND ANIMAL RIGHTS

No Animals/Humans were used for studies that are base of this research.

CONFLICT OF INTEREST

The authors declare no conflict of interest, financial or otherwise.

ACKNOWLEDGEMENTS

We appreciate the assistance provided by the staff of the Microbiology Department of CHUVI, Vigo, for this study.

REFERENCES

[1]　Kirby T. HIV pre-exposure prophylaxis: A tale of two countries. Lancet Infect Dis 2017; 17: 32-3.
[http://dx.doi.org/10.1016/S1473-3099(16)30562-X]

[2]　Bruneau J, Roy É, Demers N, Cox J. Some PWID communities are ready for PreP, so what's next? Addiction 2016; 20(Dec): 582-4.
[http://dx.doi.org/10.1111/add.13686] [PMID: 27995679]

[3]　Kabbara WK, Ramadan WH. Emtricitabine/rilpivirine/tenofovir disoproxil fumarate for the treatment of HIV-1 infection in adults. J Infect Public Health 2015; 8(5): 409-17.
[http://dx.doi.org/10.1016/j.jiph.2015.04.020] [PMID: 26001757]

[4]　Beekmann SE, Mehta SR, Anderson CM, Polgreen PM. Are we prepped for pre-exposure prophylaxis (PrEP)?Provider opinions on the real-world use of PrEP in the United States and Canada. Clin Infect Dis 2014; 58: 704-12.
[http://dx.doi.org/10.1093/cid/cit796] [PMID: 24319083]

[5]　Aggarwal P, Bhattar S, Sahani SK, Bhalla P, Garg VK. Sexually transmitted infections and HIV in self reporting men who have sex with men: A two-year study from India. J Infect Public Health 2016; 9(5): 564-70.
[http://dx.doi.org/10.1016/j.jiph.2015.12.007] [PMID: 26776704]

[6]　Lal L, Audsley J, Murphy DA, et al. Medication adherence, condom use and sexually transmitted infections in Australian preexposure prophylaxis users. AIDS 2017; 31(12): 1709-14.
[http://dx.doi.org/10.1097/QAD.0000000000001519] [PMID: 28700394]

[7]   Hoornenborg E, Achterbergh RC, van der Loeff MS, *et al.* Amsterdam PrEP project team in the HIV transmission elimination AMsterdam Initiative, MOSAIC study group. MSM starting preexposure prophylaxis are at risk of hepatitis C virus infection. AIDS 2017; 31(11): 1603-10.
[http://dx.doi.org/10.1097/QAD.0000000000001522] [PMID: 28657964]

[8]   Beymer MR, Weiss RE, Sugar CA, *et al.* Are Centers for Disease Control and Prevention guidelines for preexposure prophylaxiss pecific enough? Formulation of a personalized HIV risk score for Pre-Exposure Prophylaxis initiation. Sex Transm Dis 2017; 44(1): 48-56.
[http://dx.doi.org/10.1097/OLQ.0000000000000535] [PMID: 27898570]

[9]   Calabrese SK, Magnus M, Mayer KH, *et al.* Putting prep into practice: lessons learned from early-adopting U.S. providers' first hand experiences providing HIV pre-exposure prophylaxis and associated care. PLoS One 2016; 15-1. e0157324
[http://dx.doi.org/10.1371/journal.pone.0157324]

[10]   Krakower DS, Maloney KM, Grasso C, Melbourne K, Mayer KH. Primary care clinicians' experiences prescribing HIV pre-exposure prophylaxis at a specialized community health centre in Boston: Lessons from early adopters. J Int AIDS Soc 2016; 19(1): 21165.
[http://dx.doi.org/10.7448/IAS.19.1.21165]

[11]   Fonner VA, Dalglish SL, Kennedy CE, *et al.* Effectiveness and safety of oral HIV pre exposure prophylaxis for all populations. AIDS 2016; 30(12): 1973-83.

[12]   Sheth AN, Rolle CP, Gandhi M. HIV pre-exposure prophylaxis for women. J Virus Erad 2016; 2(3): 149-55.
[PMID: 27482454]

[13]   Haberl A. [HIV pre-exposure prophylaxis in women]. MMW Fortschr Med 2017; 159(Suppl. 2): 42-4.
[http://dx.doi.org/10.1007/s15006-017-9736-9] [PMID: 28597264]

[14]   Davey DL, Bekker LG, Gorbach P, Coates T, Myer L. Delivering PrEP to pregnant and breastfeeding women in sub-Saharan Africa: The implementation science frontier. AIDS 2017.
[http://dx.doi.org/10.1097/QAD.0000000000001604] [PMID: 28723709]

[15]   Bazzi AR, Leech AA, Biancarelli DL, Sullivan M. Experiences using pre-exposure prophylaxis for safer conception among HIV serodiscordant heterosexual couples in the United States. AIDS Patient Care STDS 2017; 31(8): 348-55.
[http://dx.doi.org/10.1089/apc. 2017.0098] [PMID: 28719229]

[16]   Callahan R, Nanda K, Kapiga S, *et al.* FEM-PrEP Study Group. Pregnancy and contraceptive use among women participating in the FEM-PrEP trial. J Acquir Immune Defic Syndr 2015; 68(2): 196-203.
[http://dx.doi.org/10.1097/QAI.0000000000000413] [PMID: 25590272]

[17]   Silapaswan A, Krakower D, Mayer KH. Krakower DI, Mayer KH. Pre-exposure prophylaxis: A narrative review of provider behavior and interventions to increase PrEP implementation in primary care. J Gen Intern Med 2017; 32(2): 192-8.
[http://dx.doi.org/10.1007/s11606-016-3899-4] [PMID: 27761767]

[18]   Di Biagio A, Riccardi N, Signori A, *et al.* PrEP in italy the time may be ripebutwho'spayingthebill? A nationwidesurveyonphysicians' attitudes toward susingantiretroviralstoprevent HIV infection. PLoSOne 2017; 12(2): 192-8.
[http://dx.doi.org/10.1371/journal.pone.0181433]

[19]   Avuvika E, Masese LN. Barriers and facilitators of screening for sexually transmitted infections in adolescent girls and young women in Mombasa, Kenya: A qualitative study. PLoSOne 2017; 12: e0169388.
[http://dx.doi.org/10.1371/journal.p one.0169388]

[20]   Carmine L, Castillo M, Fisher M. Testing and treatment for sexually transmitted infections in adolescents--what's new? J Pediatr Adolesc Gynecol 2014; 27(2): 50-60.
[http://dx.doi.org/10.1016/j.jpag.2013.06.005] [PMID: 24119658]

[21]   Momeni Z, Sadraei J, Kazemi B, Dalimi A. Trichomoniasis in older individuals: A preliminary report from Iran. J Parasit Dis 2016; 40(4): 1597-600.
[http://dx.doi.org/10.1007/s12639-015-0737-2] [PMID: 27876991]

[22]   Kelly C, Johnston J, Carey F. Evaluation of a partnership between primary and secondary care providing an accessible Level 1 sexual health service in the community. Int J STD AIDS 2014; 25(10): 751-7.
[http://dx.doi.org/10.1177/0956462413519430] [PMID: 24469970]

[23]   Rajalakshmi R, Kalaivani S. Prevalence of asymptomatic infections in sexually transmitted diseases attendees diagnosed with bacterial vaginosis, vaginal candidiasis, and trichomoniasis. Indian J Sex Transm Dis 2016; 37(2): 139-42.
[http://dx.doi.org/10.4103/0253-7184.192121] [PMID: 27890946]

[24]   Hidalgo-Tenorio C, Ramírez-Taboada J, Gil-Anguita C, *et al.* Safety and immunogenicity of the quadrivalent human papillomavirus (qHPV) vaccine in HIV-positive Spanish men who have sex with men (MSM). AIDS Res Ther 2017; 14(1): 34.
[http://dx.doi.org/10.1186/s12981-017-0160-0] [PMID: 28720147]

[25]   Rahimzadeh S, Naderimagham S, Rohani-Rasaf M, *et al.* Burden of sexually transmitted infections in Iran from 1990 to 2010: Results from the global burden of disease study 2010. Arch Iran Med 2016; 19(11): 768-73.
[PMID: 27845545]

[26]   Wetten S, Mohammed H, Yung M, Mercer CH, Cassell JA, Hughes G. Diagnosis and treatment of chlamydia and gonorrhoea in general practice in England 2000-2011: A population-based study using data from the UK Clinical Practice Research Datalink. BMJ Open 2015; 5(5):

e007776.
[http://dx.doi.org/10.1136/bmjopen-2015-007776] [PMID: 26022269]

[27]   Vázquez F, Lepe JA, Otero L, Blanco MA, Aznar J. [Microbiological diagnosis of sexually-transmitted infection (2007)]. Enferm Infecc Microbiol Clin 2008; 26(1): 32-7.
[http://dx.doi.org/10.1157/13114393] [PMID: 18208764]

[28]   WHO guidelines approved by the guidelines review committee WHO guidelines for the treatment of *Chlamydia trachomatis*. Geneva: World Health Organization 2016.

[29]   Smith L, Angarone MP. SexuallyTransmitted Infections. Urol Clin North Am 2015; 42(4): 507-18.
[http://dx.doi.org/10.1016/j.ucl.2015.06.004] [PMID: 26475947]

[30]   Girometti N, Gutierrez A, Nwokolo N, McOwan A, Whitlock G. High HIV incidence in men who have sex with men following an early syphilis diagnosis: Is there room for pre-exposure prophylaxis as a prevention strategy? Sex Transm Infect 2017; 93(5): 320-2.
[http://dx.doi.org/10.1136/sextrans-2016-052865] [PMID: 28729516]

[31]   Sauerbrei A. Optimal management of genital herpes: Current perspectives. Infect Drug Resist 2016; 9: 129-41.
[http://dx.doi.org/10.2147/IDR.S96164] [PMID: 27358569]

[32]   de Voux A, Kent JB, Macomber K, *et al.* Notes from the Field: Cluster of Lymphogranuloma Venereum cases among men who have sex with men - Michigan, August 2015-April 2016. MMWR Morb Mortal Wkly Rep 2016; 65(34): 920-1.
[http://dx.doi.org/10.15585/mmwr.mm6534a6] [PMID: 27583686]

[33]   Tamer E, Çakmak SK, İlhan MN, Artüz F. Demographic characteristics and risk factors in Turkish patients with anogenital warts. J Infect Public Health 2016; 9(5): 661-6.
[http://dx.doi.org/10.1016/j.jiph.2015.12.009] [PMID: 26776703]

[34]   Workowski KA, Bolan GA. Centersfor Disease Control and prevention Sexually transmitted disease morbidity and mortality weekly report (2015) Treatment guideline Morbidity and Mortality Weekly Report (MMWR) 2015; 64(RR3): 1-137.

[35]   Hayon R. Gender and sexual health: Care of transgender patients. FP Essent 2016; 449: 27-36.
[PMID: 27731969]

[36]   Tan WS, Chen M, Ivan M, *et al.* Partner notification out comes for men who have sex with men diagnosed with syphilis referred to partner notification officers, Melbourne, Australia. Sex Transm Dis 2016; 43(11): 685-9.
[http://dx.doi.org/10.1097/OLQ.0000000000000512] [PMID: 27893597]

14

Assessment of Dietary Supplementation in the Treatment of Vitiligo

Mallory K. Smith[1], Tasneem F. Mohammad[2] and Iltefat H. Hamzavi[2,*]

[1]*Wayne State University School of Medicine, Detroit, MI, USA*
[2]*Department of Dermatology, Henry Ford Hospital, Detroit, MI, USA*

Abstract:

Background:

Vitiligo is the most common acquired pigmentary disorder in the world. Due to alterations in physical appearance, vitiligo is a psychologically devastating disease. Although treatment options exist, a cure for this disease has yet to be discovered. Of recent interest in vitiligo is the relationship between diet and disease.

Objective:

To review various dietary modifications and supplementation used in the management of vitiligo.

Materials and Methods:

A thorough evaluation of recent literature using the keywords "vitiligo, diet, supplement, antioxidant, vitamin, mineral, zinc, copper, gluten-free, celiac disease, alternative medicine" in the NCBI PubMed search function was performed.

Results:

A total of 39 relevant articles were reviewed and critically evaluated.

Conclusion:

Initial studies regarding the treatment of vitiligo through dietary modification are promising, although further studies are needed in multiple populations to explore the therapeutic value of these interventions.

Keywords: Diet, Vitiligo, Supplementation, Antioxidant, Repigmentation, Management.

I. INTRODUCTION

Vitiligo is the most common acquired pigmentary disorder, with an estimated prevalence of 1% worldwide [1]. The disease is characterized by the development of depigmented macules and patches due to the loss of functioning melanocytes [2, 3]. Vitiligo is classified into two broad categories, segmental and non-segmental, with the latter being more common. Segmental vitiligo lesions are generally stable, unilateral, and present in a localized or dermatomal distribution. Non-segmental vitiligo is classically characterized by a waxing and waning course with depigmentation in a symmetric, bilateral pattern, and includes the generalized, acrofacial, and universal variants [4]. The pathogenesis of the disease has yet to be fully elucidated, although an impaired response to oxidative stress, autoimmunity, inflammatory, and neurogenic components may all play a role [2, 4]. The association between vitiligo and other autoimmune diseases, such as thyroid disease, psoriasis, and inflammatory bowel disease has been established, supporting an autoimmune etiology [5]. Other studies have proposed the relationship between free radicals and an

* Address correspondence to this author at the Department of Dermatology, Henry Ford Health System, 3031 West Grand Boulevard, Suite 800, Detroit, MI 48202, USA; Tel: (313) 916-6964; Email: ihamzav1@hfhs.org

impaired response of melanocytes to oxidative stress in the pathogenesis of vitiligo [2, 6].

Although there is no cure, a variety of treatment options exist for patients with vitiligo, each with different mechanisms of repigmentation and varying success. These include topical medications such as corticosteroids or immunomodulators, phototherapy, oral medications, autologous melanocyte or epidermal transplant, surgery, and depigmentation [7]. While these therapies are important components in the treatment of vitiligo, the role of dietary modification and supplementation is often overlooked [1, 8]. Recent studies have shown that alterations in dietary intake and oral supplementation can be beneficial in the treatment of many diseases, including vitiligo. This article aims to review the various types of dietary modifications and supplementation used in the management of vitiligo.

II. MATERIALS AND METHODS

The literature review process was carried out using the keywords "vitiligo, diet, supplement, antioxidant, vitamin, mineral, zinc, copper, gluten free, celiac disease, alternative medicine" in the NCBI PubMed search function. This review utilized articles published within the past ten to fifteen years to obtain recent information and developments. Each article was critically appraised to determine applicability to the topic at hand.

III. RESULTS

A total of 44 recent, relevant publications were identified within the scope of this review. Additionally, recent textbooks, as well as USDA and U.S. Department of Health and Human Services online resources were used for reference in the formulation of the discussion and conclusions sections of this article.

IV. DISCUSSION

A. Antioxidants

There is evidence to support an imbalance between oxidants and antioxidants in individuals affected by vitiligo. It has been proposed that an overproduction of reactive oxygen species (ROS), in combination with the inherent sensitivity of melanocytes to oxidative stress, may be a mechanism for melanocyte damage and death in vitiligo [9]. Yildirim et al. showed that activity levels of oxidative stress markers such as superoxide dismutase (SOD), glutathione peroxidase (GPx), and malondialdehyde (MDA) were significantly elevated in tissue samples of vitiligo patients [10]. SOD and GPx are enzymes involved in the breakdown of ROS, whereas MDA is produced via lipid peroxidation, often caused by the accumulation of ROS. Other studies observed significantly elevated serum levels of MDA and significantly lower serum levels of SOD, GPx, Vitamins C and E, and overall antioxidant activity in patients with this disease. Serum antioxidant levels were likely lower due to their use in quenching free radicals, whereas MDA was elevated due to the presence of ROS [11].

Imbalances in ox-redox status in vitiligo led to the use of antioxidant supplementation as adjuvant therapy. Oral supplementation with an antioxidant blend of *Phyllanthus emblica* fruit extracts, vitamin E, and carotenoids, combined with standard topical treatments and/or narrowband ultraviolet B (NBUVB) phototherapy, showed statistically significant increases in repigmentation compared to topical treatment and/or NBUVB alone. Lower levels of serum inflammatory markers were detected in the antioxidant treatment group as well [12].

Alpha-lipoic acid, an over the counter supplement, has also been shown to be beneficial as an adjuvant supplement. This substance acts as a free radical scavenger, lipoxygenase inhibitor, glutathione synthesis promoter, and a factor in the recycling of other antioxidants, such as vitamins C and E [13]. Similarly to the study above, a combination of vitamins C and E, alpha-lipoic acid, and polyunsaturated fats was used as antioxidant supplementation along with NBUVB phototherapy. A statistically significant increase in repigmentation and decrease in serum reactive oxygen species (ROS) was noted compared to NBUVB phototherapy alone [13].

Supplementation with vitamin E, an antioxidant known to prevent lipid peroxidation, has also been used as an adjunct to NBUVB phototherapy. Study results from Elgoweini et al. reported 72.7% repigmentation in the vitamin E-NBUVB group (n=12), compared to 55.6% repigmentation in the NBUVB phototherapy group (n=12). In particular, the average number of treatments required to achieve 50% repigmentation was significantly lower in the vitamin E supplementation group than the control group, indicating a more rapid repigmentation with the supplement [14]. Additionally, a significantly lower level of serum MDA was observed in the vitamin E group at the end of the study compared to the beginning, further supporting the value of antioxidant supplementation with traditional phototherapy treatment regimens for vitiligo [14]. Common foods high in vitamin E include sunflower seeds, almonds, hazelnuts, peanuts, oils from the aforementioned plants, and breakfast cereals [15]. Caution should be observed in using and recommending this supplement, as vitamin E has antiplatelet properties and should be used with care in patients with bleeding diathesis or recent surgical procedures. Additionally, vitamin E is lipid soluble, and overdose is a concern due to the complex metabolism and storage in the body. The recommended daily allowance and upper intake limit for vitamin E is found in Table **5** below.

Polypodium leucotomos extract (PLE) is another antioxidant used to treat dermatologic diseases. Derived from a fern native to Central and South America, this over the counter supplement has been used in the management of conditions including photodermatoses, vitiligo, pigmentary disorders, and as a photoprotectant [16]. PLE contains numerous phenolic compounds with potent antioxidant, anti-inflammatory, and photoprotective properties [17 - 19]. The combination of NBUVB and oral PLE provided statistically significant increases in repigmentation in 50 patients with generalized vitiligo, compared to placebo with NBUVB phototherapy alone. The study concluded that 44% of the PLE treated patients experienced repigmentation, compared to 27% in the placebo group. In addition, decreased levels of IL-2, IFN-γ, and TNF-α were noted in the PLE group, indicating a downregulating effect on cell-mediated immunity [19]. This highlights the interplay between oxidative stress and autoimmunity in the pathogenesis of vitiligo, as well as the utility of oral PLE in disease management. Other studies have shown efficacy in repigmentation with PLE supplementation as well. Pacifico *et al.* supplemented NBUVB therapy with 480 mg oral *P. leucotomos* daily for 6 months, and reported increased repigmentation in the PLE group compared to phototherapy alone [20]. In addition, Reyes *et al.* studied the use of PLE with Psoralen and ultraviolet A (PUVA) treatment, and found that skin repigmentation was significantly higher in the PLE + PUVA group compared to the placebo + PUVA group [21]. Of note, a study by Nestor *et al.* evaluated the safety of PLE in twenty patients taking 240 mg of PLE daily, and reported an excellent safety profile for this dose range. Gastrointestinal discomfort and pruritus were the most commonly noted side effects [22].

Ginkgo biloba, a supplement available over the counter, is another antioxidant used in the treatment of vitiligo. Parsad *et al.* studied the efficacy of *G. biloba* oral supplementation in patients with slowly developing vitiligo lesions. The treatment group took 40 mg of *G. biloba* three times daily for a period of six months. The results indicated that *G. biloba* supplements significantly arrested disease progression compared to placebo, and increased repigmentation with few side effects [23]. A more recent open-label pilot study by Szczurko *et al.* showed significant improvement in Vitiligo Scoring Index (VASI) scores with 60 mg of *G. biloba* twice daily for 12 weeks in a total of 12 patients [24]. Additional studies are needed on a larger scale to replicate these findings and provide a better understanding of the mechanism and application of *G. biloba* in the treatment of vitiligo, although initial findings are promising. Of note to patients and physicians, serious side effects include intracranial hemorrhage and bleeding diathesis, due to the substance's antiplatelet effect. *G. biloba* has also been known to interfere pharmacologically with anticoagulation medications. Clinical judgment and care should be used in the initiation of this treatment option [25].

For pediatric patients and those who do not desire supplementation in the form of a capsule, increased intake of foods with high antioxidant content is reasonable. Top dietary sources of antioxidants, modified by Wu *et al.* and reported by Hamzavi *et al.* are shown below (Table 1) [26, 27]. Although there is limited data correlating antioxidant consumption with health outcomes, these antioxidant-rich foods may be beneficial adjuncts in the treatment of vitiligo.

Table 1. Top 30 foods ranked according to total antioxidant capacities and serving measurements *in vitro* (C, cooked; g, gram; R, raw. TAC, total antioxidant capacity; umol of TE, micromoles of Trolox equivalents; umol of TE/g, micromoles of Trolox equivalents per gram) [26].

Rank	Food name	TAC (umol of TE/g)	Serving size (g)	TAC/serving (umol of TE)
1	Small red bean	149.21	Half cup (92)	13,727
2	Wild blueberry (lowbush)	92.60	One cup (145)	13,427
3	Red kidney bean	144.13	Half cup (92)	13,259
4	Pinto bean	123.59	Half cup (96)	11,864
5	Cultivated blueberry	62.20	One cup (145)	9019
6	Cranberry	94.56	One cup whole (95)	8983
7	Artichoke (C)	94.09	One cup (84)	7904
8	Blackberry	53.48	One cup (144)	7701

(Table 1) contd.....

Rank	Food name	TAC (umol of TE/g)	Serving size (g)	TAC/serving (umol of TE)
9	Prune	85.78	Half cup (85)	7291
10	Raspberry	49.25	One cup (123)	6058
11	Strawberry	35.77	One cup (166)	5938
12	Red Delicious and Granny Smith apple	42.75	One fruit (138)	5900
13	Pecan	179.40	One oz (28.4)	5095
14	Russet potato	13.23	One potato (369)	4882
15	Sweet cherry	33.61	One cup (145)	4873
16	Plum (black)	73.39	One fruit (66)	4844
17	Black bean	80.40	Half cup (52)	4181
18	Gala apple	28.28	One fruit (138)	3903
19	Walnut	135.41	One oz (28.4)	3846
20	Golden delicious and Fuji apples	26.70	One fruit (138)	3685
21	Deglet Noor dates	38.95	Half cup (89)	3467
22	Avocado (Haas)	19.33	One fruit (173)	3344
23	Pear, Green and Red Anjou cultivars	19.11	One fruit (166)	3172
24	Hazelnut	96.45	One oz (28.4)	2739
25	Raab broccoli (R)	30.84	Fifth bunch (85)	2621
26	Navel orange	18.14	One fruit (140)	2540
27	Fig	33.83	Half cup (5)	2537
28	Raisin	30.37	Half cup (82)	2490
29	Red cabbage (C)	31.46	Half cup (75)	2359
30	Red potato	10.98	One potato (213)	2339

With permission from Hamzavi *et al.* (2016).

B. Gluten-free Diet

Autoimmune diseases often co-exist with vitiligo, as reported by Gill *et al.* [5]. A relationship between vitiligo and celiac disease has been proposed, although evidence has been controversial and incomplete.

Seyhan *et al.* analyzed children and adolescents with celiac disease, reporting that 9.1% of the patients were also diagnosed with vitiligo [28]. Following this evidence, Seyhan *et al.* observed that in a group of 61 patients with vitiligo (40 adults and 21 children), there was an 18% prevalence of concomitant celiac disease seropositivity, with a positivity of 23% in children and 15% in adults. However, the relationship was not statistically significant [29]. Additional studies of vitiligo and celiac disease have shown a statistically significant relationship between celiac disease autoantibodies in patients with vitiligo, although further evaluation is needed as this topic is highly controversial at this time [30].

Case reports have provided interesting, although limited, information regarding repigmentation of patients with vitiligo upon the initiation of a gluten-free diet. In one case report, a 9-year old child with celiac disease experienced extensive repigmentation over three years following the initiation of a gluten-free diet. Seven years later, with the continuation of the gluten-free diet, the repigmentation was maintained [31]. Another case report indicated that a 22-year old female with acrofacial vitiligo experienced significant repigmentation following the initiation of a gluten-free diet, even though she did not have celiac disease. After numerous topical medications and phototherapy failed to induce repigmentation, the elimination of gluten from her diet, in combination with previously initiated oral dapsone, led to rapid repigmentation, the majority of which occurred in the first month [32].

To manage patients with concomitant celiac disease and vitiligo, a gluten-free diet is recommended for the treatment of the celiac disease, and potential repigmentation of vitiligo. In cases of vitiligo where other treatment options have been exhausted, it may be reasonable to initiate a gluten-free diet.

C. Minerals: Zinc and Copper

The role of supplementation with minerals, such as Zinc (Zn) and Copper (Cu), is another area of interest in vitiligo, although results are controversial. Zinc is a trace element required for homeostasis, with a variety of roles in growth and development, immunomodulation, wound healing, behavior, and taste. It also plays a role in the protection against free radial damage and oxidant-antioxidant balance, as Zn is a required cofactor for SOD [33]. Copper is also an important mineral in homeostasis, with a similarly broad listing of roles in the body. Copper is also considered an antioxidant, as it acts as a coenzyme with antioxidant properties. Both Zn and Cu may also be involved in melanogenesis through the catalysis of eumelanin production [34]. Zinc may further contribute, as deficiencies in the Zn-α2-Glycoprotein (ZAG) have been reported in people with vitiligo. ZAG is involved in melanocyte proliferation and maturation, with decreased ZAG levels leading to melanocyte detachment. Additionally, treatment with topical corticosteroids, which causes repigmentation, has the ability to increase ZAG activity. Finally, ZAG has been linked to chromosome 7, which contains mutations in certain patients with generalized vitiligo [35, 36]. This theory has provided an additional basis for the study of Zn supplementation in patients with vitiligo.

Previous studies, such as that by Shameer *et al.*, evaluated serum Zn levels in vitiligo patients, and found a significant relationship between low Zn levels and patients with the disease compared to controls [33]. A meta-analysis of Chinese vitiligo patients by Zeng *et al.* further explored the relationship between both Zn and Cu levels in this population of patients. Serum Cu and Zn were compared between the control and vitiligo patients, with vitiligo patients having significantly lower serum levels of both Cu and Zn compared to controls [34]. Although both of these studies indicate some relationship between serum Zn levels and vitiligo, other findings have determined no significant difference between Zn levels in vitiligo patients compared to controls, leaving this topic controversial [37].

With respect to treatment using oral Zn, Yaghoobi *et al.* studied a group of 86 patients with vitiligo, half of whom were treated with topical corticosteroid alone, while the other half was treated with topical corticosteroid plus oral zinc sulfate. A greater improvement in repigmentation was observed in the treatment group, although it was not statistically significant. Overall, this work provided evidence that the combination of topical corticosteroid and Zn sulfate supplementation was not superior to topical corticosteroid alone, although a positive correlation was observed [38]. Future studies should be continued with larger sample sizes to further understand this potential relationship, in addition to looking at the role Cu supplementation may play in the treatment of vitiligo. The recommended daily allowance and upper intake limits for Cu and Zn are found in Table **5**, as well as foods rich in Cu and Zn in Tables **2** and **3**.

Table 2. Selected foods rich in Copper [15].

Foods	Measure	Copper, Cu (mg) per measure	% RDA (0.9 mg/day)	% UL (10 mg/day)
Beef variety meats and by-products, cooked	1.0 slice	11.816	1312	118
Lamb liver, cooked	3.0 oz	11.390	1265	114
Lamb variety meats and by-products, cooked	3.0 oz	8.356	928	84
Seaweed, spirulina	1.0 cup	6.832	759	68
Mollusks, oyster, cooked	3.0 oz	4.851	539	49
Beef sweetbread, cooked	3.0 oz	4.335	481	43
Cocoa, dry powder, unsweetened	1 cup	3.258	362	33
Cashew nuts, dry roasted	1.0 cup, halves and whole	3.041	338	30
Sunflower seed kernels, toasted	1.0 cup	2.458	273	25
Buckwheat	1.0 cup	1.870	207	19

Table 3. Selected foods rich in Zinc [15].

Foods	Measure	Zinc, Zn (mg) per measure	% RDA (8 mg/day)	% UL (10 mg/day)
Mollusks, oyster, eastern, canned	3.0 oz	77.31	966	773
Beef, bottom sirloin	1.0 roast (690g raw meat)	26.57	332	267
Cereals (ready-to-eat)	0.75-1.0 cup	15.0	188	150
Wheat germ	1.0 cup	14.13	177	141
Turkey breast, cooked	1.0 breast	13.12	164	131
Sesame seed kernels, toasted	1.0 cup	13.09	163	131
Lamb, foreshank, cooked	1.0 piece, cooked	11.38	142	114
Ground Turkey	1.0 lb	10.66	133	107
Crustaceans, crab, cooked	1.0 leg	10.21	127	102
Peanuts, oil roasted	1.0 cup	9.47	118	95

D. Vitamin D

Vitamin D plays a variety of roles in the human body, including calcium and bone homeostasis, cell proliferation and growth, and melanogenesis. It is theorized that vitamin D plays an active role in melanogenesis, as this hormone is synthesized within the skin after exposure to UVB light, and perhaps involved in the maturation of melanocytes to produce melanin and undergo appropriate differentiation [39]. Vitamin D is also thought to play a role in immunomodulation, although the mechanism is not well understood. Studies have indicated the use of vitamin D in the treatment of autoimmune diseases such as systemic lupus erythematosus, diabetes mellitus, rheumatoid arthritis, and multiple sclerosis, although this topic is highly controversial [40].

In particular, Silverberg *et al.* studied the relationship between serum 25-hydroxyvitamin D levels and the presence of autoimmune diseases. It was found that very low 25-hydroxyvitamin D level (<15 ng/mL) in patients with vitiligo was associated with comorbid autoimmune disease, such as thyroid disease, Sjögren syndrome, rheumatoid arthritis, alopecia areata, and inflammatory bowel disease [41].

Looking at serum levels of vitamin D in vitiligo from a different perspective, Sehrawat *et al.* analyzed the levels of 25-hydroxyvitamin D in Indian patients with vitiligo throughout a 12-week phototherapy treatment consisting of three NBUVB sessions per week. Interestingly, all of the patients had sub-normal levels of serum 25-hydroxyvitamin D at the start of the study, but throughout the course of NBUVB treatment, serum 25-hydroxyvitamin D levels increased. Additionally, this group reported a significant improvement in VASI scores as repigmentation occurred throughout the treatment. Although the increasing trend of serum vitamin D levels was insignificant, this study provided interesting insight into the potential role of vitamin D in the repigmentation of vitiligo lesions, perhaps through the regulation of photo-induced melanogenesis [42].

Additional studies by Finamor *et al.* supported this theory, as they assessed the effect of long-term administration of 25-hydroxyvitamin D in the treatment of patients with vitiligo and psoriasis. Sixteen vitiligo patients were treated with 35,000 IU of 25-hydroxyvitamin D daily for six months, and as expected, measured serum levels of vitamin D increased significantly throughout the study. Additionally, eleven out of the sixteen patients with vitiligo experienced 25-75% repigmentation during this time period [43]. Increases in serum vitamin D levels were associated with corresponding repigmentation. This study raises the possibility of vitamin D supplementation as a treatment option for patients with vitiligo [43]. However, further studies are needed for a more complete understanding of the mechanism and clinical utility of vitamin D supplementation, as this topic is controversial and in need of further evidence. Of note, vitamin D is a fat-soluble vitamin, which can reach toxic levels if ingested in excess. Toxicity is defined as vitamin D levels higher than 150 ng/mL, or the presence of associated symptoms such as hypercalcemia, nausea, constipation, or weakness. Although daily recommendations are controversial, toxicity is unlikely in an adult when taking doses less than 10,000 IU daily. Additionally, a safe daily limit, as recommended by the Institute of Medicine, is 4,000 IU daily for individuals older than 8 years of age [44, 45]. Table **4** and **5** lists the recommended daily allowance for vitamin D as well as foods rich in vitamin D.

Table 4. Selected foods rich in Vitamin D [15].

Foods	Measure	Vitamin D (D2 + D3) (ug) per measure	% RDA (600 IU or 15 ug)	% UL (40,000 ug/day)
Mushrooms – brown, Italian or crimini (raw)	1.0 cup	27.8	185	0.70
Salmon, canned	3.0 oz	18.3	122	0.46
Smoked whitefish	1.0 cup	17.4	116	0.43
Mushrooms – portabella, grilled	1.0 cup sliced	15.9	106	0.40
Salmon, cooked	3.0 oz	14.1	94	0.35
Swordfish, cooked	3.0 oz	14.1	94	0.35
Rainbow trout, cooked	1.0 fillet	13.5	90	0.34
Tuna, canned	1.0 cup	9.8	65	0.25
Milk (whole), added vitamin D	0.25 cup	3.4	23	0.23
Hardboiled egg	1.0 cup	3.0	20	0.07

E. Alternative Medicine

A variety of alternative treatment practices have been used as therapeutic remedies for vitiligo, although there is a paucity of clinical studies in the literature. Many of these treatments utilize herbs and extracts with photosensitizing properties in conjunction with natural sunlight to induce repigmentation. These practices include Ayurvedic, Unani, and Traditional Chinese medicine (TCM) techniques [26].

Ayurvedic medicine was developed in India thousands of years ago and is still practiced today. This form of medicine takes a holistic approach toward the patient, incorporating spirit, body, mind, and emotions and often involves dietary modifications. Dietotherapy for vitiligo includes Saman Chikitsa, which consists of two parts, Kastha Aushadhi and Saman Chikitsa. Kastha Aushadhi uses herbal supplements as photosensitizing and blood-purifying treatments, whereas Rasa Shastra is a method of formulating combinations of herbs and minerals for immunosuppression. The list of herbs used in both is extensive, and the dosing and regimens are often Ayurvedic practitioner and pharmacy dependent, making it difficult to provide exact regimens. An additional form of Ayurvedic treatment for vitiligo is Sodhan Chikitsa, a method of purification of the body through the use of vomiting, purgation, enemas, and bloodletting. This practice involves the use of laxatives, bran, flaxseed, fruits, and many other dietary agents [26].

Unani medicine is derived from influences of Greek, Islamic, and Arabic cultures, and is practiced today in many parts of the Middle East, South Africa and regions of Asia. According to this practice, the human body is composed of the following four components: air, water, fire, and earth. An imbalance of these elements is thought to be the causative factor in illness and disease. Treatment regimens were developed surrounding this ideology. In addition to Iiaj Nafansi (psychotherapy), Unani medicine recommends the use of Iiaj Bil Ghiza (dietotherapy) for the treatment of vitiligo. Helpful foods according to this practice are listed as follows; warm, easily digestible foods, goat and bird meat, and digestive aids with meals. Additionally, the avoidance of fresh fish, fruits, vegetables, and foods high in fat is recommended, as these foods are theorized to cause an imbalance in the elements of the body [26].

Traditional Chinese Medicine (TCM), which was developed and practiced in China, views the human body as a combination of two opposing but complementary forces, the Ying and Yang. An imbalance in the Ying and Yang is thought to produce illness and disease. This practice uses a holistic approach in patient management, by combining physical, oral, and acupuncture practices in the management or prevention of disease. In particular, TCM dietary treatments for vitiligo include the use of herbal supplements, such as Golden Serpent fern extract in combination with NBUVB, *Ginkgo biloba*, and Xiaobai Mixture, a blend of walnut, flowers, black sesame, black beans, duckweed, Sweetgum fruit, and plums [26]. Chen et al. assessed the effectiveness of a combination of oral TCM with NBUVB therapy compared to NBUVB alone in a systematic review with meta-analysis of randomized controlled trials. This study determined that in regards to repigmentation, CHM combined with phototherapy was superior to phototherapy alone in the treatment of vitiligo (p<0.00001) [46].

Supplementation regimens in these practices are difficult to quantify and not commonly used in the United States. Future studies are necessary and may further elucidate the role of alternative medicine in the management of vitiligo.

CONCLUSION

Vitiligo is a complex disease with a multitude of components contributing to its pathogenesis. Alterations in the diet may target many of these components, and recent evidence suggests that dietary modifications and supplementation can be beneficial in the treatment of vitiligo, especially as adjuvant therapies to phototherapy or topical regimens. Although initial findings with these supplements are promising, further studies in multiple populations are needed to explore the therapeutic value of these interventions and further develop these options to optimize the management of this psychologically devastating disease.

Table 5. Compiled list of Recommended Dietary Allowances (RDA) and Upper Intake Level (UL) of discussed vitamins and minerals [47].

Substance	RDA: 19-30 years, 30-50 years, and 50-70 years	UL: 19-30 years, 30-50 years, and 50-70 years
Copper	900 ug/day	10,000 ug/day
Vitamin C	Males: 90 mg/day, Females: 75 mg/day	2,000 mg/day
Vitamin D	600 IU/day	4,000 IU/day
Vitamin E	15 mg/day	1,000 mg/day
Zinc	Males: 11 mg/day, Females: 8 mg/day	40 mg/day

CONFLICT OF INTEREST

Dr. Hamzavi is an investigator for Estee-Lauder, Ferndale, Johnson and Johnson, and Allergan, and has received equipment from Johnson and Johnson. Dr. Mohammad is a subinvestigator for Estee-Lauder, Ferndale, and Allergan. Ms. Smith has no conflicts of interest to report.

ACKNOWLEDGEMENTS

Declared none.

REFERENCES

[1]   Ezzedine K, Eleftheriadou V, Whitton M, van Geel N. Vitiligo. Lancet 2015; 386(9988): 74-84.
        [http://dx.doi.org/10.1016/S0140-6736(14)60763-7] [PMID: 25596811]

[2]   Alikhan A, Felsten LM, Daly M, Petronic-Rosic V. Vitiligo: A comprehensive overview Part I. Introduction, epidemiology, quality of life,
        diagnosis, differential diagnosis, associations, histopathology, etiology, and work-up. J Am Acad Dermatol 2011; 65(3): 473-91.
        [http://dx.doi.org/10.1016/j.jaad.2010.11.061] [PMID: 21839315]

[3]   Gauthier Y, Cario Andre M, Taïeb A. A critical appraisal of vitiligo etiologic theories. Is melanocyte loss a melanocytorrhagy? Pigment Cell
        Res 2003; 16(4): 322-32.
        [http://dx.doi.org/10.1034/j.1600-0749.2003.00070.x] [PMID: 12859615]

[4]   Taïeb A, Picardo M. Clinical practice. Vitiligo. N Engl J Med 2009; 360(2): 160-9.
        [PMID: 19129529]

[5]   Gill L, Zarbo A, Isedeh P, Jacobsen G, Lim HW, Hamzavi I. Comorbid autoimmune diseases in patients with vitiligo: A cross-sectional study.
        J Am Acad Dermatol 2016; 74(2): 295-302.
        [http://dx.doi.org/10.1016/j.jaad.2015.08.063] [PMID: 26518171]

[6]   Güntaş G, Engin B, Ekmekçi OB, et al. Evaluation of advanced oxidation protein products, prooxidant-antioxidant balance, and total
        antioxidant capacity in untreated vitiligo patients. Ann Dermatol 2015; 27(2): 178-83.
        [http://dx.doi.org/10.5021/ad.2015.27.2.178] [PMID: 25834357]

[7]   Sisti A, Sisti G, Oranges CM. Effectiveness and safety of topical tacrolimus monotherapy for repigmentation in vitiligo: A comprehensive
        literature review. An Bras Dermatol 2016; 91(2): 187-95.
        [http://dx.doi.org/10.1590/abd1806-4841.20164012] [PMID: 27192518]

[8]   Felsten LM, Alikhan A, Petronic-Rosic V. Vitiligo: a comprehensive overview Part II: treatment options and approach to treatment. J Am
        Acad Dermatol 2011; 65(3): 493-514.
        [http://dx.doi.org/10.1016/j.jaad.2010.10.043] [PMID: 21839316]

[9]   Xie H, Zhou F, Liu L, et al. Vitiligo: How do oxidative stress-induced autoantigens trigger autoimmunity? J Dermatol Sci 2016; 81(1): 3-9.
        [http://dx.doi.org/10.1016/j.jdermsci.2015.09.003] [PMID: 26387449]

[10]   Yildirim M, Baysal V, Inaloz HS, Can M. The role of oxidants and antioxidants in generalized vitiligo at tissue level. J Eur Acad Dermatol
        Venereol 2004; 18(6): 683-6.
        [http://dx.doi.org/10.1111/j.1468-3083.2004.01080.x] [PMID: 15482295]

[11]   Khan R, Satyam A, Gupta S, Sharma VK, Sharma A. Circulatory levels of antioxidants and lipid peroxidation in Indian patients with
        generalized and localized vitiligo. Arch Dermatol Res 2009; 301(10): 731-7.
        [http://dx.doi.org/10.1007/s00403-009-0964-4] [PMID: 19488773]

[12]   Colucci R, Dragoni F, Conti R, Pisaneschi L, Lazzeri L, Moretti S. Evaluation of an oral supplement containing Phyllanthus emblica fruit
        extracts, vitamin E, and carotenoids in vitiligo treatment. Dermatol Ther (Heidelb) 2015; 28(1): 17-21.
        [http://dx.doi.org/10.1111/dth.12172] [PMID: 25285994]

[13]   DellAnna ML, Mastrofrancesco A, Sala R, et al. Antioxidants and narrow band-UVB in the treatment of vitiligo: a double-blind placebo
        controlled trial. Clin Exp Dermatol 2007; 32(6): 631-6.
        [http://dx.doi.org/10.1111/j.1365-2230.2007.02514.x] [PMID: 17953631]

[14]   Elgoweini M, Nour El Din N. Response of vitiligo to narrowband ultraviolet B and oral antioxidants. J Clin Pharmacol 2009; 49(7): 852-5.
        [http://dx.doi.org/10.1177/0091270009335769] [PMID: 19553407]

[15]   USDA Food Composition Databases Available from: https://ndb.nal.usda.gov/ndb/nutrients/index 2016 [09/15/2016];

[16]   Choudhry SZ, Bhatia N, Ceilley R, et al. Role of oral Polypodium leucotomos extract in dermatologic diseases: A review of the literature. J
        Drugs Dermatol 2014; 13(2): 148-53.
        [PMID: 24509964]

[17]   Berman B, Ellis C, Elmets C. Polypodium LeucotomosAn Overview of Basic Investigative Findings. J Drugs Dermatol 2016; 15(2): 224-8.
        [PMID: 26885792]

[18]   Nestor M, Bucay V, Callender V, Cohen JL, Sadick N, Waldorf H. Polypodium leucotomos as an Adjunct Treatment of Pigmentary
        Disorders. J Clin Aesthet Dermatol 2014; 7(3): 13-7.
        [PMID: 24688621]

[19]   Middelkamp-Hup MA, Bos JD, Rius-Diaz F, Gonzalez S, Westerhof W. Treatment of vitiligo vulgaris with narrow-band UVB and oral
        Polypodium leucotomos extract: a randomized double-blind placebo-controlled study. J Eur Acad Dermatol Venereol 2007; 21(7): 942-50.
        [http://dx.doi.org/10.1111/j.1468-3083.2006.02132.x] [PMID: 17659004]

[20]   Pacifico AI, Paro Vidolin A, Leone G. Combined treatment of narrowband ultraviolet B light (NBUVB) phototherapy and oral polypodium
        leucotomos extract versus NB UVB phototherapy alone in the treatment of patients with vitiligo. J Am Acad Dermatol 2009; 60.

[21]   Reyes E, Jaén P, de las Heras E, *et al.* Systemic immunomodulatory effects of Polypodium leucotomos as an adjuvant to PUVA therapy in
        generalized vitiligo: A pilot study. J Dermatol Sci 2006; 41(3): 213-6.
        [http://dx.doi.org/10.1016/j.jdermsci.2005.12.006] [PMID: 16423508]

[22]   Nestor MS, Berman B, Swenson N. Safety and efficacy of oral polypodium leucotomos extract in healthy adult subjects. J Clin Aesthet
        Dermatol 2015; 8(2): 19-23.
        [PMID: 25741399]

[23]   Parsad D, Pandhi R, Juneja A. Effectiveness of oral Ginkgo biloba in treating limited, slowly spreading vitiligo. Clin Exp Dermatol 2003;
        28(3): 285-7.
        [http://dx.doi.org/10.1046/j.1365-2230.2003.01207.x] [PMID: 12780716]

[24]   Szczurko O, Shear N, Taddio A, Boon H. Ginkgo biloba for the treatment of vitilgo vulgaris: an open label pilot clinical trial. BMC
        Complement Altern Med 2011; 11: 21.
        [http://dx.doi.org/10.1186/1472-6882-11-21] [PMID: 21406109]   .

[25]   Ernst E. The risk-benefit profile of commonly used herbal therapies: Ginkgo, St. Johns Wort, Ginseng, Echinacea, Saw Palmetto, and Kava.
        Ann Intern Med 2002; 136(1): 42-53.
        [http://dx.doi.org/10.7326/0003-4819-136-1-200201010-00010] [PMID: 11777363]

[26]   Hamzavi IH. BH, Isedeh PN Handbook of Vitiligo. London: JP Medical Ltd. 2016.

[27]   Wu X, Beecher GR, Holden JM, Haytowitz DB, Gebhardt SE, Prior RL. Lipophilic and hydrophilic antioxidant capacities of common foods
        in the United States. J Agric Food Chem 2004; 52(12): 4026-37.
        [http://dx.doi.org/10.1021/jf049696w] [PMID: 15186133]

[28]   Seyhan M, Erdem T, Ertekin V, Selimoğlu MA. The mucocutaneous manifestations associated with celiac disease in childhood and
        adolescence. Pediatr Dermatol 2007; 24(1): 28-33.
        [http://dx.doi.org/10.1111/j.1525-1470.2007.00328.x] [PMID: 17300645]

[29]   Seyhan M, Kandi B, Akbulut H, Selımoğlu MA, Karincaoğlu M. Is celiac disease common in patients with vitiligo? Turk J Gastroenterol
        2011; 22(1): 105-6.
        [http://dx.doi.org/10.4318/tjg.2011.0169] [PMID: 21480124]

[30]   Shahmoradi Z, Najafian J, Naeini FF, Fahimipour F. Vitiligo and autoantibodies of celiac disease. Int J Prev Med 2013; 4(2): 200-3.
        [PMID: 23543680]

[31]   Rodríguez-García C, González-Hernández S, Pérez-Robayna N, Guimerá F, Fagundo E, Sánchez R. Repigmentation of vitiligo lesions in a
        child with celiac disease after a gluten-free diet. Pediatr Dermatol 2011; 28(2): 209-10.
        [http://dx.doi.org/10.1111/j.1525-1470.2011.01388.x] [PMID: 21504457]

[32]   Khandalavala BN, Nirmalraj MC. Rapid partial repigmentation of vitiligo in a young female adult with a gluten-free diet. Case Rep Dermatol
        2014; 6(3): 283-7.
        [http://dx.doi.org/10.1159/000370303] [PMID: 25685131]

[33]   Shameer P, Prasad PV, Kaviarasan PK. Serum zinc level in vitiligo: a case control study. Indian J Dermatol Venereol Leprol 2005; 71(3):
        206-7.
        [http://dx.doi.org/10.4103/0378-6323.16243] [PMID: 16394417]

[34]   Zeng Q, Yin J, Fan F, *et al.* Decreased copper and zinc in sera of Chinese vitiligo patients: a meta-analysis. J Dermatol 2014; 41(3): 245-51.
        [http://dx.doi.org/10.1111/1346-8138.12392] [PMID: 24517587]

[35]   Mohammed GF, Gomaa AH, Al-Dhubaibi MS. Highlights in pathogenesis of vitiligo. World J Clin Cases 2015; 3(3): 221-30.
        [http://dx.doi.org/10.12998/wjcc.v3.i3.221] [PMID: 25789295]

[36]   Hassan MI, Waheed A, Yadav S, Singh TP, Ahmad F. Zinc alpha 2-glycoprotein: a multidisciplinary protein. Mol Cancer Res 2008; 6(6):
        892-906.
        [http://dx.doi.org/10.1158/1541-7786.MCR-07-2195] [PMID: 18567794]

[37]   Arora PN, Dhillon KS, Rajan SR, Sayal SK, Das AL. Serum Zinc Levels in Cutaneous Disorders. Med J Armed Forces India 2002; 58(4):
        304-6.
        [http://dx.doi.org/10.1016/S0377-1237(02)80083-1] [PMID: 27407419]

[38]   Yaghoobi R, Omidian M, Bagherani N. Original article title: Comparison of therapeutic efficacy of topical corticosteroid and oral zinc sulfate-
        topical corticosteroid combination in the treatment of vitiligo patients: a clinical trial. BMC Dermatol 2011; 11: 7.
        [http://dx.doi.org/10.1186/1471-5945-11-7] [PMID: 21453467]

[39]   Parsad D, Kanwar AJ. Topical vitamin D analogues in the treatment of vitiligo. Pigment Cell Melanoma Res 2009; 22(4): 487-8.
        [http://dx.doi.org/10.1111/j.1755-148X.2009.00579.x] [PMID: 19422605]

[40]   AlGhamdi K, Kumar A, Moussa N. The role of vitamin D in melanogenesis with an emphasis on vitiligo. Indian J Dermatol Venereol Leprol
        2013; 79(6): 750-8.
        [http://dx.doi.org/10.4103/0378-6323.120720] [PMID: 24177606]

[41]   Silverberg JI, Silverberg AI, Malka E, Silverberg NB. A pilot study assessing the role of 25 hydroxy vitamin D levels in patients with vitiligo
        vulgaris. J Am Acad Dermatol 2010; 62(6): 937-41.
        [http://dx.doi.org/10.1016/j.jaad.2009.11.024] [PMID: 20466170]

[42]   Sehrawat M, Arora TC, Chauhan A, Kar HK, Poonia A, Jairath V. Correlation of Vitamin D Levels with Pigmentation in Vitiligo Patients Treated with NBUVB Therapy. ISRN Dermatol 2014; 2014: 493213.
[http://dx.doi.org/10.1155/2014/493213] [PMID: 25006488]

[43]   Finamor DC, Sinigaglia-Coimbra R, Neves LC, *et al.* A pilot study assessing the effect of prolonged administration of high daily doses of vitamin D on the clinical course of vitiligo and psoriasis. Dermatoendocrinol 2013; 5(1): 222-34.
[http://dx.doi.org/10.4161/derm.24808] [PMID: 24494059]

[44]   Reddy KK, Gilchrest BA. Iatrogenic effects of photoprotection recommendations on skin cancer development, vitamin D levels, and general health. Clin Dermatol 2011; 29(6): 644-51.
[http://dx.doi.org/10.1016/j.clindermatol.2011.08.027] [PMID: 22014986]

[45]   Holick MF. Vitamin D deficiency. N Engl J Med 2007; 357(3): 266-81.
[http://dx.doi.org/10.1056/NEJMra070553] [PMID: 17634462]

[46]   Chen YJ, Chen YY, Wu CY, Chi CC. Oral Chinese herbal medicine in combination with phototherapy for vitiligo: A systematic review and meta-analysis of randomized controlled trials. Complement Ther Med 2016; 26: 21-7.
[http://dx.doi.org/10.1016/j.ctim.2016.02.009] [PMID: 27261977]

[47]   Recommendations N. Nutrient Recommendations: Dietary Reference Intakes (DRI): U.S. Department of Health and Human Services; [Available from: https://ods.od.nih.gov/Health_Information/Dietary_Reference_Intakes.aspx 2016.

15

The Role of Dermoscopy in Assessment of the Activity and Scarring Response in Discoid Lupus Erythematosus

Khitam Al-Refu[*]

Department of Internal Medicine, Mutah University, Karak, Jordan

Abstract:

Background:

The diagnosis of Discoid Lupus Erythematosus (DLE) is usually made by clinical examination and by histopathology. Recently, dermoscopy has become an integral part in diagnoses of many inflammatory disorders and one of these is DLE.

Aims:

This research emphasizes the utility of dermoscopy in the assessing lesions of DLE from the point of activity of the disease.

Patients and Methods:

Thirty-one patients diagnosed with DLE were included in this study. The total number of examined lesions was 125 lesions. All of the lesions were assessed by dermoscopy at different stages of the activity of the diseases.

Results:

The dermoscopic features of DLE vary according to the stage of activity of the disease. There are characteristic dermoscopic features for the lesions of the scalp different from that of the body. In the active and early phase, the most common dermoscopic features were the presence of lesional and perilesional scales, follicular keratotic plugging, telangiectasia, arborized blood vessels, follicular red dots and perifollicular scales. In addition, there are less common dermoscopic features such as pigmentary changes, white rosettes and pinpoint white dots. For active scalp lesions, the follicular plugging and perifollicular scales were more prominent than that of the body DLE lesions. For inactive and late DLE lesions, the most significant dermoscopic changes were perifollicular whitish halos, variable patchy whitish hypopigmented areas, and the presence of white colored structureless areas.

Conclusion:

The present study provides new insights into the dermoscopic variability of DLE lesions at different levels of activity.

Keywords: Discoid lupus erythematosus, Dermoscopy, Lesions, Perifollicular, Papule, Scarring.

1. INTRODUCTION

Discoid Lupus Erythematosus (DLE) is the chronic form of the cutaneous type of lupus erythematosus [1]. It represents the most common subtype of cutaneous lupus erythematosus, and commonly affected females [2]. It may occur at any age, but most frequently at middle age. This is a scarring disease that can cause permanent scarring if treatment is inadequate or ineffective. Patients with DLE are often divided into two subtypes: localized (lesions occur only on the head or neck) and generalized (occurs below the chin with or without lesions present above this level). Clinically, the DLE patients present with a fairly defined, erythematous patches and plaques with adherent scale. Early

[*] Address Correspondence to this author at the Department of Internal Medicine, Mutah University, Karak, Jordan; Tel: 00962797401149; E-mail: alrefukhi@yahoo.com

lesions present as a well-demarcated round or oval purplish macule or papule with little scaling. By the time, some of these lesions progress to annular lesions that enlarge into a patch with follicular plugging, erythema, and adherent scaling. The old and end-stage disease is characterized by fibrotic and atrophic patches that may be hypo- or hyperpigmented without follicular ostia. Scarring alopecia occurs in the scalp and other hairy areas in about one-third of patients and is usually permanent [3, 4]. The diagnosis is based on direct immunofluorescence, and histopathology [5]. By histopathology, early DLE showed prominent perivascular and periadnexal lymphohistiocytic, an interface dermatitis, basal layer degeneration, and marked thickening of the basement membrane. In well-established lesions, there may be marked follicular plugging and acanthosis.

Recently, dermoscopy has become an integral part of diagnosing many inflammatory disorders [6] and one of these is DLE. It is very helpful in the diagnosis of various general dermatological disorders, including scalp/hair diseases [7]. It has been shown to be an effective tool to differentiate the scalp DLE from other causes of scarring alopecia such as lichen planopilaris [8]. In addition, there were reports [9 - 14] documented specific dermoscopic features of DLE in other locations, such as the face. These features included follicular plugging, telangiectasias, arborizing vessels, honeycomb pigmented network, variable scaling, and perifollicular whitish halo. Also, rosettes and structure-less white and brown areas have been reported by others [13, 14]. All of the previous dermoscopic features were correlated well with histopathological findings.

This research emphasizes the utility of dermoscopy in the assessing lesions of DLE at different stages of activity. Dermoscopy may be a good tool in assessing the lesions of DLE at different stages of the activity of the disease (active and new lesions, active edge of old or new lesions, perilesional skin, and old scarred lesions.). In addition, it will be a good way to follow up the patients with DLE and to assess the response to treatment. Patients with discoid lupus erythematosus diagnosed initially by histopathology and immunofluorescence, and they are followed up and assessed subjectively by clinical features. Dermoscopy may help in making follow up for these cases by objective means looking for features of activity of the disease. In addition, the previous reports published on dermoscopy of DLE lesions in the past few years, have been mainly carried on western countries and Indian population. The patients of the study were from Jordan (one of the Arab Middle East countries).

2. PATIENTS AND METHODS

This was an out-patient clinic-based study done in dermatology clinics (Mutah University Medical Center, Jordan) from January 2015 to April 2018. The ethical committee approved the study protocol. Informed consent was obtained from the patients before enrolment in the study.

All patients diagnosed with discoid lupus erythematosus (based on clinical, physical and histopathological examinations) were included in this study. All DLE lesions located on the scalp, face, trunk, and extremities were examined by dermoscopy. The intention was to examine DLE lesions at a different stage of activities: active and new lesions, active edge of old or new lesions, perilesional skin, and old scarred lesions. A dermoscopic examination of all cases was performed using a hand-held dermoscope (Dermlite DL3, Gen, USA) application which captured images with iPhone, and then was evaluated as saved photos on a computer screen. This dermoscopy can block light reflection from the skin surface without immersion gels or alcohol. The Characteristics and specifications of the DermLiteDL3 dermoscope used in the study were 20x and 40x magnification with focusing optics. The dates and times of capturing photos were automatically stored. Selection of the dermoscopic variables included in the evaluation process was based on data in the available literature on DLE of the scalp and our preliminary observations.

3. RESULTS

Thirty-one patients diagnosed with DLE were included in this study. All of the patients were diagnosed clinically and confirmed by histopathological means (Fig. 1). Four of the cases were males with a mean age of 34 years. The females were with a mean age of 28 years. Two of the cases (males) had exclusive scalp involvement. 29 of cases had mixed scalp and body involvement by discoid lesions. Three cases (females) has generalized DLE. The total number of examined lesions by dermoscopy was 125 lesions from 31 patients. The clinical data were summarized in Table 1.

All of the DLE lesions were assessed clinically and dermoscopically at different stages of the activity of the diseases (active and new lesions, active edge of old or new lesions, perilesional skin, and old scarred lesions). Clinically, the active DLE lesions of the scalp were characterized clinically by being indurated erythematous plaques with slight scales. These scales were mild, adherent, and some were perifollicular. Follicular plugging was a common finding in most of the scalp lesions; these plugs were more pigmented in patients with skin type IV. The marginal skin was indurated and erythematous. The perilesional skin was slightly more erythematous. Older lesions in the scalp were scarred with central loss of pigmentation (white patches), atrophic, and with loss of hair ostium. Some of the edges of plaques showed marginal hyperpigmentation especially in older lesions (Fig. 2).

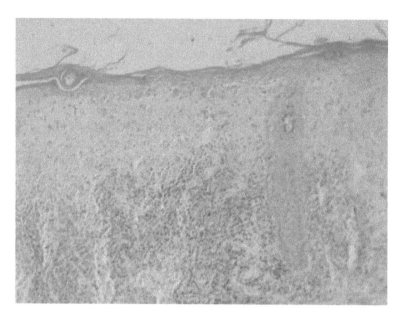

Fig. (1). DLE section shows hyperkeratosis, follicular plugging, epidermal atrophy and patchy superficial and deep perivascular and perifollicular lymphoid cell infiltrate.

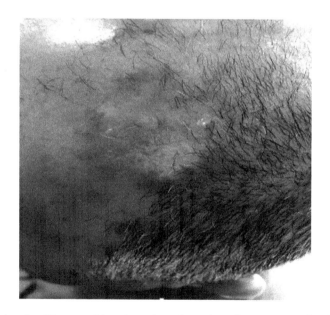

Fig. (2). DLE lesion of a scalp of a 38 -year-old male patient showed erythematous patch; there is central atrophy (hypopigmentation), the active edge is more dark and hyper-pigmented than the surrounding skin.

Table 1. Characteristic features of the DLE patients.

	Clinical Data	
1.	Number of the patients	31 patients
2.	Sex	4 males and 27 females
3.	The mean age	males (34 years) females (28 years)

(Table 1) contd.....

4.	The clinical types of DLE	Two cases had exclusive scalp lesions 29 cases had mixed scalp and body DLE lesions
5.	The total number of examined DLE lesions	125 lesions were examined by dermoscopy
6.	The scalp DLE lesions	56 were active lesions 13 were old and inactive lesions
7.	DLE lesions on the body	40 were active lesions 16 were old and inactive scarred lesions

Similarly, the presentation of active lesions of the DLE of the body (including face, trunk, and extremities) was as an erythematous papule or plaques with slight-to-moderate scales (Fig. **3a**). Some of the lesions showed more thickened and adherent scales. The active edges were more indurated and erythematous compared to the perilesional skin which also showed some erythema. The older lesions were atrophic and sclerotic. These burnt-out DLE lesions were commonly hyperpigmented (Fig. **3b**).

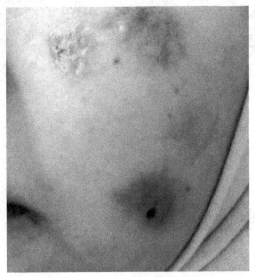

Fig. (3a). Active DLE lesion on a cheek of a female patient showed well-demarcated erythematous plaque with scales.

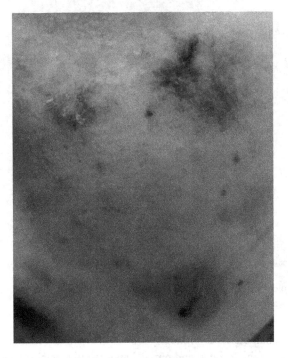

Fig. (3b). An old lesions on a face of a patient, the skin looks atrophic and hyperpigmented.

Dermoscopically, the presence of keratotic follicular plugging was a common finding especially in active and early DLE lesions of the scalp; they have been seen in 52 lesions (93%) of DLE. They have been observed in active DLE lesions from the face and trunk but to a lesser degree (22 lesions (55%)). These keratotic plugs appeared as dark yellow-brown dots and were very numerous from scalp lesions compared to these from face or trunk (Fig. **4**). These follicular pluggings have been seen uncommonly in four old inactive scalp DLE lesions (31%) and two inactive lesions facial lesions (13%). For older lesions, these follicular plugging was replaced with follicular whitish halo (Fig. **5**) with lost hair ostium and loss of follicular opening. This had been observed in all old scarred lesions from the scalp and body and occasionally from 6 active lesions of the scalp (11%) and four lesions from the trunk (11%).

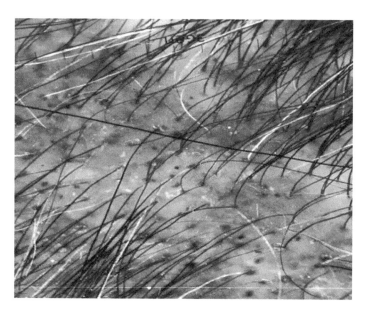

Fig. (4). A dermoscopy view of an early active DLE lesions showed prominent follicular plugging, with diffuse patchy honeycomb pigmentation. In addition, there are no prominent scars.

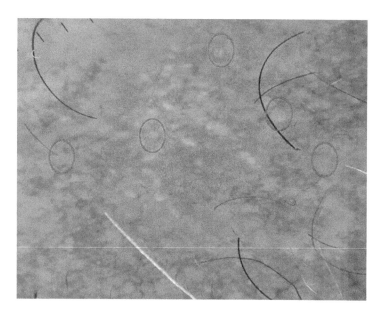

Fig. (5). A dermoscopy view for an old DLE lesion from the frontal area of a scalp of DLE patient showed multiple whitish follicular halos (blue circles) in a whitish (scar) and erythematous back ground.

Clinically the active DLE characterized clinically as erythematous lesions, and this has been observed dermoscopically by the abundance of the lesional and perilesional telangiectasia and thick branching blood vessels (Fig. **6**). This has been seen in 50 active DLE lesions of the scalp (89%), and with similar frequency from 38 lesions from face and trunk (95%). Even in old and scarred lesions, these arborized blood vessels have been seen but at a lesser degree and more blurred (60% of the scalp and 50% from the face and trunk).

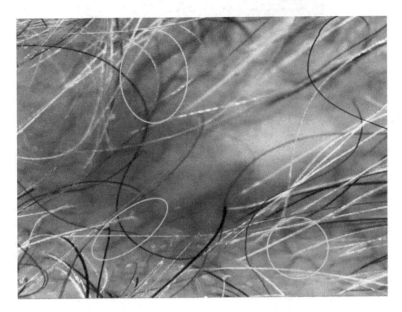

Fig. (6). A dermoscopy view showed thick arborized blood vessels (surrounded by yellow circles) was prominent within the lesions of DLE of the scalp lesion of a patient.

It has been common to see the scaling in new and active lesions, these have been diffuse within the plaques of DLE (Fig. **7a**). This was seen in all new active lesions of the scalp, face and truncal lesions. The active edges also demonstrated these scaling and in the perilesional skin. For old and inactive lesions, these scales were seen only in perilesional skin and at the active edge. Particularly, in the active scalp lesions, some hair follicular demonstrated perifollicular scaling (42 lesions (75%)), these were occasionally seen from nine lesions of body DLE (23%) (Fig. **7b**).

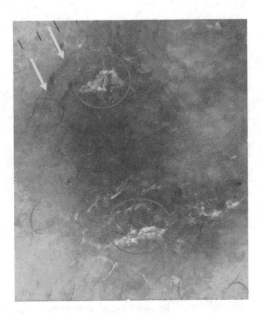

Fig. (7a). Dermoscopy of an early active DLE, showed erythematous plaque, with prominent branching blood vessels at the active edge of the lesion (yellow arrows), variable scaling (red circles).

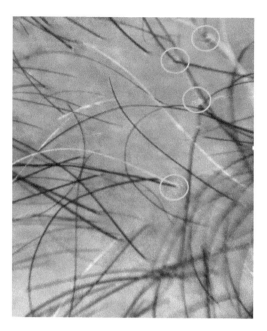

Fig. (7b). An early active DLE of the scalp showed perifollicular scaling (yellow circles).

Follicular red dots were a common finding in active DLE; it has been seen in 37 lesions (66%) and 70% of facial lesions (12 lesions). They appear as an erythematous and concentric structure around the hair follicle (Fig. **8**). These are non-exclusive in new lesions; as has been in some scarred lesions (6 lesions from the scalp and body).

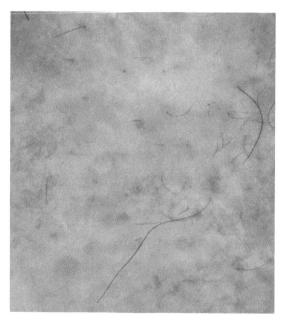

Fig. (8). Concentric erythema around hair follicles in facial DLE lesion.

Pin-point white dots (Fig. **9**) were another common dermoscopic features; they are white dots distributed throughout the plaques of DLE lesions between hair follicles. This was a common finding in 37 active scalp lesions (66%) and 28 body lesions (70%). They appear smaller than these of whitish halos which surrounded the hair follicles. In addition, it has been seen in the perilesional skin of some old DLE lesions of the scalp (38%) and facial skin (38%).

White rosettes were another but uncommon dermoscopic features in the patients of the study. These were shiny white structures seen as four oval-shaped points that come together in the center. They had been observed in only three active lesions of scalp DLE but was more common from DLE of the trunk and face (10 lesions). They have also been seen even in old hyperpigmented lesions especially in old scarred lesion especially from the trunk (4 lesions) (Fig. **10**).

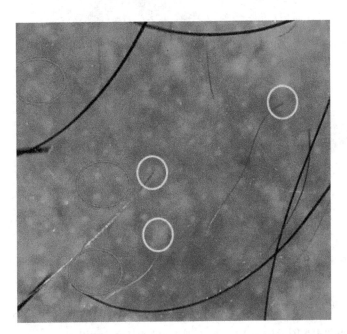

Fig. (9). Prominent pin-point white dots as shown by blue circles and perifollicular hypopigmentation in active DLE lesions (yellow circles).

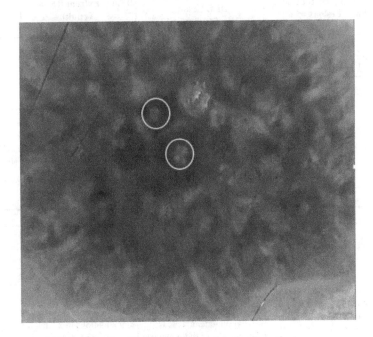

Fig. (10). White rosette (yellow circle) in an inactive DLE lesion from a trunk of a patient.

Pigmentary changes (Fig. **11**) in DLE lesions were common, especially in old inactive lesions. Patchy honey comp pigmentations were seen in 19 active scalp lesions (34%). Perifollicular hyperpigmentation was seen in 8 active scalp DLE lesions (14%). Regarding the old and scarred lesions, the most characteristic finding was follicular whitish halo and variable patchy whitish hypopigmented areas. The margin of these plaques was hyperpigmented. Similar pigmentary changes were recorded from active DLE of the face and trunk as scattered dark-brown pigmentations in active lesions (55%). Old lesions of body DLE (16 lesions) characterized by the presence of white colored structureless areas, hyperpigmentation in the form of a honeycomb network, and blurred telangiectasia. These dermoscopic features were seen characteristically in all old discoid lupus erythematous lesions.

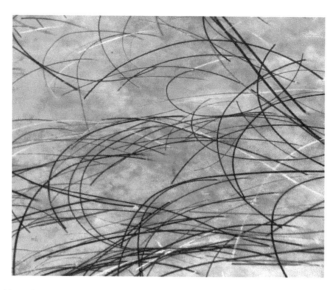

Fig. (11). Dermoscopy of an old scalp DLE lesions showed prominent whitish fibrosed areas (White and milky red areas) lacking follicular openings.

Table **2** summarized all of these dermoscopic features in active and old scarred DLE lesions.

Table 2. Dermoscopic features in 125 DLE lesions (scalp, face, trunk and extremities)

Dermoscopic Feature	Active Scalp DLE Lesions No of Lesions =56	Inactive and Old Scalp DLE Lesions No of Lesions =13	Active DLE Lesions (Face, Extremities, and Trunk) NO of Lesions =40	Inactive and Old DLE Lesions (Face, Extremities, and Trunk) No of Lesions =16
Follicular keratotic plug	52/56 (93%) Vey numerous, yellow-dark brown	4/13 (31%) Few in numbers, more keratotic	22/40 (55%) Numerous, Yellow in color	2/16 (13%) Few in numbers, more keratotic
Follicular whitish halo	6/56 (11%) Very few	13/13 (100%) Numerous	7/40 (11%) Very few	16/16 (100%) Numerous
Telangiectasia and arborized blood vessels	50/56 (89%) Lesional and perilesional	8/13 (60%) The blood vessels and telangiectasia more blurred	38/40 (95%) Lesional and perilesional	8/16 (50%) The blood vessels and telangiectasia more blurred
Scales	All of lesions (lesional and perilesional)	prominent at the active edge of all lesions	All of lesions (lesional and perilesional)	prominent at the active edge of all lesions
Perifollicular scales	42/56 (75%)	Occasional One case	9/40 (23%)	None of the cases
Follicular red dots	37/56 (66%)	3 lesions (23%)	28/40 (70%)	3 lesions (19%)
Pin-point white dots	34/56 (61%) In the lesional and perilesional skin	5 (38%) In the perilesional skin	28 (70%) In the lesional and perilesional skin	6 (38%) In the perilesional skin
White rosettes	3/56 (5%)	1 lesion (8%)	10/40 (25%)	6 (38%)
Pigmentary changes	Patchy honey comp pigmentations were seen in 19 lesions (34%). Perifollicular hyperpigmentation was seen in 8 lesions (14%).	Follicular whitish halo, Variable patchy whitish hypopigmented areas. The margin of these plaques was hyperpigmented.	Scattered dark-brown pigmentations in 22 active lesions (55%)	Presence of white colored structureless areas, Hyperpigmentation in the form of a honeycomb network,

4. DISCUSSION

DLE is a chronic inflammatory disease with liability to scar formation. The lesions of DLE develop initially as erythematous-to-violaceous, inflamed papules and patches with crusting and scaling appearance. Follicular plugging is a common feature in these early and active lesions. Later on, the center of these patches or plaques may appear lighter in color, that often results in scarring and atrophy with an edge darker than the normal skin. When lesions occur in hairy areas such as the scalp or beard area, permanent scarring and hair loss can occur.

Early recognition and treatment improve the prognosis [15]. This current report documents the dermoscopic features in DLE at different stages of disease activity. The aim was to describe dermoscopic criteria observed in a series of patients with DLE had their lesions on the scalp and body, at active and inactive disease activity. The patients of the study were from Jordan (one of the Arab Middle East countries). The skin type of the patients of the study was mainly with a Fitzpatrick skin type of III and IV. The previous reports published on dermoscopy of DLE lesions have been mainly carried on western countries and Indian population.

Thirty-one patient with DLE (diagnosed clinically and by histopathology) were examined by dermoscopy. The total number of the lesions was 125 (including active, inactive and old scarred lesions from scalp and body (trunk and extremities)). Clinically, active and new lesions from the scalp and body look similar. All lesions were erythematous and indurated plaques. Scales were prominent in the lesional and perilesional skin and mainly perifollicular in scalp lesions. In addition, follicular plugging was a common finding in lesions from the scalp and hairy areas; they are darker in patients with skin type IV than those of type III. Older lesions in all sites were scarred with central loss of pigmentation (white patches), atrophic, and with loss of hair ostium. The marginal skin was indurated and erythematous. In addition, some lesions showed hyperpigmented pigmentary changes that developed within the old scarred patches and at the active borders.

The dermoscopic features in DLE vary according to the stage of activity of the disease. In addition, there are characteristic dermoscopic features for the lesions of the scalp. The results showed that different dermoscopic features were seen according to the localization of DLE lesions, disease duration and the activity of the disease. In the active and early phase, the most common dermoscopic features were the presence of lesional and perilesional scales, follicular keratotic plugging, telangiectasia and arborized blood vessels, follicular red dots and perifollicular scales. In addition, there are less common dermoscopic features such as pigmentary changes, white rosettes and pinpoint white dots. For active scalp lesions, the follicular plugging and perifollicular scales were more prominent than that of the body DLE lesions. For inactive and late DLE lesions, the most significant dermoscopic changes were perifollicular whitish halos, variable patchy whitish hypopigmented areas and the presence of white colored structureless areas. The active edge of these latent lesions showed blurred telangiectasias and marginal hyperpigmentation.

The most common dermoscopic features for early and active DLE lesions was the presence of scales (lesional and perilesional skin). This was a common feature for all DLE lesions from the scalp and body. For old and inactive DLE lesions, these scales were localized at the active edge and perilesional skin. The presence of the scales at the perifollicular areas was a common and characteristic feature for active DLE from the scalp; it had been seen in two-thirds of cases compared to active lesions from face and body which had been seen in 23% of cases. In addition, this perifollicular scaling was absent from all inactive and old lesions of DLE from the scalp or body; so it can be considered as a sign of activity of the disease.

Follicular plugging was another common and important dermoscopic features of DLE lesions from the scalp (93%) of lesions. They were numerous and yellow to dark brown in color. It has been observed but to a lesser degree from the facial and body lesions (55%). Follicular keratotic plugs were considered as a marker of DLE [16] and correlate with the hyperkeratosis and plugging of the follicular ostia with a keratotic material. And this is expected in a disease like DLE in which the process of inflammation targets the skin and follicular structures [17]. For old and inactive lesions from the scalp and body, the follicular plugging was uncommon finding. They have been replaced by fibrosis and this was seen dermoscopically as follicular whitish halos which has been seen in all of inactive and scarred DLE lesions from the scalp and body and occasionally in inactive lesions (11%). The presence of these halos can be considered as a characteristic feature for a late and inactive disease.

Characteristically, the active lesions of DLE are erythematous one, even for late and inactive lesions. The margins are red and the perilesional skin more erythematous than uninvolved skin. This was visualized dermoscopically in all lesions as lesional and perilesional telangiectasia with the presence of thick arborizing vessels even at the margin of old and late lesions. These vessels are significantly wider than that of arborizing vessels in the normal scalp or seborrheic dermatitis [18, 19]. These vessels were seen similarly in indistinguishable from those in basal cell carcinoma. This vascular network, which is visible through the thinned atrophic epidermis may explain the milky red (pink) fibrosis that seen in DLE fibrotic lesions and not as an ivory white, as in most other types of cicatricial alopecia. This results from the vascular network, which is visible through the thinned atrophic epidermis [19].

A novel dermoscopic feature observed in DLE by Tosti *et al.* [12]. was a red follicular pattern and was considered as a specific feature of scalp lesions of active lupus erythematosus of the scalp. These dots correspond to widened infundibula with dense perivascular lymphocytic in filtrates, dilated vessels, and extravasated erythrocytes [11, 20]. The loss of this pattern in DLE may be a sign of hair follicle damage with poor prognosis [20]. Recognition of this distinctive dermoscopic pattern may help the clinician to differentiate DLE from other diseases causing cicatricial alopecia [12] This has been in the patients of this study as multiple red dots, which are regularly distributed in and around the follicular ostia. This has been seen nearly in two third of active lesions of DLE from the scalp and body. It was seen uncommonly in few inactive lesions. Their presence in these old lesions may be associated with a good prognostic factor for hair regrowth [12].

Another feature was seen in active DLE lesions of this study was the presence of dark-brown discoloration of the skin in both DLE lesions from the scalp and body. The localization and distribution of melanin and haemoglobin pigment in skin layers reflect these characteristic patterns of altered pigmentation which is visualized using dermoscopy [21]. This finding corresponds to pigment incontinence on histopathology [22]. Dark brown to blue-grey pigment pattern is seen in DLE affecting the interfollicular area unlike in LPP where it is concentrated around the follicles. For longstanding inactive DLE lesions, the prominent pigmentary change was the presence of presence of structureless pink or white areas and follicular whitish halos. The hyperpigmentation was seen mainly at the advancing active edges.

A new report of white rosettes in discoid lupus erythematosus has been reported recently [13]. They are shiny white points seen under polarized dermoscopy. They vary in size from 0.2 mm to 0.5 mm, and they can be oriented in the same or in different angulations [23]. Many authors believe that it is due to the optical effect of polarized light. It is postulated that rosettes are formed by narrowing of infundibula or blockage by keratin [24]. Others suggested that rosettes correspond to an alternating focal hyperkeratosis and normal corneal layer and keratin-filled acrosyringeal openings. These rosettes were occasionally seen in this study; only a few lesions of active DLE lesions, but seen more in old and latent DLE lesions of the body (38%). The rosettes may be may be attributed to concentric perifollicular fibrosis. White rosettes are not specific dermoscopic patterns to any particular condition as has been seen in other types of scarring alopecia and skin diseases [23, 24]. In addition to these whitish rosettes, there were pin-point whitish dots distributed through the lesional and perilesional DLE patches and plaques. They have been seen in all lesions but to a lesser degree than latent lesions. These represent the opening of eccrine glands and are not specific for DLE as has been described in other types of scarring alopecia and in normal scalp [25, 26], so they are not specific for DLE nor the activity of the disease.

The above dermoscopic features of DLE lesions may reflect the dynamic process of the disease its self. There were specific features indicated the activity of the disease and were seen to a lesser degree as the disease became more late and inactive. There were some features that can be considered as specific if combined with other dermoscopic features such as the presence of keratotic follicular plugging and erythematous follicular dots within a background of lesional telangiectasia and scales. Some of the dermoscopic features were not specific such as rosettes sign and pinpoint white dots. Presence of perifollicular white halos may be an impending sign of progression of the disease to a fibrosis and scar formation. The present study provides new insights into the dermoscopic variability of DLE located on the face, trunk, and extremities at different levels of activity of the disease.

HUMAN AND ANIMAL RIGHTS

No Animals were used in this research. All human research procedures followed were in accordance with the ethical standards of the committee responsible for human experimentation (institutional and national), and with the Helsinki Declaration of 1975, as revised in 2013.

CONFLICT OF INTEREST

The authors declare no conflict of interest, financial or otherwise.

ACKNOWLEDGEMENTS

Declared none.

REFERENCES

[1]   Gilliam JN, Sontheimer RD. Distinctive cutaneous subsets in the spectrum of lupus erythematosus. J Am Acad Dermatol 1981; 4(4): 471-5.
        [http://dx.doi.org/10.1016/S0190-9622(81)80261-7] [PMID: 7229150]

[2]   Walling HW, Sontheimer RD. Cutaneous lupus erythematosus: Issues in diagnosis and treatment. Am J Clin Dermatol 2009; 10(6): 365-81.
        [http://dx.doi.org/10.2165/11310780-000000000-00000] [PMID: 19824738]

[3]   Wilson CL, Burge SM, Dean D, Dawber RP. Scarring alopecia in discoid lupus erythematosus. Br J Dermatol 1992; 126(4): 307-14.
        [http://dx.doi.org/10.1111/j.1365-2133.1992.tb00670.x] [PMID: 1373948]

[4]   Al-Refu K, Goodfield M. Scar classification in cutaneous lupus erythematosus: Morphological description. Br J Dermatol 2009; 161(5):
        1052-8.
        [http://dx.doi.org/10.1111/j.1365-2133.2009.09313.x] [PMID: 19624543]

[5]   Bharti S, Dogra S, Saikia B, Walker RM, Chhabra S, Saikia UN. Immunofluorescence profile of discoid lupus erythematosus. Indian J Pathol
        Microbiol 2015; 58(4): 479-82.
        [http://dx.doi.org/10.4103/0377-4929.168850] [PMID: 26549071]

[6]   Errichetti E, Stinco G. The practical usefulness of dermoscopy in general dermatology. G Ital Dermatol Venereol 2015; 150(5): 533-46.
        [PMID: 26086412]

[7]   Miteva M, Tosti A. Hair and scalp dermatoscopy. J Am Acad Dermatol 2012; 67(5): 1040-8.
        [http://dx.doi.org/10.1016/j.jaad.2012.02.013] [PMID: 22405573]

[8]   Duque-Estrada B, Tamler C, Sodré CT, Barcaui CB, Pereira FB. Dermoscopy patterns of cicatricial alopecia resulting from discoid lupus
        erythematosus and lichen planopilaris. An Bras Dermatol 2010; 85(2): 179-83.
        [PMID: 20520933]

[9]   Lallas A, Apalla Z, Lefaki I, et al. Dermoscopy of discoid lupus erythematosus. Br J Dermatol 2013; 168(2): 284-8.
        [http://dx.doi.org/10.1111/bjd.12044] [PMID: 22985425]

[10]   Jha AK, Sonthalia S, Sarkar R. Dermoscopy of discoid lupus erythematosus. Indian Dermatol Online J 2016; 7(5): 458.
        [http://dx.doi.org/10.4103/2229-5178.190493] [PMID: 27730061]

[11]   Lopez-Tintos BO, Garcia-Hidalgo L, Orozco-Topete R. Dermoscopy in active discoid lupus. Arch Dermatol 2009; 145(3): 358.
        [http://dx.doi.org/10.1001/archdermatol.2008.585] [PMID: 19289790]

[12]   Tosti A, Torres F, Misciali C, et al. Follicular red dots: A novel dermoscopic pattern observed in scalp discoid lupus erythematosus. Arch
        Dermatol 2009; 145(12): 1406-9.
        [http://dx.doi.org/10.1001/archdermatol.2009.277] [PMID: 20026850]

[13]   Ankad BS, Shah SD, Adya KA. White rosettes in discoid lupus erythematosus: A new dermoscopic observation. Dermatol Pract Concept
        2017; 7(4): 9-11.
        [http://dx.doi.org/10.5826/dpc.0704a03] [PMID: 29214102]

[14]   Liebman TN, Rabinovitz HS, Dusza SW, Marghoob AA. White shiny structures: Dermoscopic features revealed under polarized light. J Eur
        Acad Dermatol Venereol 2012; 26(12): 1493-7.
        [PMID: 22035217]

[15]   Panjwani S. Early diagnosis and treatment of discoid lupus erythematosus. J Am Board Fam Med 2009; 22(2): 206-13.
        [http://dx.doi.org/10.3122/jabfm.2009.02.080075] [PMID: 19264946]

[16]   Lanuti E, Miteva M, Romanelli P, Tosti A. Trichoscopy and histopathology of follicular keratotic plugs in scalp discoid lupus erythematosus.
        Int J Trichology 2012; 4(1): 36-8.
        [http://dx.doi.org/10.4103/0974-7753.96087] [PMID: 22628989]

[17]   Rudnicka L. Atlas of Trichoscopy: Dermoscopy in Hair and Scalp Disease. Springer London Heidelberg New York Dordrecht 2012.
        [http://dx.doi.org/10.1007/978-1-4471-4486-1]

[18]   Rakowska A, Slowinska M, Kowalska-Oledzka E, et al. Trichoscopy of cicatricial alopecia. J Drugs Dermatol 2012; 11(6): 753-8.
        [PMID: 22648224]

[19]   Rudnicka L, Olszewska M, Rakowska A, Slowinska M. Trichoscopy update 2011. J Dermatol Case Rep 2011; 5(4): 82-8.
        [http://dx.doi.org/10.3315/jdcr.2011.1083] [PMID: 22408709]

[20]   Pirmez R, Piñeiro-Maceira J, Almeida BC, Sodré CT. Follicular red dots: A normal trichoscopy feature in patients with pigmentary disorders?
        An Bras Dermatol 2013; 88(3): 459-61.
        [http://dx.doi.org/10.1590/abd1806-4841.20132555] [PMID: 23793216]

[21]   Bowling J. Non-melanocytic lesionsBowling J (ed), Diagnostic dermoscopy- The illustrated guide (2012) 1st edition West Sussex: Wiley-
        Blackwell. 59-91.

[22]   Khadatkar AS, Ghodake NB. Trichoscopic findings in cicatricial alopecias and hair shaft disorders and its application in histopathology. Int J
        Res Med Science 2017; 5(12): 5254.
        [http://dx.doi.org/10.18203/2320-6012.ijrms20175435]

[23]   González-Álvarez T, Armengot-Carbó M, Barreiro A, et al. Dermoscopic rosettes as a clue for pigmented incipient melanoma. Dermatology

(Basel) 2014; 228(1): 31-3.
[http://dx.doi.org/10.1159/000356822] [PMID: 24356536]

[24]   Haspeslagh M, Noë M, De Wispelaere I, *et al.* Rosettes and other white shiny structures in polarized dermoscopy: Histological correlate and optical explanation. J Eur Acad Dermatol Venereol 2016; 30(2): 311-3.
[http://dx.doi.org/10.1111/jdv.13080] [PMID: 25786770]

[25]   Kossard S, Zagarella S. Spotted cicatricial alopecia in dark skin. A dermoscopic clue to fibrous tracts. Australas J Dermatol 1993; 34(2): 49-51.
[http://dx.doi.org/10.1111/j.1440-0960.1993.tb00856.x] [PMID: 8311827]

[26]   Abraham LS, Piñeiro-Maceira J, Duque-Estrada B, Barcaui CB, Sodré CT. Pinpoint white dots in the scalp: Dermoscopic and histopathologic correlation. J Am Acad Dermatol 2010; 63(4): 721-2.
[http://dx.doi.org/10.1016/j.jaad.2009.12.011] [PMID: 20846575]

16

A Review of Prevalent Methods for Automatic Skin Lesion Diagnosis

Damilola A Okuboyejo* and Oludayo O Olugbara

ICT and Society Research Group, Durban University of Technology, Durban, South Africa

Abstract:

Background:

Skin cancer has been reported to be one of the most predominant forms of cancer diseases, especially amongst Caucasian descendant and light-skinned people. In particular, the melanocytic skin lesion has been judged to be the most deadly amongst three prevalent skin cancer diseases and the second most common form amongst young adults ranging from 15-29 years of age. These concerns have propelled the need to provide automated systems for medical diagnosis of skin cancer diseases within a strict time window towards reducing the unnecessary biopsy, increasing the speed of diagnosis and providing reproducibility of diagnostic results.

Objective:

This paper is aimed at using a comparative analysis method to review and compare the existing novel approaches for automating the diagnostic procedures of melanocytic skin lesion, including their success and shortcomings. This task is particularly valuable for decision makers to consider tradeoffs inaccuracy of diagnostic procedure versus complexity.

Methods:

A comparative study was carried out on selected literature from different accessible digital libraries of skin lesion research, especially cancerous moles in regard to the convention used, assumptions made, success recorded and noticeable gaps that need to be adequately filled by further study.

Conclusion:

Image standardization should be embraced in the medical research community to ensure the reproducibility of findings. Moreover, efforts should be made to have a large image library of varying skin lesion samples with categories based on lesion types and making these accessible to researchers to ensure proper benchmarking of research results.

Keywords: Computer-assisted dermoscopy, Skin lesion segmentation, Pattern recognition, Remote health diagnosis, Medical image analysis, Computational intelligence, Melanoma skin disease, Automated diagnosis.

1. INTRODUCTION

Skin cancer has been reported to be one of the most predominant forms of cancer disease, especially amongst the Caucasian descendant and light-skinned people. In particular, the melanoma has been judged to be the most deadly form of skin cancer among the three prevalent skin cancer diseases and equally adjudicated as the fifth most common cancer occurring among males, seventh most commonly occurring form of cancer diseases in females and second most common form of cancer diseases amongst young adults ranging from 15-29 years of age. These concerns have compelled the need to provide medical diagnosis within a very strict time frame through the application of advances in telecommunications-based services. Moreover, this application has been geared towards reducing unnecessary biopsy, increasing the speed of diagnosis and providing reproducibility of diagnostic results.

* Address correspondence to this author at the ICT and Society Research Group, Durban University of Technology, P.O. Box 1334, 4000, Durban, South Africa; E-mail: d.okuboyejo@gmail.com

This study reviews the state-of-the-art approaches for achieving an automated skin lesion image diagnosis. Section 2 provides an overview of the anatomy of the skin in relation to the focus of the paper. The analysis of medical imaging in fostering a good decision-making process for skin diagnosis is discussed in Section 3. The computer-aided diagnostic system for the development of automated skin lesion diagnosis process is illustrated in Section 4. Current and state-of-the-art skin lesion diagnostic methods for assisting the diagnosis of melanocytic lesions are reviewed in Section 5. Homogenous skin lesion diagnostic procedures frequently used in the research community are comprehensively discussed in Section 6. We conclude our findings with the proposed recommendation in Section 7.

2. HUMAN SKIN

The surface of human skin is a detailed landscape with complex geometry and local optical properties. The skin is the largest organ of the human body and consists of three principal layers which are the epidermis (see **2.1 Epidermis**), the dermis (see **2.2 Dermis**) and the subcutaneous layer (see **2.3 Subcutaneous**). Skin features depend heavily on many essential variables such as body location (forehead or cheek), subject parameters (age or gender), imaging parameters (lighting or camera) and the direction from which it is viewed and illuminated. Bacterial and viral skin infections generally affect the human skin by decolourizing and distorting the pigmented skin areas which make the automation of medical image analysis difficult [1].

2.1. Epidermis

The epidermis is a layered scale-like tissue which serves as a protection against external belligerences (extreme radiation, wounds and contaminations). The epidermis consists of four types of cells, which are Keratinocytes, Melanocytes, Langerhans and Merkel cells.

2.2. Dermis

The dermis is composed of collagen and elastic fibres. The dermis has two primary sub-layers which are the Papillary dermis (thin layer) that acts as a glue to hold the epidermis, and the dermis and Reticular dermis (thick layer) that supplies energy and nutrition to the epidermis. It contains nerve endings, sweat glands, hair follicles, blood vessels and lymph vessels. In addition, it is responsible for healing and sense of touch.

2.3. Subcutaneous

The subcutaneous layer is responsible for supplying nutrients to the other two layers. The subcutis, being made of made of fat and connective tissue that helps to cushion and insulate the body.

3. MEDICAL IMAGING OF THE SKIN

The principal aim of image analysis is to use image processing techniques to provide a machine interpretation of an image, typically in a format that could foster effective decision-making process. Interestingly, while the merit of medical imaging is getting popular, the World Health Organization (WHO) reported in one of its findings that three quarters of the entire world population is yet to have access to medical imaging, which is an essential technique in the new age of telemedicine such as in automation of skin disease diagnosis [2]. Hitherto, medical imaging has contributed immensely towards advancing medical procedures. However, one notable challenge is that interpretation and analysis of medical imaging results are still heavily dependent on medical experts whose availability is low or non-existent for developing and underserved regions (especially rural settings).

The fundamental task of medical imaging of the human skin is the segmentation of a mole that provides essential output for the mole feature extraction and mole classification. A mole is a skin lesion that essentially results from the local proliferation of pigment cells (melanocytes). Due to its root in melanocytes, it can sometimes be referred to as melanocytic nevus (naevus). Typically, a mole can be congenital or acquired. Congenital melanocytic nevi are present at birth and sometimes referred to as a birthmark in some regions. Congenital moles are often classified based on size. Three main types of congenital moles include small-size nevi, medium-sized nevi and giant-sized (garment) nevi. Acquired melanocytic nevi generally appears at a later stage in childhood or adult life because of several reasons such as unprotected exposure to sun radiation, immune status, genetic factors and at times from unpredictable adverse event from medication [3]. Mole transformation from nevi into cutaneous melanoma has been reported in the literature to increase with age, especially the dysplastic nevi [4, 5]. A benign mole might grow to be cutaneous for 1 in every 200000 male and female under the age of 40, as well as for 1 in 33000 for males older than 20 years of age [4]. While most moles occurring in adolescents might not transform into cutaneous melanoma [4], it has been reported that precautions need to be taken for scheduled examination on suspicious moles because some malignant melanoma might masquerade clinically as benign lesions [6, 7].

A skin lesion could also be categorised as pigmented or non-pigmented, based on its colour resulting from melanin, blood or exogenous pigment. While most Pigmented Skin Lesions (PSL) are melanocytic (benign moles or malignant), some have been reported to be non-melanocytic [8, 9]. Most moles could be said to be benign (not harmful). A cancerous mole, however, is malignant (life-threatening). Some reports have argued that a number of malignant melanomas stem from the preexisting benign nevi [4, 10].

Pathologically, melanocytic nevi are often classified based on the location reference of the nevi cells in the skin. Dermal or intradermal nevi are associated with nevus cells located in the dermis. Junctional nevus refers to a flat mole affiliated with nevus cells located at the junction of the epidermis and dermis. Compound nevi have nevus cells at the epidermal-dermal junction and equally within the dermis. The usage of dermoscope in the process of dermatoscopy has introduced the classification based on pigment patterns. A starburst nevus reflects radial lines around the periphery of a skin lesion. Blue nevi refer to uniform but structure less skin lesions that are steel blue in colour. Other common nevi include spitz, reticular, globular, eclipse, dysplastic (atypical), fried egg, lentiginous and cockade nevus.

Early detection of malignant moles is one of the essential keys to prevent untimely death resulting from skin cancer diseases [11 - 28]. The three prevalent skin cancers, according to the literature are Basal Cell Carcinoma (BCC), Squamous Cell Carcinoma (SCC) and Melanoma. The incidence of skin cancer diseases such as BCC, SCC and Melanoma has also been seen to increase rapidly throughout the world and it is gradually becoming one of the predominant forms of cancer diseases, especially in Caucasian population countries and among fair-skinned people [29 - 31]. Skin cancer incidence is on the order of 10 to 12 in Europe, 18 to 20 in the United States, and 30 to 40 in Australia per 100000 subjects [32]. The Australian Institute of Health and Welfare (AIHW) and Australian Association of Cancer Registries (AACR) detailed that more people have had skin cancer disease than all other cancer diseases combined in the past three decades [33]. Robinson [34], reported that 1 in 5 Americans develops skin cancer in the course of a lifetime. It has been reported that approximately 40%-50% of Americans who live up to the age of 65 have a high risk of having either BCC or SCC at least once [35].

Melanoma is a skin cancer typically resulting from an unpredictable disorder in the melanocytic cells, thus causing improper synthesis of the melanin. While melanoma might account for the least amongst the three aforementioned skin cancer types, it has, however, been umpired to account for 75-79% of skin cancer related deaths [29, 36]. The literature records that Melanoma is the fifth most common cancer occurring amongst males, seventh most commonly occurring cancer in females, and second most common form of cancer amongst young adults ranging from 15-29 years of age [37, 38]. Melanoma, which is currently the third prevalent cancer in Australia, was reported to occur in 61.7 for every 100000 Australian men and 40.0 for every 100000 women [33]. In the same study, melanoma of the skin was judged to have accounted for 22800 Disability-Adjusted Life Years (DALYs) in Australia. DALYs depict years of healthy life lost either because of premature death or through living with illness or injury-bound disability. The study made by American Cancer Society (ACS) [36] has revealed that at least 1 person would likely die every hour as a result of melanoma. Similarly, the study [33] reported that melanoma of the skin accounts for 22800 DALYs in Australia. DALYs refer to years of healthy life that have otherwise been lost either as a result of illness or premature death. It has been projected that melanoma would have caused 10130 deaths in the year 2016 [36] and 9730 deaths are predicted for 2017 [39].

The incidence of cutaneous melanoma in Caucasian patients has been reported to increase historically in most parts of the world over the decades [40 - 42]. In Europe for instance, it has been reported that malignant melanoma incidence is steadily increasing by 5% year-on-year, and it is responsible for 91% of skin cancer deaths [31]. Amazingly, most incidents are reported in the literature among Caucasians, but some reports state that black Africans and Asians account for 20% of the world melanoma [43, 44]. Tuma et al. [45], however, argued that the African descendant population is rarely affected by melanoma because an average of 1.1 out of 100,000 persons per year has an incidence of melanoma. Though most reports of melanoma have majorly reflected an infection rate among Caucasians, the overall five-year melanoma survival rate for African-Americans and other people of colour is only 77% compared to 91% for Caucasians [46]. A fact sheet report compiled by Cancer Association of South Africa (CASA) [47] has stated that South Africa has the second highest incidence of skin cancer in the world after Australia.

Gruesome reports as highlighted above have led to many advances in computer-aided systems towards assisting dermatologists to administer the diagnosis of skin-related diseases. The development of automated diagnosis systems that are capable of performing some level of remote diagnosis of skin cancer diseases such as melanoma and basal cell carcinoma and equally assisting physicians in various imaging tasks have gained tremendous attention in the bioinformatics and computer vision research [48].

The efforts towards the automation of diagnostic procedures are geared mainly to improve the speed of diagnosis and to increase reproducibility of results. The automated diagnosis has helped in reducing the first-time diagnostic errors, which sometimes could be as much as 40% [49, 50].

4. COMPUTER-AIDED DIAGNOSTIC SYSTEMS

In the past decades, the literature has reported advances in computer-aided diagnostic systems that provide a more manageable solution. These propositions are geared towards the development of automated systems that are less prone to possible bias and that are often introduced in the process of diagnosis by medical experts, whose availability is low and sometimes do not exist in underserved communities [51 - 53]. A strong impulse has been seen in the literature to be given to the development of automated systems capable of assisting physicians in medical imaging tasks [48]. However, the presence of noise, masking structures, variability of biological shapes and tissues, and imaging system anisotropy make the automated analysis of medical images a hard task [42, 48, 51].

One of the best approaches to overcome the aforementioned challenges in automating medical imaging diagnosis is to exploit some kind of hypothetical information about the imaged structures. The information about the structures to be analysed can be anatomical knowledge about their typical appearance (such as shape and grey levels) and position or it can be statistical knowledge of their properties such as grey level of the tissues included in those structures. The images can then be classified using their morphological structure, colour, fractal and texture properties. Laws [54], transformed digital images to identify regions of interest and provided an input data set for segmentation and features detection operation. In the same study [54], operations such as thresholding, morphological analysis and texture detection were used in order to divide a digital image into individual objects to perform a separate analysis of each region.

Over the years, it has been reported that an automatic data analysis used for melanoma showed a higher diagnostic performance compared to an observation by a physician in terms of sensitivity (proportion of true positives), though lower in terms of specificity (proportion of true negatives) [29, 55 - 57]. (Fig. 1) highlights the frequently used evaluation metrics to determine the effectiveness of the diagnostic results. A common technique used for the foregoing automated data analysis is Dermoscopy or Epiluminiscence Light Microscopy (ELM). It is an in-vivo, non-invasive technique that in recent years has disclosed a new dimension of the clinical morphological features of Pigmented Skin Lesions (PSLs) using different light magnification systems [29]. Dermoscopy can be based on non-polarized light techniques that require liquid interface or direct skin contact or polarized light techniques [58]. For the past decades, dermoscopy has been a major tool used by the dermatologists to proffer early detection of skin cancer-related cases, thus lowering the number of excisions and consequently impacting the clinical management of PSLs [59]. Dermoscopy provides dermatologists with a higher accuracy for detecting suspicious cases than it is possible with popular practice of naked-eye inspection [56, 60]. In addition, dermoscopy has been observed to aid the diagnosis of several other skin tumours such as Angiomas, Basal Cell Carcinomas, Cylindromas, Seborrheic Keratosis, and Hematomas, just to mention a few. In relation to the malignancy classification of melanocytic images, the ELM has been a great tool for dermatologists distinguish between life-threatening (malignant) and benign melanocytic lesions. The trend identified in the literature is the increase in the adoption of dermoscopy, primarily because of its ease of use, non-invasive approach, and slow adoption of other advance diagnostic technologies by many dermatologists. A recurring challenge, however, with the usage of dermoscopy is the complexity and subjectivity that characterize the interpretation of its results [41, 42, 57, 61, 62]. The poor reproducibility of an analysis made with the usage of the technique is also a concern.

The development of automated diagnostic systems for skin lesion screening has provided promising reproducibility of diagnostic results, and an increase in the speed of diagnosis procedures [42, 63, 64]. In addition, the application of automated diagnosis has assisted to reduce the first-time diagnostic error which can be as much as 40% [49, 50] and mis-pathology cancerous analysis [65]. Proposed automated diagnosis techniques in the literature are essentially based on different diagnostic checklists and rules such as the Asymmetry, Border Irregularity, Colour (ABCD) variation and diameter of lesion [14], modified ABC-point list of dermoscopy [66], pattern analysis [67], ELM 7-Point checklists [15], and Menzies score [68].

- ➡ True Positive (TP) - correctly identified subject against a particular criteria in a given set of subjects
- ➡ False Positive (FP) - incorrectly identified subject against a particular criteria in a given set of subjects
- ➡ True Negative (TN) - correctly rejected subject against a particular criteria in a given set of subjects
- ➡ False Negative (FN) - incorrectly rejected subject against a particular criteria in a given set of subjects
- ➡ Sensitivity (S_n) - statistical measurement of the percentage of proportion of true positive

$$S_n = \frac{TP}{TP+FN} \times 100\%$$

- ➡ Specificity (S_p) - statistical measurement of the percentage of proportion of true negative

$$S_p = \frac{TN}{TN+FP} \times 100\%$$

- ➡ Likelihood Ratio Positive: $LR+ = \frac{S_n}{1-S_p}$
- ➡ Likelihood Ratio Negative: $LR- = \frac{1-S_n}{S_p}$
- ➡ Positive Predictive Value: $+PV = \frac{TP}{TP+FP}$
- ➡ Negative Predictive Value - $PV = \frac{TN}{TN+FN}$

		Ground Truth			
		Positive	Negative		
Test Result	Positive	True +	False +	=	$+PV$
	Negative	False -	True -	=	$-PV$
		‖	‖		
		S_n	S_p		

- ➡ Diagnostic Accuracy: $DA = \frac{TP+TN}{TP+TN+FP+FN}$

- ➡ Jaccard Index (J): Statistically compares similarity and diversity between Training data set (Tr_D) and Test data set (Ts_D)

$$J(Tr_D, Ts_D) = \frac{Tr_D \cap Ts_D}{|Tr_D| + |Ts_D| - (Tr_D \cap Ts_D)} = \frac{TP}{TP+FP+FN}$$

- ➡ Dice Coefficient (DSC): Statistically compares similarity between Training data set (Tr_D) and Test data set (Ts_D)

$$DSC(Tr_D, Ts_D) = \frac{2(Tr_D \cap Ts_D)}{|Tr_D| + |Ts_D|} = \frac{2TP}{2TP+FP+FN}$$

NOTE:
❶ High Sensitivity and Specificity indicates high performance of a given method
❷ Likelihood Positive ratio greater than 1 with Likelihood Negative ratio less than 1 reflect the subject associate well with the specified criteria (such as classification or segmentation)
❸ High Positive and Negative Predictive Value indicates high-performance of a given method

Fig. (1). Evaluation Metrics.

5. SKIN LESION DIAGNOSTIC METHODS

The literature generally shows that several methods for skin lesion diagnostic have been proposed to assist in the diagnosis of melanocytic lesions over the years. Prominent among these methods are Pattern Analysis for Microscopic Images (PAMI) [67], the ABCD criteria for macroscopic images [11], the ABCD rule of dermoscopy [14] for microscopic images, the ABCDE criteria [19] for macroscopic images, ABCDE rule [12], Glasgow 7-point checklists

[13, 69] for macroscopic images, ELM 7-point checklists [70] for microscopic images, Menzies score [68] for microscopic images, 7 features for melanoma [71], Modified ABC-Point (MABCP) list of Dermoscopy [66] and Colour, Architecture, Symmetry, and Homogeneity (CASH) algorithm [72, 73].

The quantitative pattern analysis proposed by Pehamberger et al. [67], is based on detailed qualitative assessment of the numerous individual ELM criteria and typically requires a significant degree of formal training. Pattern analysis categorises specific patterns as global (reticular, globular, homogeneous, parallel) or local (pigmented network, dots, streaks, globules, blotches). The ABCD criteria proposed by Friedman et al. [11] employs a semi quantitative counting classification based on the evaluation of asymmetry of overall lesion shape, border irregularity, colour variation and diameter of lesion of minimum of 6mm. The ABCD rule of dermoscopy initially suggested by Stolz et al. [14] and later standardized in Argenziano et al. [52] uses similar measures in relation to the criteria defined by Friedman et al. [11], although different. Stolz et al. [14] have highlighted the key features of diagnosing a skin lesion. These features include asymmetry properties of the specific lesion (contour, colour and structures), unexpected border sharpness, colour variegation of 1 to 6 predefined colours (white, red, light brown, dark brown, blue-grey, black) and the inclusion of 5 differential dermoscopic structures (network, structure-less or homogeneous areas, branched streaks, dots, and globules). It was recommended that white colour should be only counted if the area is lighter than the adjacent skin. A Total Dermoscopic Score (TDS) of 4.75 or less signifies a benign melanocytic lesion, a score ranging from 4.8 to 5.45 denotes a suspicious lesion, and a TDS of more than 5.45 symbolizes malignancy.

Blum et al. [66] debated the need to simplify the criteria used in identifying malignant lesions. The simplified procedure termed as ABC-point (ABCP) list was formulated based on the concept of the ABCD rule of dermoscopy [14], Menzies score [68], and the modified ABCD rule by Kittler [56]. The simplicity of the ABC-point list for lesion evaluation is a great benefit, however, there exist some concerns about its sensitivity and accuracy. The CASH algorithm for dermoscopy proposed by Henning et al. [72] suggested that architectural order of lesion could be the most important features in distinguishing between malignant and benign melanocytic lesions. The comparative study carried out for CASH and state-of-the-art methods (Menzies score, ABCD rule of dermoscopy and ELM 7-point checklists) reported a comparable result [73].

Recently, a modified 4-points algorithm designed on the success of ABC-point list has been proposed, whose accuracy is similar to the CASH algorithm and similar in simplicity to the 3-point checklist [74]. The 4-point algorithm uses the existing criteria from the ABC-point list and adds another criterion by doubling the symmetry parameter criterion. The algorithm certainly looks promising, it might however be difficult to really ascertain the superiority of the algorithm over the ABC-point list and CASH, given the small sample size on which it was tested. Moreover, the validation of this new algorithm is yet to be discussed in the literature.

The Glasgow 7-point checklists which was first discussed by Mackie [13] before being popularized [69] uses change in shape, size and colour of skin lesions as its major criteria, while lesion inflammation, crusting or oozing, sensory change or Pruritus and minimum diameter of 7mm were used as minor criteria. While the Glasgow 7-point checklist has shown good adoption in clinical practice, there have been some concerns about its application in early lesion detection as well as its sensitivity and capability [15, 75]. Walter et al. [76] argued that the application of weighted revised version of the 7-points checklist, with a cut-off score of 4 rather than 3 performs considerably better and could thus be applied in general practice towards supporting recognition of clinically significant lesions as well as early identification of melanoma. ELM 7-point checklist proposed by Argenziano et al. [70] and endorsed in Malvehy et al. [61] uses 3 major criteria and 4 minor criteria, with each major criterion having a score of 2 points, whereas each minor criterion is given 1 point. A minimum total score of 3 is required for the diagnosis of melanoma. The major criteria used in the ELM 7-point checklists include atypical pigment networks, atypical vascular patterns and blue-white veil, while the minor criteria consist of irregular streaks, irregular globules or dots, irregular blotches and regression structures.

Contrary to the general adoption of the ABCD criteria for macroscopic image evaluation, there have been a number of concerns regarding the unwarranted biopsy because of misdiagnosis resulting from morphological overlap with dysplastic nevi. The relevance of the metrics such as Diameter (D) identifier from the ABCD criteria on melanoma having diameters less than 6mm or on thin melanoma (≤1 mm) has also been questioned [19, 77 - 82]. Whiteman et al. [83] recently validated this assumption by arguing that more melanoma deaths were attributable to thin tumours (≤1 mm) than thick tumours (>4 mm) in Queensland, Australia.

The discussions by Zaharna & Brodell [84] as well as by Liu et al. [85] reasoned that change in lesion characteristics is one of the most important diagnostic features reported by patients towards early detection of melanoma. This inference further validates the choice of variegation in size, shape, and colour as major criteria for Glasgow 7-point checklists. The literature has thus seen various proposals for additional measures to complement the ABCD criteria. Fitzpatrick et al. [12] discussed the importance of expanding the ABCD criteria to ABCDE by studying the elevation (E) of lesion for early melanoma detection. The study by Rigel & Friedman [86] and Thomas et al. [87] agreed on the need for the addition of identifier E to represent enlargement of lesion relative to other neighbouring lesion for optimizing the sensitivity and specificity of lesion diagnosis. Hazen et al. [16], equally suggested yet another similar criterion: E for evolutionary changes in lesion colour, including surrounding erythema and hyper-pigmented halo, size, pruritus, pain, surface characteristics, bleeding, symmetry and tenderness. To avoid misinterpretation of terms and to further ease distinguishing between melanoma and benign pigmented lesions, Abbasi et al. [19] proposed a more encompassing and simple criterion named evolving (E) to emphasize changes in lesion characteristics over time. Abbasi et al. [19] argued that the usage of E to represent lesion elevation (proposed by Fitzpatrick et al [12]) would be misleading since substantial elevation might not be apparent especially in early melanomas. In addition, there has been a recent discussion on the replacement of Diameter (D) in the ABCDE with lesion darkness (D) for early melanoma detection [26].

The Ugly Duckling (UD) sign introduced by Grob & Bonerandi [88] has also been seen as a major insignia for spotting the possible presence of melanoma. The UD sign signifies suspected lesions that appear different from other benign lesions examined in the same patient. The validity of the UD sign was inspected in Grob et al. [89] as a useful tool for lesion expert towards second diagnosis opinion as well as for general population when performing self-examination. The UD sign has influenced a number of research efforts towards early detection of malignant lesions. Hazen et al. [16] used the basis of UD sign to argue that it is beneficial to add another criterion of F (funny looking lesions) to the established ABCDE criteria. Similar argument to expand ABCDE to ABCDEF was recently discussed by Jensen & Elewski [90] to improve patient self-screening examination, which has been applied as a useful tool for physicians in identifying worrisome melanocytic lesions. The progressive increase in letter addition to the established ABCD criteria has been seen to have contributed to the handling of edge case skin lesion diagnosis as highlighted above. However, it has also been sometimes criticized [91].

The 7 features for melanoma developed by Dal Pozzo et al. [71] include dermoscopic features that can aid screening of pigmented skin lesions. 4 of these features are considered major, each with the score of 2, while the remaining 3 features are classified as minor features with a score of 1. The major features include regression erythema (white-pinkish depigmented area), radial streaming, grey blue veil, and irregularly distributed pseudopods. Inhomogeneity of two or more dermoscopic features, irregular pigment network and sharp margin all constitute the minor features. The 7 features for melanoma use a scoring system similar to ELM 7-point checklists however differ in the criteria.

Menzies et al. [68], discussed 11 features required to successfully diagnose a skin lesion. 2 of the features are tagged negative, while the remaining 9 are positive. The negative features include symmetry of patterns and singular colour (either of black, grey, blue, dark brown, tan and red). The positive features include blue-white veil, multiple brown dots, pseudopods, radial streaming, scar-like depigmentation, peripheral black dots/globules, multiple (5-6) colours, multiple blue or grey dots and broadened network. According to Menzies' score, a lesion is considered melanoma if it contains 1 or more of the positive features and none of the negative features.

In a bid to effectively recognize acral melanoma that does not exhibit the parallel ridge pattern, Lallas et al. [92] recently proposed irregular Blotch, parallel Ridge pattern, Asymmetry of structures, Asymmetry of colours, parallel Furrow pattern and Fibrillar pattern (BRAAFF) as a new checklist to improve diagnostic sensitivity of the acral melanoma. The BRAAFF checklist is composed of four positive of irregular blotches, ridge pattern, asymmetry of structures and asymmetry of colours and two negative predictors of furrow pattern and fibrillar pattern.

A comparative analysis made by Annessi et al. [93] on three of the algorithmic methods (Pattern Analysis, ABCD rule and 7-Point Checklists) using 198 equivocal melanocytic lesions revealed that Pattern Analysis was the most sensitive (85.4%) and specific (79.4%) in identifying Thin Melanoma (TM), followed by ABCD rule. Comparative performance of 4 dermoscopic algorithms (pattern analysis, the 7-point checklist, the ABCD rule, and the Menzies method) by non-experts for the diagnosis of melanocytic lesions lauded Menzies method for producing the highest diagnostic accuracy [94]. Over the years, dermatologists have been using both ABCD criteria as well as the ABCD rule as a standard for classifying Pigmented Skin Lesion (PSL) as benign, suspicious or life threatening (malignant) primarily because of their simplicity and efficient approach [66, 95, 96].

It is important to note that the rules that target microscopic (dermoscopic) images differ from that of macroscopic (clinical) images even in the areas where similar terms are shared. The ABCD criteria [11] for macroscopic images differ from ABCD rule of dermoscopy [14] for microscopic images. The identifier 'B' in the study of Friedman *et al.* [11] refers to border irregularity, whereas the same identifier reflects border sharpness in the study of Stolz *et al.* [14]. In addition, identifier 'D' refers to differential structure for microscopic images, whereas it generally represents diameter greater or equal to 6mm in macroscopic images. These consequently filter down to the popular ABCDE criteria [19] and likewise the ABCDE rule [12]. Similarly, the different criteria highlighted above for both macroscopic bound Glasgow 7-point checklists discussed by Mackie & Doherty [69] and the microscopic bound ELM 7-Points checklists proposed by Malvehy *et al.* [61] showed a clear distinction between criteria and checklists used in both the procedures.

Most articles in the literature generally use either of aforementioned methods in speculating lesion classifications. This speculation is often accompanied with the assumptions that malignant moles are pigmented. However, there has been an increase in the reports of non-pigmented skin tumours [97 - 100]. This suggests a more careful approach and systems that need to be instituted to resolve such cases to curtail potential fatality. It should also be noted that some types of melanoma (amelanotic) have been reported to be clinically and dermoscopically featureless resulting in misdiagnosis during both clinical examination and dermoscopy screening [101].

6. HOMOGENOUS SKIN LESION DIAGNOSTIC PROCEDURES

To achieve a reproducible diagnosis, the research community has frequently used a number of standard automated procedures for improved diagnosis of Pigmented Skin Lesions (PSL) and its non-pigmented counterpart. These procedures include skin lesion image acquisition and preprocessing; lesion segmentation from surrounding healthy skin, extraction of selected features and classification of skin lesions.

6.1. Skin Lesion Image Acquisition and Preprocessing

Results of diagnosis reported in the literature have been judged to be highly dependent on the volume and quality of images used [29, 102, 103]. Often, variations in devices used in capturing lesion images and conditions under which these images are acquired have been observed to adversely affect the results of automated skin lesion diagnosis. In the time past, the source of image data for lesion screening was colour slides. However, over the past decades, it has been proven that quality and accurate diagnosis can be achieved using digitized lesion images [104 - 106]. The two predominant dermatological image types are macroscopic (clinical) and microscopic (dermoscopic) images. While the use of digitised dermoscopic images is on the increase, some reports have argued that pertinent distinguishing image features (diminishing textures and pored) are easily examined using macroscopic images rather than under dermoscopic images [107].

The literature has reported several imaging techniques that could assist in the acquisition and screening of skin lesion images [108 - 110]. One of such popular technique is dermoscopy which provides in-vivo, non-invasive imaging of skin lesion using different light magnification systems [14, 17, 45, 52, 56, 58 - 61, 66, 67, 111 - 131]. Other notable imaging techniques include digital photography [108, 110, 131 - 134], radiography [110, 135], confocal microscopy [80, 108, 115, 133, 136 - 148], tomography such as computed tomography, positron emission tomography, photoacoustic tomography, optical coherence tomography and magnetic resonance imaging [108, 110, 149 - 172], ultrasound imaging [108, 110, 173 - 180], multispectral imaging [108, 181, 182] and thermal imaging (thermography) [183 - 186]. A review of non-invasive imaging techniques was recently discussed by Menge & Pellacani [109], detailing the application of various imaging techniques and the accompanying shortfalls. Arguably, due to slow adoption of advances in diagnostic technology by many dermatologists, the trend noticed in the literature is a growing increase of the usage of dermatoscopy (Dermoscopy). Recently, the usage of dermatoscope with mobile phone camera has also been discussed in some studies for making acquisition of lesion images easier [28, 187, 188]. Reflectance microscopy has equally been dubbed to give good result against the light coloured melanoma lesions [80].

While each individual imaging method has produced a promising result in the screening of lesions, there has been a rise in the mixture of imaging methods to enhance sensitivity, specificity and accuracy of lesion screening [151, 152, 189, 190]. This is further validated by Mohr *et al.* [191] and Reinhardt *et al.* [153] and recently by Bourgeois *et al.* [170] that the combination of Positron Emission Tomography and Computed Tomography (PET/CT) revealed a better sensitivity in staging of malignant tumours. Wang *et al.* [173] equally argued that integrating photoacoustic tomography with ultrasound has yielded a better specificity when compared to when either method was used in isolation. The combination of confocal and photo thermal microscopy was recently discussed by He *et al.* [192] for noninvasive and label free 3-D imaging of melanoma. A good review was conducted by Dancey *et al.* [110] to compare various techniques used in imaging melanoma, and consequently recommended a choice of imaging techniques based on their applicability, accuracy and cost. In the review [110], it has been suggested that ultrasound imaging (ultrasonography) is the most effective mode of screening in the absence of sentinel lymph node biopsy. A similar view was shared by Xing *et al.* [189] during the comparison made between the usage of ultrasonography, CT, PET and PET/CT in staging and surveillance of melanoma patients.

In image processing, commonly used colour spaces include Red-Green-Blue (RGB and sRGB), Commission Internationale de l'Eclairage (CIE L*a*b, CIE L*u*v and CIE X*Y*Z), Luma plus chrominance (Y'CbCr, Y'PbPr, Y'UV and YIQ) and Hue-Saturation-Intensity-Value-Luminance (HSI, HSV/B and HSL). Most digitized lesion images are commonly generated as RGB. However, because of device dependency of RGB colour space, digitized lesion images are often converted to greyscale or blue channel for single channel (scalar) processing in order to represent the intensity of the image. In a bid to ease the accuracy of classification, Dobrescu *et al.* [48] converted each image used in their study to 256 grey levels image of the same size as a form of preprocessing of the image in Hue Saturation Value (HSV) colour space. Multichannel (vector) processing can equally be used to take advantage of the original colour information of the lesion. The main challenge, however, with the use of vector images is the computational requirement. Gómez *et al.* [193] argued that it is implausible that a particular colour space is optimal across different dermoscopic images acquired via different systems, even though the images have similar prognosis. Some reports [194 - 196], however, revealed that CIE L*a*b colour space produced a convincing result compared to its counterparts (CIE L*u*v and CIE X*Y*Z) and the popular YCbCr colour space when performing preprocessing of multichannel microscopic lesion images.

The term preprocessing in lesion image diagnostic procedures usually encompasses lesion image enhancement, image restoration with neighbourhood pixels and artefact removal [197]. The conditions surrounding the acquisition of lesion images generally influence possible discriminating features that can be extracted from such images for the purpose of automated diagnosis. Rahman *et al.* [198] reasoned that retrieval and the classification tasks of lesion could be challenging when images collected from separate data sets are captured by different devices under varying conditions (such as lightening). This creates a non-uniform illumination pattern, thus confusing diagnostic procedures. Colour calibration of image acquisition device has been one of the approaches proposed in the literature to resolve such challenges [199 - 205]. Low contrast of lesion images could also make isolation of lesion a very difficult task [206]. Abbas *et al.* [195] proposed enhancing lesion image contrast by adjusting and mapping the intensity values of the lesion pixels in the specified range in CIE L*a*b colour space. One major flaw of contrast enhancement is over amplification of noise in the region having relatively small intensity range. The use of Contrast Limited Adaptive Histogram Equalization (CLAHE) might be applied to address such limitations [207, 208]. (Figs. **2** and **3**) respectively illustrate the normal and filled histogram of the image shown in (Fig. **4** and **5**) shows an equalized histogram of the same image in (Fig. **4**) for better noise removal resolution.

A major hindrance to a successful diagnosis in medical skin imaging is the presence of artefacts, typically referred to as noise. Artefacts such as hair shaft (Figs. **6** and **7**), dermoscopic gels, thin blood vessel, shadows, ruler marking, specular reflections, vignetting and air bubble can confuse diagnosis and impede achievement of better accuracy in automated diagnosis process [107, 209 - 211]. To resolve the challenges posed by these artefacts, the literature report the use of a number of approaches which consist primarily of artefact detection (Fig. **5**) and subsequent artefact removal (Fig. **4**). Methods used for aiding the detection of artefact include filtering (curvilinear matched, Prewitt, Gaussian, median and bilateral), derivative of Gaussian, morphology operations (closed based top hat) and anisotropic diffusion. Filtering is a popular method to smooth a lesion image before detecting artefacts. Bilateral filtering has been seen to perform very well amongst other types of filtering because of its edge-preserving smoothing operation on the lesion images, especially on microscopic images [194]. Karkunen-Loéve is another method often used to preserve artefact edges during image smoothening. Prominent among the artefact removal methods is the linear interpolation [212, 213]. This was popularized in the demonstration of the system named DullRazor that was proposed by Lee *et al.* [213] to remove hair artefacts from a given lesion image. Other commonly used artefacts removal methods include inpainting (partial differential equation, exemplar-based, fast marching) [214 - 219] and region growing [107, 220]. A promising method called lacunarity algorithm which is a measure of transitional invariance for computing aspects of patterns exhibiting scale-invariant changes in the structure was equally proposed by Gilmore *et al.* [96] to avoid the need for a more sophisticated method.

The hair shafts and ruler marking appear to be the most common artefacts reported in the literature [210, 214, 221 - 226]. In our study, we observed that much effort has been given to the removal of hair shaft and ruler markings from lesion images [107, 209, 210, 213, 214, 220, 225, 227]. An excellent review by Abbas *et al.* [55] discussed a comparative study of the state-of-the-art algorithms for automatic detection of hair and restoration, vis-à-vis their applicability to the texture-part of lesion images. A novel algorithm comprising of morphological and fast marching schemes was also suggested in a study [55]. Similar procedure of using fast marching inpainting was discussed by Okuboyejo *et al.* [194] towards improving the speed of preprocessing of dermoscopic lesion images. Toossi *et al.* [228] also suggested the usage of multi-resolution coherence transport inpainting based on wavelet-based structure for the removal of hair artefacts in dermoscopic images. The algorithm proposed in a study [228] combines simple coherence transport inpainting with a wavelet decomposition and reconstruction method in an iterative and multi-resolution structure.

6.2. Lesion Image Segmentation

The successful segmentation of skin lesion from the healthy surrounding skin is a pertinent requirement for a workable lesion diagnostic process. The analysis of a number of the dermoscopic features (asymmetry, border sharpness) and clinical features (asymmetry, border irregularity) is only as accurate as the estimated lesion boundary. The variations in human interpretation of manual lesion boundary tracing have equally influenced the automation of lesion segmentation procedure [229, 230]. According to the literature, the estimation of lesion border by dermatologists has been reported to depend upon higher-level knowledge, leading to poor reproducibility of segmentation results [231]. However, Silletti *et al.* [232] argued that with exception of the Fuzzy C-Means (FCM), some state-of-the-art automatic segmentation methods performed poorly when compared with segmentation carried out by expert dermatologists. In Fig. **8**), an example is shown on a segmented lesion image that has been localized from its surrounding healthy skin.

The segmentation task has sometimes been referred to as one of the most difficult tasks in medical imaging. Among other concerns, the difficulty can be attributed to low-contrasts surrounding the skin, fuzzy borders, the existence of artefacts and irregular structures characterizing lesion images [48, 65, 211, 233 - 235]. Readers can refer to the previous section detailing preprocessing techniques for image contrast enhancement and removal of occluding artefacts typically found in both macroscopic and microscopic images. Some reports in the literature have equally suggested that tumour areas manually extracted by dermatologists have been discovered to be sometimes characterized with inconsistency [232, 236 - 238], validating the need for an automated lesion segmentation approach that can aid reproducibility of results. In recent times, the literature has seen a great improvement in automating lesion image segmentation from the surrounding healthy skin parts for the purpose of achieving automated diagnosis of such lesion images. However, Chang *et al.* [239] argued that it is impractical to perform fully automatic segmentation on all skin lesion images due to reasons such as complexities surrounding acquisition of lesion images.

Most segmentation approaches incorporate some forms of image preprocessing to reduce or eliminate image noises such as air bubbles, ruler marking, hair shafts that could confuse segmentation. An example of this is the application of combined spline and B-spline by Abbas *et al.* [240] to enhance the quality of dermoscopic images before segmentation. The Karkunen-Loéve Transform (KLT) also known as Principal Component Analysis/Transform (PCA/T) was used to enhance the edges of the lesion image for better segmentation result in some studies [20, 57, 193, 241, 242]. The top-hat and bottom-hat transformations were applied in a study [243] to maximize the contrast of lesion images in order to achieve a comparable lesion segmentation using ensemble methods. The literature has chronicled the numerous lesion localization (border detection) approaches that can help to segment pigmented skin lesion from the neighbouring region in an automated mode. A number of lesion segmentation algorithms (including edge based, region based and thresholding) have equally been proposed in the literature. In the course of our study, we observed that most of the reported segmentation methods in the literature are based on the colour information of the lesion being examined arguably due to the simplicity of the representation of lesion colour properties. Some reports [244 - 249] have equally used texture properties of skin lesions to estimate lesion boundaries. Commonly adopted texture feature methods used in segmenting skin lesion areas include Grey Level Co-occurrence Matrix (GLCM) [245], Gabor functions [248], Laws texture energy masks [54], Markov Random Field (MRF) models [246, 250]. Glaister *et al.* [244] equally proposed a texture oriented lesion segmentation algorithm called Texture Distinctive Lesion Segmentation (TDLS). The TDLS algorithm uses joint statistical information to characterise skin and lesion textures as representative texture distributions. Maeda *et al.* [251] combined colour and texture features in a proposed Fuzzy-based hierarchical algorithm to achieve a perceptual segmentation of dermoscopic lesion images.

The edge based segmentation methods essentially use metadata about edges of a given lesion image in addition to related post-processing techniques to estimate the boundary of a lesion [219, 234, 252, 253]. The implementation of edge-based lesion segmentation often requires the use of the established edge operators such as Canny [254 - 256], Prewitt [257], Sobel [258], Kirsch [259] and Laplacian of Gaussian (LOG) [260]. An edge-based segmentation method based on dynamic programming using CIE L*a*b* colour space was proposed by Abbas et al. [233, 234]. However, the major challenge in the application of dynamic programming is its inability to accurately detect outline of lesion in scenarios where areas belonging to the lesion are divided into multiple tumours.

Region-based methods use a seed-based approach that groups the regions according to common image properties and relative information of the neighbouring pixels [236, 261 - 267]. Popular region-based methods include Fuzzy-Based Split and Merge (FBSM), J-Image Segmentation (JSEG) [262, 268], Statistical Region Merging (SRM) [269, 270], Iterative Stochastic Region Merging (ISRM) [266] and watershed [226, 271]. At this juncture, we would like to state that though there exists a similarity between edge-based lesion segmentation and region-based lesion segmentation, but both are different. Essentially, region-based segmentation methods require closed boundary to properly estimate lesion borders, whereas such requirement is not essential for edge-based segmentation. It has been argued that region-based lesion segmentation sometimes leads to over-segmentation [272]. Over-segmentation can occur when the interior of a lesion exhibits multi-coloured areas. Many advances have been recorded in the literature to resolve the aforementioned challenges, thus yielding effective region-based lesion segmentation. Ma & Tavares [273] recently proposed an algorithm built on deformable model methods to define speed function on the lightness, saturation, and colour information of a given dermoscopic image in order to estimate its lesion boundary. Geometric deformable models have been posed to implicitly represent the moving curve evolution in a way that helps to obtain desirable features (such as regions and the boundaries of the skin lesions) for shape and colour analysis simultaneously [273]. Similarly, a saliency-based segmentation method was proposed by Ahn et al. [274] via measurement of sparse reconstruction errors against image backgrounds to estimate contrast discrimination between the lesion part of a given image and the surrounding healthy skin. Saliency-based segmentation techniques help to resolve the problem of target localization, such as the difficulties in segmenting lesion image with multi-coloured objects, as well as lesion images having similar colour between the foreground and background region. The approach proposed by Olugbara et al. [275] utilized a perceptual colour difference saliency with morphological analysis to achieve a compelling segmentation result of lesions. A good future research would be to investigate how saliency segmentation can be used on lesion images with multiple saliency-regions.

In general, contour segmentation methods can be either region-focused or edge-focused. Edge related contour segmentation typically applies edge detectors to estimate stopping function for terminating contours at distinct edges, making it unusable for fuzzy edges. Region related contour segmentation computes region energy based on the mean value of lesion image intensity and consequently uses global image information to terminate contours even for indistinguishable edges. Most contour-oriented lesion segmentation techniques are more or less similar to their region-based segmentation method counterparts. The similarity is due to the usage of seed-based approach in categorising image region according to the common criteria between both methods. Contour oriented segmentation is often referred to as snakes [219]. Frequently used contour-oriented methods include adaptive snake, robust snake [276], Gradient Vector Flow (GVF) snake [277, 278], Mean-Shift based GVF [279 - 282], level set [263, 264, 276, 283, 284] and radial search [285, 286]. Mete & Sirakov [287] discussed enhancing active contour model with optimum parameters, including high boost filtering to achieve comparable segmentation results with other state-of-the-art segmentation methods. Similarly, Ivanovici & Stoica [288] suggested that a diffusion model for colour images can be used as external energy for active contours in order to achieve lesion segmentation by independently computing diffusion at various scales. The study reported by Yuan et al. [284] equally introduced a region-fusion-based segmentation framework by combining graph partitioning methods with chan-vese level set to achieve a comparable lesion segmentation result. In addition, Kasmi et al. [289] recently proposed a geodesic active contour (GAC) based lesion segmentation method that employs an automatic contour initialization close to the actual lesion boundary. This approach was lauded to address the sticking challenge at minimum local energy spots typically caused by noise artefacts such as hair shaft. Fig. (5) displays an example of result after applying contour-based techniques called Line Segmentation Detection (LSD) [290] on an image in order to segment occludinh hair artefacts.

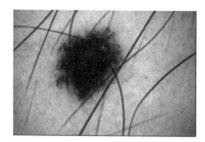

Fig. (2). Original Image.

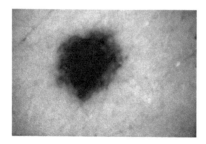

Fig. (3). Preprocessed.

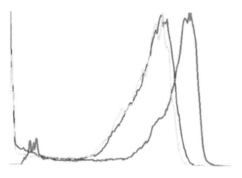

Fig. (4). Histrogram.

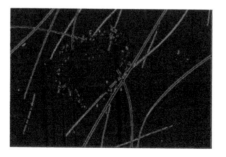

Fig. (5). Noise image.

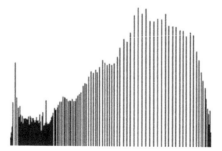

Fig. (6). Equalised Histrogram.

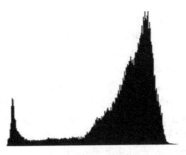

Fig. (7). Filled Histrogram.

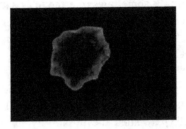

Fig. (8). Segmented Image.

Given a grey level co-occurrence matrix GLCM $\rightarrow C_{i,j}$

➡ *Entropy* - measures the unpredictability of grey level distribution
$$\sum_i \sum_j C_{i,j} \log(C_{i,j})$$

➡ *Energy* - measures the sum of squared elements in GLCM. It is also referred to as angular 2nd moment
$$\sum_i \sum_j C_{i,j}^2$$

➡ *Contrast* - measures the local variation in the greylevel co-occurrence matrix
$$\sum_i \sum_j (i-j)^2 C_{i,j}$$

➡ *Correlation* - measures the joint possibility of specified pixel points occurrence
$$\sum_{i,\ j=0}^{k-1} C_{i,j} \left[\frac{(i-\mu_i)(j-\mu_j)}{\sqrt{\sigma_i^2 \sigma_j^2}} \right]$$

➡ *homogeneity*: measures closeness of the distribution of elements in GLCM, relative to its diagonals
$$\sum_i \sum_j \frac{C_{i,j}}{1+|i-j|}$$

Fig. (9). Textual feature descriptors.

The thresholding technique is adjudged to be the most adopted approach in the literature for lesion segmentation using the computation of image intensity [198, 206, 207, 221, 240, 247, 291 - 299]. The discussion of thresholding in this section addresses segmentation of the lesion image rather than its usage in preprocessing of images. Typically, thresholding technique involves a non-linear process of producing a binary image such as by assigning two levels to pixels below or above a specified threshold value. Thresholding can be categorised based on the parameter usage as either parametric or non-parametric. Parametric thresholding uses a set of parameters to control fitness of the model while non-parametric thresholding estimates thresholds by optimizing objective functions such as variance-based functions (cluster variance) or entropy-based functions (cross entropy). Non-parametric thresholding can be further categorised either as global thresholding based on whether thresholding is performed on an entire lesion image using a single value or as local thresholding if a lesion image is partitioned into sub images, with each image region having their respective threshold value. Most thresholding approaches discussed in the literature are seen to be global. Global thresholding can be further classified as either a point dependent, if the threshold value is determined using grey level of each pixel of the lesion image or as a region dependent if the threshold value is determined from the local property in the neighbourhood of each pixel of the lesion image. According to the literature, the implementation of a particular thresholding technique could be based on region entropy, local lesion property, histogram shape, spatiality, image attribute similarity as well as clustering [300]. Notable thresholding techniques reported in the literature for lesion image segmentation are based on popular thresholding algorithms such as Otsu [294, 301 - 306], type-2 fuzzy logic [297, 307], random walker [308], Kapur [304, 305, 309], Kittler [310], Ridler [311] and Sahoo [312].

In relation to image processing, clustering is sometimes referred to as a multidimensional extension of thresholding. Clustering based lesion segmentation techniques generally adopt unsupervised erudition to identify a finite set of clusters to which image pixels would be grouped. Notable clustering methods vis-à-vis skin lesion image segmentation include fuzzy c-means (FCM) [20, 238, 313, 314], k-means [193, 215, 315 - 317], g-means [248], density-based spatial clustering [229, 230, 318 - 320], grid-based spatial clustering [318], wavelet transform [313, 321, 322] and Markov random field (MRF). Recently, Khalid *et al.* [321] proposed an implementation of dynamic wavelet transform based on Cohen–Daubechies–Feauveau Biorthogonal to segment lesion images. The Independent Histogram Pursuit (IHP) algorithm proposed by Gómez *et al.* [193] revealed the possibility of segmenting lesion images using K-means clustering technique that is agnostic of colour space of the image and the number of image bands. Kockara *et al.* [323] used a graph clustering segmentation technique based on the soft kinetic data structure to estimate lesion border of microscopic images and consequently segmenting the lesion images. Mete el al [230]. proposed a border-driven density-based framework to identify skin lesion border by expanding regions at borders of a cluster. This approach was further improved [229] by removing preprocessing dependency. Castillejos *et al.* [313] proposed an ensemble of clustering based methods to segment lesion image by exploring all colour channels. Melli *et al.* argued in a comparison study [324] that mean shift clustering can outperform other colour clustering algorithms (median cut, k-means and fuzzy-c means) in terms of sensitivity and specificity as the number of clusters increases. Kockara *et al.* [325] argued that density-based clustering produces a high precision and recall rate, with low border error when used to estimate lesion image border leading to a superior result when compared to the FCM. Recently, Lemon *et al.* [320] advanced the usage of density clustering by proposing a skin lesion border detection method based on web computing language (WebCL) parallel density. The approach [320] takes advantage of Graphical Processing Unit (GPU) computing power of web browsers to provide quick skin lesion border detection for dermoscopic images.

The usage of morphology and statistical information, together with clustering based approaches has equally been reported in the literature. This technique involves the use of morphological features to estimate discontinuity in lesion image structures [193, 261, 326 - 328]. Popular morphological based clustering methods include normalized cut [328], Principal Component Analysis (PCA) [20, 57, 193, 242], linear component analysis (LDA) [329], median cut [324] and grabcut [207].

There has been a growing need to advance lesion segmentation via machine learning system. This has led to the application of several expert systems to aid segmentation of lesion images from surrounding healthy skin [238, 322, 327, 330 - 332]. Application of machine learning for lesion segmentation typically involves the use of expert systems to process small areas of an image for the purpose of classification. Subsequently, the network system then classifies different areas of the image based on classifications recognized by the system. Xie *et al.* [331] proposed a lesion segmentation algorithm for dermoscopic images by combining Self Generating Neural Network (SGNN) with Genetic Algorithm (GA). Frequently used neural network systems recorded in the literature for lesion segmentation include Radial Basis Function (RBF), Back Propagation Network (BPN), Extreme Learning Machine (ELM), Markov Random Field (MRF) [250, 327], Wavelet Network (WN), Multi-Layer Perceptron (MLP) [326] and Bayesian [327].

The literature has equally reported attempts to use ensemble of methods to improve lesion image segmentation, such as using multiple thresholding algorithms, multiple clustering approaches, region-based segmentation with neural networks or combining thresholding with region-based methods [20, 226, 240, 243, 295, 303 - 305, 313, 315, 331, 333 - 335]. In a study [48], variable threshold (based on binary imaging) and contour extraction were used to detach the shapes of the masses before determining border outline of the lesion. A study [51] utilized Laplacian filter to localize the lesion area, while zero-crossing algorithm helped the author to perform automatic outline of the lesion border. The study [41] used both pixel-based and region-based approaches to develop an algorithm, which is referred to as

Dermatologists-like Tumour Area Extraction Algorithm (DTEA) to discriminate the actual tumour area from the surrounding skin. The combination of statistical clustering of the lesion colour space and hierarchical region-growing algorithm was used in a study [336] as a segmentation technique. In another study [65], segmentation was performed using a combination of bimodal histogram based on fuzzy sets region growing. Three segmentation algorithms (global thresholding, dynamic thresholding and a 3D colour clustering concept), together with fusion strategy were used [337] to obtain binary segmentation of the lesion. Pennisi *et al.* [272] proposed a fully automatic lesion segmentation procedure that combined edge based method (Canny) with region-based method (Delaunay triangulation) to resolve the segmentation of lesion areas.

A number of good reviews have discussed and compared notable automated lesion segmentation approaches. In the comparison study conducted by Mete & Sirakov [287], it was argued that density-based clustering performs better than Active Contour Models (ACM) when segmenting noisy lesion images. However, the ACM was adjudged to perform better when used with an optimum parameter. Celebi *et al.* [338] used a normalized probabilistic rand index to evaluate five different lesion segmentation approaches which include Orientation-Sensitive Fuzzy C-means Method (OSFCM) [314, 339], Dermatologist-like Tumour Extraction Algorithm (DTEA) [40, 41], mean shift clustering method [324], modified J-image Segmentation (JSEG) method [262, 268], and Statistical Region Merging (SRM) [269]. The evaluation reported the prowess of SRM as well as the consistency of DTEA across varying lesion image types. Recently, a comprehensive lesion border detection was surveyed by Celebi *et al.* [340] and some of the unresolved border detection issues were discussed. The latest review by Oliveira *et al.* [221] on computational methods for segmenting lesion images discussed several lesion boundary techniques. In the review, edge-based segmentation for lesion image was discouraged due to the fact that edge-based segmentation doesn't consider closed boundary, and as such may produce segmented images that are not completely closed. The comparative evaluation carried out by Mendonça *et al.* [276] adjudged adaptive thresholding to produce the most favorable automatic segmentation of lesions, while robust snake was said to have produced a more consistent result. Silveira *et al.* [283] however, argued that adaptive thresholding as well as vector-valued Chan-Vese level set [341] yielded the least satisfactory result in their comparative work. In the same study [283], a proposed extension of Chan-Vese level set, called Expectation-Maximization Level Set (EM-LS) method which uses probability density functions to model lesion intensity assumptions, was observed to produce robust skin lesion segmentation result. This inconsistency in the reported evaluation could be attributed to several factors, including varying data set used as well as different comparative evaluation metrics.

It is sometimes difficult to properly analyse different automatic border detection methods for lesion images without subjective opinions resulting from the evaluation of the parameters used. Celebi *et al.* [338] suggested a Normalized Probabilistic Rand Index (NPRI), which takes into account the variations in the ground-truth images when evaluating different skin lesion segmentation methods. In the study [338], NPRI was adjudged to outperform the commonly used exclusive OR (XOR) measure. Garnavi *et al.* [342] equally proposed a weighted performance index for objective evaluation of five automated border detection methods for dermoscopy images. The weighted index was computed from six standard evaluation metric (sensitivity, specificity, accuracy, precision, border error, and similarity). The approach was further optimized in a study [343] by applying constrained non-linear multivariable optimization method in the computation of the weights.

We observed that most reported work in the literature on lesion image segmentation has been on microscopic (dermoscopic) images. From the literature, only a few efforts have been recorded in the usage of clinical (macroscopic) images for evaluating automatic lesion area segmentation approaches [249, 261, 298, 306, 335, 344]. This arguably could be attributed to the increased adoption of dermoscope in the evaluation of skin lesion images. Cavalcanti *et al.* [335] proposed an Independent Component Analysis (ICA) based ensemble methods to estimate lesion areas from healthy surrounding skin. In the same study [335], ensemble of thresholding and level set methods were then applied for the actual lesion boundary detection and segmentation thereof. Recently, Flores & Scharcanski [249] proposed an unsupervised dictionary learning method called Unsupervised Information Theoretic Dictionary Learning (UITDL) for estimating lesion area in macroscopic images.

The analysis made from the reports discussed in the literature suggests that a number of past works in the lesion segmentation efforts have focused on the development of algorithms based on colour information in the non-uniform space. There's however a growing need towards optimizing segmentation algorithms in order to reduce computation time. In a bid to resolve the later, Okuboyejo *et al.* [207] proposed a Fast Image Segmentation (FIS) method based on the notable Contrast-Limited Adaptive Histogram Equalization (CLAHE), morphological operations, thresholding and grabcut techniques to localize lesion area from the surrounding healthy skin in a recorded time.

While most of the segmentation techniques discussed above yielded considerable promising results, the main problem with most of the approaches is that the computer-extracted regions sometimes were often smaller than the dermatologist-drawn ones (segmentation ground truth). Consequently, this makes some areas surrounding the tumour which are important features in the diagnosis to be excluded from the subsequent analysis [96, 103]. There are indications from the literature that many existing segmentation systems have high sensitivity rates towards effective diagnosis, they however experience high computing time [41, 57]. The usage of more than one algorithm for segmentation is one of the major causes of the non-realistic computing time as highlighted in a study [57]. It has also been noted that numerous past works have focused significantly on developing algorithms based on colour information in non-uniform colour spaces (disregarding the role of textural information). This has been reported to sometimes yield unsatisfactory segmentation results [234]. Another unresolved concern is the development of clinically oriented evaluation methods that can adapt variations in multiple manual borders [340]. While future research most likely would continue to use the mixture of algorithms due to increasing success rate of such approaches, more efforts should be made towards optimizing these algorithms to reduce their computing time. We would also like to suggest that the comparison of segmentation algorithms should be done on the same set of lesion images to ensure proper accuracy measure.

6.3. Feature Extraction

The primary objective of feature extraction is to quantify the macroscopic (clinical) or microscopic (dermoscopic) signs used in determining the malignancy of a skin lesion by a set of finite numerical features. Isolation of discriminating features in a given lesion image is an essential step towards effective automated lesion image classification. However, the vast variety of dermoscopic images and highly subjective definition of features characterizing these images have made the extraction of needful features a tedious task [40, 64, 96, 345, 346]. Skin distortion caused by bacterial and viral skin infections also makes analysis of features very difficult. In addition, variables such as body location, subject parameters (age), imaging parameters (lightening or camera), and direction from which lesion image is viewed and illuminated, greatly influence the resulting features that can possibly be extracted for classification purpose. These challenges typically add some overheads towards achieving automatic screening and diagnosis of medical images, especially skin lesions.

There have been numerous attempts reported in the literature to solve some of the above-mentioned challenges. One of the best approaches to address these aforementioned challenges in automating medical imaging diagnosis is to simplify the objective of the analysis and exploit some kinds of hypothetical information about the image structures. The information about the structures to be analysed can be anatomical knowledge about their typical appearance (shape, grey levels and position) or statistical knowledge of their properties (such as the greylevel of the tissues included in those structures). The images can then be classified using their morphological properties such as colour, shape, edges and texture.

The familiarity and potential discriminating power of the previously mentioned lesion diagnostic algorithm methods (such as ABCD rule of dermoscopy, ABCD criteria and Pattern analysis) have led to their usage in feature quantification. These feature descriptors can be dermoscopic, clinical or simply morphological in nature. Most reports discussed in the literature derived various discriminating lesion feature descriptors from these diagnostic algorithms, especially from the ABCD rule for dermoscopic images and ABCD criteria for clinical images. Feature descriptors used in the discrimination of skin lesion can favourably be categorised mostly as either photometric or textural. In the literature, it has been observed as common practice to use an amalgamation of various descriptors for lesion discrimination. Essentials features with corresponding discriminating properties used across the reviewed literature has been listed in Table 1.

Photometric has been seen to constitute the majority of the properties used in the literature when examining descriptors that could be used in classifying skin lesions. Photometric features include colour, island of colour, colour homogeneity & colour histogram etc. Barata et al. [64] argued that photometric features, when used with textual descriptors, yield a good result, however, the photometric features were observed to outperform the textual features if used in isolation. Stoecker et al. [347] equally suggested in his work that greater separation of melanoma from benign lesions is achieved using relative colour than using absolute colour.

Texture-based descriptors are yet another set of features that reflect the structural pattern of lesion surfaces irrespective of the colour or illumination characterizing the lesion. Texture descriptors can be categorised as spatial frequency based, statistical based, geometric based or model based. Spatial frequency based texture features are frequently associated with wavelet and ridgelet transformations. Statistical based descriptors include co-occurrence matrices and Fourier properties for describing lesion's local neighbourhood properties. Geometric features describe skin lesion characteristics that include shape, border, symmetry, area, diameter, variance, perimeter, circularity and anisotropy. Model based textual descriptors are frequently associated with fractals and Markov random fields. Due to simplicity and ease of feature retrieval, commonly used texture descriptors include co-occurrence texture features, wavelet features and fractal-based texture features.

Table 1. Essential features.

Features	Properties	References
Asymmetry	asymmetry index	[27, 32, 40, 57, 62, 65, 130, 252, 253, 291, 298, 336, 344, 363, 382, 387, 388]
	circularity factor	[40, 51, 62, 267, 291, 337, 344, 349, 366, 382, 386, 388 - 391]
	skewness	[103, 392]
Border irregularity	edge abruptness	[57, 65, 130, 252, 291, 351]
	lesion areas and perimeters	[62, 252, 253, 337, 363, 366, 367, 379, 382]
	radial distance	[267, 369]
	bounding box	[267, 344, 369, 377, 382, 390]
	mean and variance of lesion boundary magnitude	[40, 57, 337, 344, 366, 393]
Border Sharpness	compactness index	[27, 57, 65, 252, 337, 344, 351, 379, 382, 394]
	fractal dimension	[48, 57, 65, 96]
Colour	colour homogeneity	[51, 57, 65, 252, 347, 351, 363]
	island of colour	[40, 51, 58, 103, 130, 366, 382, 391]
	colour histogram	[28, 64, 198, 292, 299, 345, 366, 370, 376, 377, 379, 382, 395 - 398]
	RBG statistics (such as ratio, chromaticity, spectral)	[57, 103, 252, 253, 291, 337, 344, 367, 382, 385, 392, 393]
Diameter	lesion diameter	[51, 57, 168, 252, 344, 369]
Differential Structures	pigmented network (typical/atypical)	[17, 21, 28, 52, 58, 93, 94, 121, 127, 190, 242, 291, 347, 358, 371, 373, 376, 399 - 406]
	homogeneous areas	[61, 382, 407]
	branched streaks globules	[17, 52, 93, 94, 345, 400, 405, 406, 408]
	structure-less areas (such as dots, globules, blotches)	[17, 52, 93, 94, 121, 291, 345, 357, 358, 376, 400, 402, 405, 406, 408 - 410]
	blue-white veil	[17, 52, 58, 121, 291, 372, 400, 403]
Lesion Surface Structures	co-occurrence texture features	[40, 48, 51, 103, 291, 344, 347, 351, 366, 369, 376, 382, 386, 391, 392]
	wavelet texture features	[62, 64, 336, 386]
Other features	correlation index between geometry and photometry	[57, 65]
	sonography characteristics, hypo-echogenicity	[57, 108, 177, 411, 412]

Co-occurrence texture descriptors such as entropy, correlation, energy, contrast, homogeneity etc. are based on co-occurrence matrices, typically the GLCM. (Fig. **9**) detailed some of the frequently used texture descriptors, as well as corresponding computation. The GLCM [348] also known as greylevel spatial dependence matrix, is a form of statistical method of examining texture in relation to image pixels. GLCM outlines within a grey scale image, the probability of greylevel i occurring at a distance in direction θ from grey level j.

$$C_{i,j} = Pr(i, j \mid d, \theta)$$

Wavelet texture features such as wavelet energy, variance and residual energy are based on wavelet transform coefficients. Fractal based texture features such as mean fractal dimension, local connected fractal dimension and global box-counting are based on fractal dimensions. One major shortfall of local fractal dimensions and local connected fractal dimensions, however, is the dependency on the choice of the maximum window size [48]. However, while it is desirable to determine features to represent these structures directly, extracting these features is often challenging primarily due to a vast variety of dermoscopy images and the highly subjective definitions of these features [40, 41, 96].

A number of different feature selection methods have been used in the literature towards ensuring appropriate discriminating features for lesion image classification. Frequent selection methods reported in the literature include Sequential Floating Forward Selection (SFFS) [337], Sequential Floating Backward Selection (SFBS) [337], Leave-One-Out, Cross Validation (xVal), Plus-I-Take-Away-r, and Genetic algorithm. Zagrouba and Barhoumi [57] argued that relative reduction of selection features could yield 50% reduction in the processing time, as well as 65% reduction in the time required to train classifiers.

While these selectors have produced positive results and contribute positively towards classification of lesion images, there resource intensive patterns are still a concern. There is thus a growing need to improve the algorithms implemented by each of the selectors to better achieve optimal feature selection process, which in turn would help reduce complexity and time-consuming computation experienced during quantification of features [349].

6.4. Classification of Lesion

Image classification involves using selected features of an image to classify pixels of the image into one of the several classes depending on specific knowledge domain. This could be in the form of training a model using a data set and then testing the model using a data set which is disjoint from the training set. Most lesion classifications are binary in nature, distinguishing between benign and malignant moles. The classification results are typically influenced by the chosen feature descriptors and strength of the classifiers. Performance of the automated classification is equally dependent on the degree of dataset population [168].

The two main classification types as reported in the literature in relation to medical imaging are supervised classification and unsupervised classification. Supervised classification uses image analysis tool to generate a statistical categorisation (such as mean and co-variance) of the reflectance of each identified information class. The completion of the categorisation then fosters effective classification by examining the reflectance of each pixel and deciding on the best matching signatures. Decision criterion such as maximum likelihood can be used for cases of overlapping signatures in order to assign pixels to the highest probable class. Unsupervised classification typically examines a large number of unknown pixels and divides them into a number of classes based on natural groupings present in the image values using procedures such as clustering. Essentially, unsupervised classification groups values that are close together in a measurement space as a single class, thus arranging the data in different classes to be comparatively separated [350].

The literature has reported the application of several classification methods for lesion images. Frequently used among these methods are the Artificial Neural Network (ANN), Decision Trees (DT), K-Nearest Neighbour (KNN), Support Vector Machine (SVM) and Regression Analysis (RA) classifiers. Similar to the neurons of a human brain, ANN comprises of an interconnected group of nodes, otherwise termed as neurons. Neural network models typically consist of both an adaptive weight that is adjusted during model training, as well as the capability to use quantitative characterization to approximate non-linear functions of their inputs.

Popular ANN methods include Back Propagation Network (BPN) [22, 40, 292, 332, 347, 351 - 355], Auto Associative Network (AAN) [22], Multi-Layer Perceptron (MLP) [57, 168, 224, 236, 349, 351, 355 - 357], and Single Layer Perceptron (SLP) [51, 358]. In the literature, extreme Learning Machine (XLM), SLP and MLP seem to be the most commonly used Feed Forward Network (FFN) methods. Main benefits of Bayesian network include its quick training capability and insensitivity to irrelevant features [298]. Sample application of ANN for lesion classification purpose can be seen in different studies [22, 40, 51, 57, 63, 168, 236, 292, 332, 352, 353, 359]. A major challenge in the application of ANN includes the excessive time that might be required in training dataset.

Bayesian network is another frequently used classifier in the space of lesion discrimination [351]. It is a probabilistic graphical model that applies Directed Acyclic Graph (DAG) to represent a set of random variables with their corresponding conditional dependencies. It should be noted that the term Bayesian network depicts the usage of Bayes rule for probabilistic inference and not necessarily implies commitment to Bayesian statistics. One major advantage in the use of Bayesian network is its insensitivity to irrelevant features. Its drawback, however, includes sometimes undesirable assumption declaring that discriminating features are independent [298]. Application and analysis of Bayesian network can be seen in different studies [224, 360 - 364]. In the literature, Hidden Naïve Bayes (HNB) has been observed to perform better than the Bayesian network method used [62, 361]. If a set of lesion outcomes represented by a vector $v=v1, v2, ..., vn$ is to be classified to j possible classes (Cj), then the conditional posterior probability using Bayesian rule can be expressed as:

$$p\left(C_j \mid v\right) = \frac{p(C_j)\,p(v \mid C_j)}{p(v)}$$

Regression analysis is a statistical analysis for estimating the relationship between dependent (criterion) and independent variables (regression function or predictors). This typically tracks changes in the dependent variables as one of the members of the predictors is kept constant while other members of the predictors are varied. Frequently used regression analysis methods include Discriminant Function Analysis (e.g. Linear or Quadratic Regression) [40, 57, 60, 137, 253, 292, 364 - 367] and Logistic Regression [18, 75, 93, 102, 137, 368, 369].

Decision trees typically adopt a tree-like graph of possible decisions and the corresponding outcomes which could trigger another decision till a specific conclusion is reached [291, 361, 369, 370]. The major merit of using decision trees includes the speed at which it can be trained as well as its ease of use. Frequently used DT methods include C4.5 Decision Tree [291, 371 - 373], Logistic Model Tree (LMT) [291, 361, 374], Random Forest [357, 361, 370, 375], and Gradient Boosting (e.g. Adaptive Boosting: AdaBoost) [64, 291, 375 - 380]. Drawbacks seen in the usage of decision trees include difficulties in dealing with correlated features and the likelihood of over-fitting which typically results in excessive adjustments [298]. DT method was dubbed to perform the least in the comparative study described by Dreiseitl et al. [381], however, comparable to human expert.

The K-Nearest Neighbour (K-NN) is an algorithm that can also be applied as a classifier by storing the available cases and then classifying new cases based on the similar measurement in feature space [64, 198, 337, 344, 362]. The classifier input consists of k closest sample in the feature space, while its output result in class membership of objects being sampled. Contrary to some other classifiers, K-NN does not implement a decision boundary, however, uses the elements of the training set to estimate the density distribution of the data [381]. Hierarchical K-NN is an optimized subset of K-NN, however, it adopts both observation and feature space in its classification procedures.

The SVM is a non-probabilistic binary linear classifier that uses a learning module to analyse patterns within a collection of data for possible classification into one of the two categories. It adopts supervised learning for labelled data and an unsupervised clustering approach when data is not labelled. SVM also provides a unified framework in which different learning machine architectures can further be generated through an appropriate choice of kernel [382]. Applications of SVM can be seen in some studies [42, 130, 291, 354, 363, 369, 383 - 386]. In a number of studies, SVM was judged to outperform several classifiers [354, 357, 360, 363, 375]; and it is often praised for its good generalization and simplification of the non- linear data separation by means of kernel functions [298]. While the application of SVM in discriminating between melanocytic lesions has seen a number of good results, it sometimes could be very sensitive to noise hence producing a poor result. Contrary reports to the effectiveness of SVM when compared to other classifiers has equally been reported by some research works [64, 291]. SVM and MLP performed better than the counterpart classifier in the confusion matrix described in a study [357] between MLP, K-NN, Random Forest (RF) and SVM. In a similar study described by Dreiseitl et al. [381], logistic Regression, ANN and SVM produced good discriminating results for PSL compared to KNN and Decision Tree methods.

Kreutz et al. [336] argued for the need to incorporate a combination of expert systems in classifying lesion images to enable data set to be split into regions where each expert system works effectively. Results from each expert system can then be aggregated by a gating network. This is to help resolve recurrent challenges faced when training a single expert system to classify varying degrees of input space. In effect, when input space is separated and targeted, scalability and interpretability of solutions increase. Similarly, A Multiple Expert-Based Melanoma Recognition System for Dermoscopic Images of Pigmented Skin Lesions has been proposed by Rahman and Bhattacharya [198, 299] by using combination rules generated with the application of Bayes' theorem to produce a probabilistic output. The comparative study discussed by Ruiz et al. [351] equally argued that collaborative classifiers produced better classification compared to the usage of individual classifiers.

Furthermore, Dreiseitl et al. [381] suggested that linear factors contribute to a better discrimination compared to non-linear elements in the classifying models. This was proved in the comparative analysis [381] between K-NN, Logistic Regression, ANN, DT and SVM, where linear method (logistic regression) outperformed non-linear counterpart. Other remarkable classifiers as reported in the literature include Lacunarity analysis [96] and Markov Random Field MRF [246]. The literature also records the use of rule-based process for classifying skin lesion images. Frequently used rule-based procedures include Pattern Analysis, ABCD rule, ELM 7-point checklists, Menzies score, 7

Features for melanoma. Notable results have been recorded in the literature by various classification methods; however, there still exists some unresolved concerns in relation to effective lesion classification. Highlights of the issues include the great unbalance between lesion image classes, the difficulty in defining discriminating visual features and the effect of multiplicities of some lesion image classes. The execution speeds of the classification algorithms and resource intensive nature of some of these classifiers have posed a need for a more optimized approach, especially when considering mobile portability of these solutions.

CONCLUSION

The development of automated systems capable of assisting physicians in medical imaging tasks has been seen to be marred by the presence of noise such as masking structures, variability of biological shapes and tissues, and imaging system anisotropy. These noises make an automated analysis of both microscopic and macroscopic images a cumbersome task. We discussed different approaches proposed in the literature for resolving some of the doubts resulting from the automated diagnosis of microscopic (dermoscopic) as well as macroscopic (clinical) images.

Most articles in the literature often assume that malignant moles are pigmented. However, there has been an increase in the reports of non-pigmented skin tumours, as well as clinically and dermoscopic featureless moles being misdiagnosed during both clinical examination and dermoscopy screening, thus necessitating a careful approach.

Among others, subjective opinions resulting from the evaluation of parameters used in lesion segmentation were recorded as one of the difficulties encountered in the literature in an attempt to analyze different automatic border detection methods for lesion images. To achieve a proper measure of accuracy and consistent results when performing lesion localization, we would like to recommend that comparison of segmentation algorithms should be done on the same set of lesion images.

We propose that more efforts should be geared towards optimizing feature selection in order to reduce complexity and time-consuming computation. A number of the classification models proposed in the literature still exhibit some challenges such as unbalance between lesion image classes, the difficulty in defining discriminating visual features and the effect of multiplicities of some lesion image classes. We believe that given a good classification model, less emphasis could be given to the number of features required to discriminate between lesion categories.

CONFLICT OF INTEREST

The authors declare no conflict of interest, financial or otherwise.

ACKNOWLEDGEMENTS

Declared none.

REFERENCES

[1]   Tushabe F, Mwebaze E, Kiwanuka FN. An image-based diagnosis of virus and bacterial skin infections The International Congress on Complications in Interventional Radiology (ICCIR).

[2]   World Health Organization. (2007, Jan 5, 2012). Report: Essential Health technologies Strategy 2004-2007 Available from: http://www.who.int/eht/en/EHT_strategy_2004-2007.pdf

[3]   Gençler B, Gönül M. Cutaneous side effects of BRAF inhibitors in advanced melanoma: Review of literatures. Dermatol Res Pract 2016; Vol. 2016.

[4]   Tsao H, Bevona C, Goggins W, Quinn T. The transformation rate of moles (melanocytic nevi) into cutaneous melanoma: A population-based estimate. Arch Dermatol 2003; 139(3): 282-8. [http://dx.doi.org/10.1001/archderm.139.3.282] [PMID: 12622618]

[5]   Friedman RJ, Farber MJ, Warycha MA, Papathasis N, Miller MK, Heilman ER. The "dysplastic" nevus. Clin Dermatol 2009; 27(1): 103-15. [http://dx.doi.org/10.1016/j.clindermatol.2008.09.008] [PMID: 19095156]

[6]   Grant-Kels JM, Bason ET, Grin CM. The misdiagnosis of malignant melanoma. J Am Acad Dermatol 1999; 40(4): 539-48. [http://dx.doi.org/10.1016/S0190-9622(99)70435-4] [PMID: 10188671]

[7]   Stratigos AJ, Katsambas AD. The value of screening in melanoma. Clin Dermatol 2009; 27(1): 10-25. [http://dx.doi.org/10.1016/j.clindermatol.2008.09.002] [PMID: 19095150]

[8]   Botella-Estrada R, Sanmartín O, Sevila A, Escudero A, Guillén C. Melanotic pigmentation in excision scars of melanocytic and non-melanocytic skin tumors. J Cutan Pathol 1999; 26(3): 137-44.
        [http://dx.doi.org/10.1111/j.1600-0560.1999.tb01818.x] [PMID: 10235379]

[9]   Laishram RS, Myrthong BG, Laishram S, Shimray R. A. K. K, and D. C. Sharma, "Pigmented skin lesions: Are they all of melanocytic origin? A histopathological perspective. J Pak Assoc Dermatol 2013; 23: 284-8.

[10]   Sam AH, Teo JTH. Rapid Medicine. Wiley-Blackwell 2010.

[11]   Friedman RJ, Rigel DS, Kopf AW. Early detection of malignant melanoma: The role of physician examination and self-examination of the skin. CA Cancer J Clin 1985; 35(3): 130-51.
        [http://dx.doi.org/10.3322/canjclin.35.3.130] [PMID: 3921200]

[12]   Fitzpatrick TB, Rhodes AR, Sober AJ, Mihm MC. Primary malignant melanoma of the skin: The call for action to identify persons at risk, to discover precursor lesion, to detect early melanoma. Pigment Cell Res 1988; 9: 110-7.

[13]   MacKie RM. Clinical recognition of early invasive malignant melanoma. BMJ 1990; 301(6759): 1005-6.
        [http://dx.doi.org/10.1136/bmj.301.6759.1005] [PMID: 2249043]

[14]   Stolz W, Riemann A, Cognetta A. ABCD rule of dermoscopy: A new practical method for early recognition of malignant melanoma. Eur J Dermatol 1994; 4: 521-7.

[15]   Healsmith MF, Bourke JF, Osborne JE, Graham-Brown RA. An evaluation of the revised seven-point checklist for the early diagnosis of cutaneous malignant melanoma. Br J Dermatol 1994; 130(1): 48-50.
        [http://dx.doi.org/10.1111/j.1365-2133.1994.tb06881.x] [PMID: 8305316]

[16]   Hazen BP, Bhatia AC, Zaim T, Brodell RT. The clinical diagnosis of early malignant melanoma: Expansion of the ABCD criteria to improve diagnostic sensitivity. Dermatol Online J 1999; 5(2): 3.
        [PMID: 10673456]

[17]   Argenziano G, Soyer HP. Dermoscopy of pigmented skin lesions-A valuable tool for early diagnosis of melanoma. Lancet Oncol 2001; 2(7): 443-9.
        [http://dx.doi.org/10.1016/S1470-2045(00)00422-8] [PMID: 11905739]

[18]   Lucas C R, Sanders L L, Murray J C, Myers S A, Hall R P, Grichnik J M. Early melanoma detection: Nonuniform dermoscopic features and growth J Dermatol 2003; 48
        [http://dx.doi.org/10.1067/mjd.2003.283]

[19]   Abbasi NR, Shaw HM, Rigel DS, et al. Early diagnosis of cutaneous melanoma: Revisiting the ABCD criteria. JAMA 2004; 292(22): 2771-6.
        [http://dx.doi.org/10.1001/jama.292.22.2771] [PMID: 15585738]

[20]   Zouridakis G, Doshi M, Mullani N. Early diagnosis of skin cancer based on segmentation and measurement of vascularization and pigmentation in Nevoscope images. Conf Proc IEEE Eng Med Biol Soc 2004; 3: 1593-6. [EMBS].
        [PMID: 17272004]

[21]   Geller AC, Swetter SM, Brooks K, Demierre M-F, Yaroch AL. Screening, early detection, and trends for melanoma: Current status (2000-2006) and future directions. J Am Acad Dermatol 2007; 57(4): 555-72.
        [http://dx.doi.org/10.1016/j.jaad.2007.06.032] [PMID: 17870429]

[22]   Lau HT, Al-Jumaily A. Automatically early detection of skin cancer: Study based on neural netwok classification Inter Conf Soft Comp Pattern Reco. 375-80.
        [http://dx.doi.org/10.1109/SoCPaR.2009.80]

[23]   Hoshyar AN, Sulaiman AA-JR. Review on automatic early skin cancer detection International Conference on Computer Science and Service System (CSSS). Nanjing. 2011.
        [http://dx.doi.org/10.1109/CSSS.2011.5974581]

[24]   Do T-T, Zhou Y, Zheng H, Cheung N-M. Early melanoma diagnosis with mobile imaging 36th IEEE annual international conference of the engineering in medicine and biology society (EMBC).

[25]   Perakis K, Bouras T, Kostopoulous S, Sidiropoulos K. MARK1 - A decision support system for the early detection of malignant melanoma 4th EAI International Conference on Wireless Mobile Communication and Healthcare (Mobihealth). Athens. 2014.
        [http://dx.doi.org/10.4108/icst.mobihealth.2014.257247]

[26]   Tsao H, Olazagasti JM, Cordoro KM, et al. Early detection of melanoma: Reviewing the ABCDEs. J Am Acad Dermatol 2015; 72(4): 717-23.
        [http://dx.doi.org/10.1016/j.jaad.2015.01.025] [PMID: 25698455]

[27]   Hadi S, Tumbelaka BY, Irawan B, Rosadi R. Implementing DEWA framework for early diagnosis of melanoma. Procedia Comput Sci 2015; 59: 410-8.
        [http://dx.doi.org/10.1016/j.procs.2015.07.555]

[28]   Abuzaghleh O, Barkana BD, Faezipour M. Noninvasive Real-Time automated skin lesion analysis system for melanoma early detection and prevention. IEEE J Transl Eng Health Med 2015; 3: 2900310.
        [http://dx.doi.org/10.1109/JTEHM.2015.2419612] [PMID: 27170906]

[29]   Ali A-RA, Deserno TM. A systematic review of automated melanoma detection in dermatoscopic images and its ground truth data. Society of

Photo-Optical Instrumentation Engineers. SPIE 2012.
[http://dx.doi.org/10.1117/12.912389]

[30]   Han J, Colditz G A, Hunter D J. Risk factors for skin cancer: A nested case-control study within the Nurse's health study Int J Epidemiol
          2006; 35
          [http://dx.doi.org/10.1093/ije/dyl197]

[31]   Sboner A, Blanzieri E, Eccher C, Baurer P, Cristofolini M, Zumiani G, *et al.* A knowledge based system for early melanoma diagnosis
          support, 6th IDAMAP Workshop – Intelligent Data Analysis in Medicine and Pharmacology. London, UK. 2001.

[32]   Schmid-Saugeona P, Guillodb J, Thirana JP. Towards a computer-aided diagnosis system for pigmented skin lesions. Comput Med Imaging
          Graph 2003; 27(1): 65-78.
          [http://dx.doi.org/10.1016/S0895-6111(02)00048-4] [PMID: 12573891]

[33]   Australian Institute of Health and Welfare & Australian Association of Cancer Registries. Cancer in Australia In: 2012.

[34]   Robinson JK. Sun exposure, sun protection, and vitamin D. JAMA 2005; 294(12): 1541-3.
          [http://dx.doi.org/10.1001/jama.294.12.1541] [PMID: 16193624]

[35]   National Cancer Institute.(2012, Dec 12, 2013). Sun Protection Cancer Trends Progress Report 2011-2012 Update Available from:
          http://progressreport.cancer.gov/doc_detail.asp?pid=1&did=2007&chid=71&coid=711&mid

[36]   American   Cancer   Society.   (2016,   Feb   24,   2016).   Cancer   Facts   and   Figures   Available   from:
          http://www.cancer.org/acs/groups/content/@research/documents/document/acspc-047079.pdf

[37]   Bleyer AA, O'Leary MC, Barr RD, Ries LAG. Cancer Epidemiology in Older Adolescents and Young Adults 15 to 29 Years of Age,
          Including SEER Incidence and Survival: 1975-2000 In: 2006.

[38]   American   Cancer   Society.   (2015,   Nov   13,   2015).   http://www.cancer.org/acs/groups/   content/@editorial/
          documents/document/acspc-044552.pdf

[39]   American Cancer Society. (2017, Sep 09, 2017). Cancer Facts & Figures. Available: https://www.cancer.org/content/dam/cancer-org/
          research/cancer-facts-and-statistics/annual-cancer-facts-and-figures/ 2017/cancer-facts-and-figures-2017.pdf

[40]   Iyatomi H, Oka H, Celebi ME, *et al.* An improved Internet-based melanoma screening system with dermatologist-like tumor area extraction
          algorithm. Comput Med Imaging Graph 2008; 32(7): 566-79.
          [http://dx.doi.org/10.1016/j.compmedimag.2008.06.005] [PMID: 18703311]

[41]   Iyatomi H, Oka H, Saito M, *et al.* Quantitative assessment of tumour extraction from dermoscopy images and evaluation of computer-based
          extraction methods for an automatic melanoma diagnostic system. Melanoma Res 2006; 16(2): 183-90.
          [http://dx.doi.org/10.1097/01.cmr.0000215041.76553.58] [PMID: 16567974]

[42]   Stanganelli I, Brucale A, Calori L, Gori R, Lovato A, Magi S, *et al.* Computer-aided diagnosis of melanocytic lesions in Anticancer Res.
          2005; pp. 4577-82.

[43]   Asuquo ME, Nwagbara VI, Otel OO, Bassey I, Ugbem T. Cutaneous Malignant Melanoma in Calabar, South Nigeria. University of Calabar
          Teaching Hospital 2012.

[44]   Samalia MOA, Rafindadi AH. Pattern of Cutaneous malignant melanoma in Zaria, Nigeria. Ann Afr Med 2006; 5: 16-9.

[45]   Tuma B, Yamada S, Atallah AN, Araujo FM, Hirata SH. Dermoscopy of black skin: A cross-sectional study of clinical and dermoscopic
          features of melanocytic lesions in individuals with type V/VI skin compared to those with type I/II skin. J Am Acad Dermatol 2015; 73(1):
          114-9.
          [http://dx.doi.org/10.1016/j.jaad.2015.03.043] [PMID: 25982540]

[46]   Jemal A, Siegel R, Xu J, Ward E. Cancer statistics, 2010. CA Cancer J Clin 2010; 60(5): 277-300.
          [http://dx.doi.org/10.3322/caac.20073] [PMID: 20610543]

[47]   Cancer Association Of South Africa (CANSA). (2010, May 22, 2013). http://www.cansa.org.za/files/ 2012/05/SKIN_CANCER_
          leaflet-2010.pdf

[48]   Dobrescu R, Dobrescu M, Mocanu S, Popescu D. Medical images classification for skin cancer diagnosis based on combined texture and
          fractal analysis. In: World Scientific and Engineering Academy and Society. WSEAS Transactions on Biology and Biomedicine 2010.

[49]   Kantrowitz M. (2009, Jan 16, 2014). Pathology Reports May Contain Errors. Available: http://www.kantrowitz.com/ cancerpoints/
          diagnosiserrors.html

[50]   Singh H, Sethi S, Raber M, Petersen L A. Errors in cancer diagnosis: Current understanding and future directions J Clin Oncol 2007; 5009-18.
          [http://dx.doi.org/10.1200/JCO.2007.13.2142]

[51]   Rubegni P, Cevenini G, Burroni M, *et al.* Automated diagnosis of pigmented skin lesions. Int J Cancer 2002; 101(6): 576-80.
          [http://dx.doi.org/10.1002/ijc.10620] [PMID: 12237900]

[52]   Argenziano G, Soyer HP, Chimenti S, *et al.* Dermoscopy of pigmented skin lesions: results of a consensus meeting via the Internet. J Am
          Acad Dermatol 2003; 48(5): 679-93.
          [http://dx.doi.org/10.1067/mjd.2003.281] [PMID: 12734496]

[53]   Rosendahl C, Tschandl P, Cameron A, Kittler H. Diagnostic accuracy of dermatoscopy for melanocytic and nonmelanocytic pigmented
          lesions. J Am Acad Dermatol 2011; 64(6): 1068-73.

[http://dx.doi.org/10.1016/j.jaad.2010.03.039] [PMID: 21440329]

[54]   Laws KI. Textured image segmentation. DTIC Document 1980.
        [http://dx.doi.org/10.21236/ADA083283]

[55]   Abbas Q, Celebi ME, García IF. Hair removal methods: A comparative study for dermoscopy images. Biomed Signal Process Control 2011; 6: 395-404.
        [http://dx.doi.org/10.1016/j.bspc.2011.01.003]

[56]   Kittler H. Dermoscopy of pigmented skin lesions. G Ital Dermatol Venereol 2004; 139: 541-6.

[57]   Zagrouba E, Barhoumi W. An accelerated system for melanoma diagnosis based on subset feature selection. Int J Comput Models Algorithms Med 2005; 13: 69-82.

[58]   Benvenuto-Andrade C, Dusza SW, Agero ALC, et al. Differences between polarized light dermoscopy and immersion contact dermoscopy for the evaluation of skin lesions. Arch Dermatol 2007; 143(3): 329-38.
        [http://dx.doi.org/10.1001/archderm.143.3.329] [PMID: 17372097]

[59]   Argenziano G, Soyer HP, Chimenti S, Argenziano G, Ruocco V. Impact of dermoscopy on the clinical management of pigmented skin lesions. Clin Dermatol 2002; 20(3): 200-2.
        [http://dx.doi.org/10.1016/S0738-081X(02)00234-1] [PMID: 12074853]

[60]   Zortea M, Schopf TR, Thon K, et al. Performance of a dermoscopy-based computer vision system for the diagnosis of pigmented skin lesions compared with visual evaluation by experienced dermatologists. Artif Intell Med 2014; 60(1): 13-26.
        [http://dx.doi.org/10.1016/j.artmed.2013.11.006] [PMID: 24382424]

[61]   Malvehy J, Puig S, Argenziano G, Marghoob AA, Soyer HP. Dermoscopy report: Proposal for standardization. Results of a consensus meeting of the International Dermoscopy Society. J Am Acad Dermatol 2007; 57(1): 84-95.
        [http://dx.doi.org/10.1016/j.jaad.2006.02.051] [PMID: 17482314]

[62]   Garnavi R, Aldeen M, Bailey J. Computer-Aided diagnosis of melanoma using border- and wavelet-based texture analysis. 2012.

[63]   Mittra AK, Parekh R. Automated detection of skin disease using texture features. Int J Eng Sci Technol 2011; 3(June): 2011.

[64]   Barata C, Ruela M, Francisco M, Mendonça T, Marques JS. Two systems for the detection of melanomas in dermoscopy images using texture and color features. IEEE Syst J 2013.

[65]   Zagrouba E, Barhoumi W. A preliminary approach for the automated recognition of malignant melanoma. Image Anal Stereol 2004; 23: 121-35.
        [http://dx.doi.org/10.5566/ias.v23.p121-135]

[66]   Blum A, Rassner G, Garbe C. Modified ABC-point list of dermoscopy: A simplified and highly accurate dermoscopic algorithm for the diagnosis of cutaneous melanocytic lesions. J Am Acad Dermatol 2003; 48(5): 672-8.
        [http://dx.doi.org/10.1067/mjd.2003.282] [PMID: 12734495]

[67]   Pehamberger H, Steiner A, Wolff K. In vivo epiluminescence microscopy of pigmented skin lesions. I. Pattern analysis of pigmented skin lesions. J Am Acad Dermatol 1987; 17(4): 571-83.
        [http://dx.doi.org/10.1016/S0190-9622(87)70239-4] [PMID: 3668002]

[68]   Menzies SW, Ingvar C, Crotty KA, McCarthy WH. Frequency and morphologic characteristics of invasive melanomas lacking specific surface microscopic features. Arch Dermatol 1996; 132(10): 1178-82.
        [http://dx.doi.org/10.1001/archderm.1996.03890340038007] [PMID: 8859028]

[69]   Mackie RM, Doherty VR. Seven-point checklist for melanoma. Clin Exp Dermatol 1991; 16(2): 151-3.
        [http://dx.doi.org/10.1111/j.1365-2230.1991.tb00329.x] [PMID: 1867692]

[70]   Argenziano G, Fabbrocini G, Carli P, De Giorgi V, Sammarco E, Delfino M. Epiluminescence microscopy for the diagnosis of doubtful melanocytic skin lesions. Comparison of the ABCD rule of dermatoscopy and a new 7-point checklist based on pattern analysis. Arch Dermatol 1998; 134(12): 1563-70.
        [http://dx.doi.org/10.1001/archderm.134.12.1563] [PMID: 9875194]

[71]   Dal Pozzo V, Benelli C, Roscetti E. The seven features for melanoma: A new dermoscopic algorithm for the diagnosis of malignant melanoma. Eur J Dermatol 1999; 9(4): 303-8.
        [PMID: 10356410]

[72]   Henning JS, Dusza SW, Wang SQ, et al. The CASH (color, architecture, symmetry, and homogeneity) algorithm for dermoscopy. J Am Acad Dermatol 2007; 56(1): 45-52.
        [http://dx.doi.org/10.1016/j.jaad.2006.09.003] [PMID: 17190620]

[73]   Henning JS, Stein JA, Yeung J, et al. CASH algorithm for dermoscopy revisited. Arch Dermatol 2008; 144(4): 554-5.
        [http://dx.doi.org/10.1001/archderm.144.4.554] [PMID: 18427058]

[74]   Meo N D, Stinco G, Bonin S, Gatti A, Trevisini S, Damiani G, et al. CASH algorithm versus 3-point checklist and its modified version in evaluation of melanocytic pigmented skin lesions: The 4-point checklist J Dermatol 2015; 42

[75]   Haenssle H A, Korpas B, Hansen-Hagge C, Buhl T, Kaune K M, Rosenberger A, et al. Seven-point checklist for dermatoscopy: Performance during 10 years of prospective surveillance of patients at increased melanoma risk J Am Acad Dermaatol Mar 12, 2010 2009.

[76]   Walter FM, Prevost AT, Vasconcelos J, *et al.* Using the 7-point checklist as a diagnostic aid for pigmented skin lesions in general practice: A diagnostic validation study. Br J Gen Pract 2013; 63(610): e345-53.
        [http://dx.doi.org/10.3399/bjgp13X667213] [PMID: 23643233]

[77]   Andersen WK, Silvers DN. 'Melanoma? It can't be melanoma!' A subset of melanomas that defies clinical recognition. JAMA 1991; 266(24): 3463-5.
        [http://dx.doi.org/10.1001/jama.1991.03470240085038] [PMID: 1744961]

[78]   Bergman R, Katz I, Lichtig C, Ben-Arieh Y, Moscona AR, Friedman-Birnbaum R. Malignant melanomas with histologic diameters less than 6 mm. J Am Acad Dermatol 1992; 26(3 Pt 2): 462-6.
        [http://dx.doi.org/10.1016/0190-9622(92)70073-O] [PMID: 1564154]

[79]   Braun-Falco M, Hein R, Ring J, McNutt NS. Histopathological characteristics of small diameter melanocytic naevi. J Clin Pathol 2003; 56(6): 459-64.
        [http://dx.doi.org/10.1136/jcp.56.6.459] [PMID: 12783974]

[80]   Marghoob AA, Scope A. The complexity of diagnosing melanoma. J Invest Dermatol 2009; 129(1): 11-3.
        [http://dx.doi.org/10.1038/jid.2008.388] [PMID: 19078984]

[81]   Paul SP. Micromelanomas: A review of melanomas ≤2 mm and a case report. Case Rep Oncol Med 2014; 2014: 206260.
        [http://dx.doi.org/10.1155/2014/206260] [PMID: 24716040]

[82]   Goldsmith SM, Solomon AR. A series of melanomas smaller than 4 mm and implications for the ABCDE rule. J Eur Acad Dermatol Venereol 2007; 21(7): 929-34.
        [http://dx.doi.org/10.1111/j.1468-3083.2006.02115.x] [PMID: 17659002]

[83]   Whiteman DC, Baade PD, Olsen CM. More people die from thin melanomas (□1 mm) than from thick melanomas (>4 mm) in Queensland, Australia. J Invest Dermatol 2015; 135(4): 1190-3.
        [http://dx.doi.org/10.1038/jid.2014.452] [PMID: 25330295]

[84]   Zaharna M, Brodell RT. It's time for a change in Our approach to early detection of malignant melanoma. In: Clin Dermatol. 2003; Vol. 21.

[85]   Liu W, Hill D, Gibbs AF, *et al.* What features do patients notice that help to distinguish between benign pigmented lesions and melanomas?: the ABCD(E) rule versus the seven-point checklist. Melanoma Res 2005; 15(6): 549-54.
        [http://dx.doi.org/10.1097/00008390-200512000-00011] [PMID: 16314742]

[86]   Rigel DS, Friedman RJ. The rationale of the ABCDs of early melanoma. J Am Acad Dermatol 1993; 29(6): 1060-1.
        [http://dx.doi.org/10.1016/S0190-9622(08)82059-2] [PMID: 8245255]

[87]   Thomas L, Tranchand P, Berard F, Secchi T, Colin C, Moulin G. Semiological value of ABCDE criteria in the diagnosis of cutaneous pigmented tumors. Dermatology (Basel) 1998; 197(1): 11-7.
        [http://dx.doi.org/10.1159/000017969] [PMID: 9693179]

[88]   Grob JJ, Bonerandi JJ. The 'ugly duckling' sign: identification of the common characteristics of nevi in an individual as a basis for melanoma screening. Arch Dermatol 1998; 134(1): 103-4.
        [http://dx.doi.org/10.1001/archderm.134.1.103-a] [PMID: 9449921]

[89]   Grob JJ, Wazaefi Y, Bruneu Y, Gaudy-Marqueste C, Monestier S, Thomas L, *et al.* Diagnosis of melanoma: Importance of comparative analysis and ugly duckling sign. J Clin Oncol 2012; 30: 8578.

[90]   Daniel Jensen J, Elewski BE. The ABCDEF Rule: Combining the "ABCDE Rule" and the "Ugly Duckling Sign" in an effort to improve patient self-screening examinations. J Clin Aesthet Dermatol 2015; 8(2): 15.
        [PMID: 25741397]

[91]   Weinstock MA. ABCD, ABCDE, and ABCCCDEEEEFNU. Arch Dermatol 2006; 142(4): 528.
        [http://dx.doi.org/10.1001/archderm.142.4.528-a] [PMID: 16618883]

[92]   Lallas A, Kyrgidis A, Koga H, *et al.* The BRAAFF checklist: a new dermoscopic algorithm for diagnosing acral melanoma. Br J Dermatol 2015; 173(4): 1041-9.
        [http://dx.doi.org/10.1111/bjd.14045] [PMID: 26211689]

[93]   Annessi G, Bono R, Sampogna F, Faraggiana T, Abeni D. Sensitivity, specificity, and diagnostic accuracy of three dermoscopic algorithmic methods in the diagnosis of doubtful melanocytic lesions: the importance of light brown structureless areas in differentiating atypical melanocytic nevi from thin melanomas. J Am Acad Dermatol 2007; 56(5): 759-67.
        [http://dx.doi.org/10.1016/j.jaad.2007.01.014] [PMID: 17316894]

[94]   Dolianitis C, Kelly J, Wolfe R, Simpson P. Comparative performance of 4 dermoscopic algorithms by nonexperts for the diagnosis of melanocytic lesions. Arch Dermatol 2005; 141(8): 1008-14.
        [http://dx.doi.org/10.1001/archderm.141.8.1008] [PMID: 16103330]

[95]   Day GR, Barbour RH. Automated melanoma diagnosis: where are we at? Skin Res Technol 2000; 6(1): 1-5.
        [http://dx.doi.org/10.1034/j.1600-0846.2000.006001001.x] [PMID: 11428935]

[96]   Gilmore S, Hofmann-Wellenhof R, Muir J, Soyer HP. Lacunarity analysis: A promising method for the automated assessment of melanocytic naevi and melanoma. PLoS One 2009; 4(10): e7449.
        [http://dx.doi.org/10.1371/journal.pone.0007449] [PMID: 19823688]

[97]   Detrixhe A, Libon F, Mansuy M, *et al.* Melanoma masquerading as nonmelanocytic lesions. Melanoma Res 2016; 26(6): 631-4.
[http://dx.doi.org/10.1097/CMR.0000000000000294] [PMID: 27537773]

[98]   Tashiro J, Perlyn CA, Melnick SJ, Gulec SA, Burnweit CA. Non-pigmented melanoma with nodal metastases masquerading as pyogenic granuloma in a 1-year old. J Pediatr Surg 2014; 49(4): 653-5.
[http://dx.doi.org/10.1016/j.jpedsurg.2014.01.007] [PMID: 24726130]

[99]   Diniz G, Tosun Yildirim H, Yamaci S, Olgun N. Nonpigmented metastatic melanoma in a two-year-old girl: A serious diagnostic dilemma. Case Rep Oncol Med 2015; 2015: 298273.
[http://dx.doi.org/10.1155/2015/298273] [PMID: 25763285]

[100]   Zalaudek I, Kreusch J, Giacomel J, Ferrara G, Catricala C, Argenziano G. How to diagnose nonpigmented skin tumors: a review of vascular structures seen with dermoscopy: part I Melanocytic skin tumors. J Am Acad Dermaatol 2010; Vol. 63: pp. 361-74.

[101]   Carli P, Massi D, de Giorgi V, Giannotti B. Clinically and dermoscopically featureless melanoma: When prevention fails. J Am Acad Dermatol 2002; 46(6): 957-9.
[http://dx.doi.org/10.1067/mjd.2002.120569] [PMID: 12063500]

[102]   Blum A, Luedtke H, Ellwanger U, Schwabe R, Rassner G, Garbe C. Digital image analysis for diagnosis of cutaneous melanoma. Development of a highly effective computer algorithm based on analysis of 837 melanocytic lesions. Br J Dermatol 2004; 151(5): 1029-38.
[http://dx.doi.org/10.1111/j.1365-2133.2004.06210.x] [PMID: 15541081]

[103]   Iyatomi H, Norton K, Celebi ME, Schaefer G, Tanaka M, Ogawa K. Classification of melanocytic skin lesions from non-melanocytic lesions 32nd Annual International Conference of the IEEE Engineering in Medicine and Biology Society (EMBS). Buenos Aires, Argentina. 2010.
[http://dx.doi.org/10.1109/IEMBS.2010.5626500]

[104]   Schindewolf T, Schiffner R, Stolz W, Albert R, Abmayr W, Harms H. Evaluation of different image acquisition techniques for a computer vision system in the diagnosis of malignant melanoma. J Am Acad Dermatol 1994; 31(1): 33-41.
[http://dx.doi.org/10.1016/S0190-9622(94)70132-6] [PMID: 8021369]

[105]   Green A, Martin N, Pfitzner J, O'Rourke M, Knight N. Computer image analysis in the diagnosis of melanoma. J Am Acad Dermatol 1994; 31(6): 958-64.
[http://dx.doi.org/10.1016/S0190-9622(94)70264-0] [PMID: 7962777]

[106]   Cascinelli N, Ferrario M, Tonelli T, Leo E. A possible new tool for clinical diagnosis of melanoma: the computer. J Am Acad Dermatol 1987; 16(2 Pt 1): 361-7.
[http://dx.doi.org/10.1016/S0190-9622(87)70050-4] [PMID: 3819073]

[107]   Huang A, Kwan S-Y, Chang W-Y, Liu M-Y, Chi M-H, Chen G-S. A Robust Hair Segmentation and Removal Approach for Clinical Images of Skin Lesions 35th Annual International Conference of the IEEE Engineering in Medicine and Biology Society (EMBC). 3315-8.
[http://dx.doi.org/10.1109/EMBC.2013.6610250]

[108]   Marghoob AA, Swindle LD, Moricz CZM, *et al.* Instruments and new technologies for the in vivo diagnosis of melanoma. J Am Acad Dermatol 2003; 49(5): 777-97.
[http://dx.doi.org/10.1016/S0190-9622(03)02470-8] [PMID: 14576657]

[109]   Menge TD, Pellacani G. Advances in noninvasive imaging of melanoma. Semin Cutan Med Surg 2016; 35(1): 18-24.
[http://dx.doi.org/10.12788/j.sder.2016.003] [PMID: 26963113]

[110]   Dancey AL, Mahon BS, Rayatt SS. A review of diagnostic imaging in melanoma. J Plast Reconstr Aesthet Surg 2008; 61(11): 1275-83.
[http://dx.doi.org/10.1016/j.bjps.2008.04.034] [PMID: 18694659]

[111]   Forsea AM, Tschandl P, Del Marmol V, *et al.* Factors driving the use of dermoscopy in Europe: A pan-European survey. Br J Dermatol 2016; 175(6): 1329-37.
[http://dx.doi.org/10.1111/bjd.14895] [PMID: 27469990]

[112]   Moscarella E, Tion I, Zalaudek I, Lallas A, Kyrgidis A, Longo C, *et al.* Both short-term and long-term dermoscopy monitoring is useful in detecting melanoma in patients with multiple atypical nevi. J Eur Acad Dermatol Venereol 2016.
[PMID: 27422807]

[113]   Noor O II, Nanda A, Rao BK. A dermoscopy survey to assess who is using it and why it is or is not being used. Int J Dermatol 2009; 48(9): 951-2.
[http://dx.doi.org/10.1111/j.1365-4632.2009.04095.x] [PMID: 19702978]

[114]   Braun RP, Saurat JH, French LE. Dermoscopy of pigmented lesions: A valuable tool in the diagnosis of melanoma. Swiss Med Wkly 2004; 134(7-8): 83-90.
[PMID: 15106024]

[115]   Ribero S, Marra E, Tomasini CF, Fierro MT, Bombonato C, Longo C. Confocal microscopy and dermoscopy for the monitoring of BRAF inhibitor therapy of melanoma skin metastases. Br J Dermatol 2016.
[PMID: 27515562]

[116]   Kittler H, Pehamberger H, Wolff K, Binder M. Diagnostic accuracy of dermoscopy. Lancet Oncol 2002; 3(3): 159-65.
[http://dx.doi.org/10.1016/S1470-2045(02)00679-4] [PMID: 11902502]

[117]   Stolz W, Semmelmayer U, Johow K, Burgdorf WH. Principles of dermatoscopy of pigmented skin lesions. Semin Cutan Med Surg 2003; 22(1): 9-20.

[http://dx.doi.org/10.1053/sder.2003.50001] [PMID: 12773010]

[118]   Lallas A, Apalla Z, Lazaridou E, Ioannides D. Chapter 3 - Dermoscopy In: Imaging in Dermatology, P Avci and G K Gupta, Eds, ed Boston: Academic Press. 2016; pp. 13-28.

[119]   Bafounta ML, Beauchet A, Aegerter P, Saiag P. Is dermoscopy (epiluminescence microscopy) useful for the diagnosis of melanoma? Results of a meta-analysis using techniques adapted to the evaluation of diagnostic tests. Arch Dermatol 2001; 137(10): 1343-50.
[http://dx.doi.org/10.1001/archderm.137.10.1343] [PMID: 11594860]

[120]   Tromme I, Legrand C, Devleesschauwer B, et al. Cost-effectiveness analysis in melanoma detection: A transition model applied to dermoscopy. Eur J Cancer 2016; 67: 38-45.
[http://dx.doi.org/10.1016/j.ejca.2016.07.020] [PMID: 27592070]

[121]   Crotty KA, Menzies SW. Dermoscopy and its role in diagnosing melanocytic lesions: A guide for pathologists. Pathology 2004; 36(5): 470-7.
[http://dx.doi.org/10.1080/00313020412331283851] [PMID: 15370118]

[122]   De Giorgi V, Carli P. Dermoscopy and preoperative evaluation of melanoma thickness. Clin Dermatol 2002; 20(3): 305-8.
[http://dx.doi.org/10.1016/S0738-081X(02)00224-9] [PMID: 12074872]

[123]   Ciudad-Blanco C, Avilés-Izquierdo JA, Lázaro-Ochaita P, Suárez-Fernández R. Dermoscopic findings for the early detection of melanoma: an analysis of 200 cases. Actas Dermosifiliogr 2014; 105(7): 683-93.
[http://dx.doi.org/10.1016/j.adengl.2014.07.015] [PMID: 24704190]

[124]   Ferrari A, Peris K, Piccolo D, Chimenti S. Dermoscopic features of cutaneous local recurrent melanoma. J Am Acad Dermatol 2000; 43(4): 722-4.
[http://dx.doi.org/10.1067/mjd.2000.107942] [PMID: 11004641]

[125]   de Giorgi V, Sestini S, Massi D, Maio V, Giannotti B. Dermoscopy for "true" amelanotic melanoma: A clinical dermoscopic-pathologic case study. J Am Acad Dermatol 2006; 54(2): 341-4.
[http://dx.doi.org/10.1016/j.jaad.2005.04.040] [PMID: 16443072]

[126]   Braun RP, Marghoob A. High-dynamic-range dermoscopy imaging and diagnosis of hypopigmented skin cancers. JAMA Dermatol 2015; 151(4): 456-7.
[http://dx.doi.org/10.1001/jamadermatol.2014.4714] [PMID: 25535875]

[127]   Braun RP, Oliviero M, Kolm I, French LE, Marghoob AA, Rabinovitz H. Dermoscopy: what's new? Clin Dermatol 2009; 27(1): 26-34.
[http://dx.doi.org/10.1016/j.clindermatol.2008.09.003] [PMID: 19095151]

[128]   Chappuis P, Duru G, Marchal O, Girier P, Dalle S, Thomas L. Dermoscopy, a useful tool for general practitioners in melanoma screening: a nationwide survey. Br J Dermatol 2016; 175(4): 744-50.
[http://dx.doi.org/10.1111/bjd.14495] [PMID: 26914613]

[129]   Johr RH. Dermoscopy: alternative melanocytic algorithms-the ABCD rule of dermatoscopy, Menzies scoring method, and 7-point checklist. Clin Dermatol 2002; 20(3): 240-7.
[http://dx.doi.org/10.1016/S0738-081X(02)00236-5] [PMID: 12074859]

[130]   Mete M, Sirakov NM. Dermoscopic diagnosis of melanoma in a 4D space constructed by active contour extracted features. Comput Med Imaging Graph 2012; 36(7): 572-9.
[http://dx.doi.org/10.1016/j.compmedimag.2012.06.002] [PMID: 22819294]

[131]   Taylor S, Westerhof W, Im S, Lim J. Noninvasive techniques for the evaluation of skin color. J Am Acad Dermatol 2006; 54(5)(Suppl. 2): S282-90.
[http://dx.doi.org/10.1016/j.jaad.2005.12.041] [PMID: 16631969]

[132]   Menzies SW. Cutaneous melanoma: Making a clinical diagnosis, present and future. Dermatol Ther 2006; 19(1): 32-9.
[http://dx.doi.org/10.1111/j.1529-8019.2005.00054.x] [PMID: 16405568]

[133]   Psaty EL, Halpern AC. Current and emerging technologies in melanoma diagnosis: The state of the art. Clin Dermatol 2009; 27(1): 35-45.
[http://dx.doi.org/10.1016/j.clindermatol.2008.09.004] [PMID: 19095152]

[134]   Silveira CEG, Silva TB, Fregnani JHGT, Vieira RAC, Haikel RL, Syrjänen K, et al. Digital photography in skin cancer screening by mobile units in remote areas of Brazil. BMC Dermatol 2014; Vol. 14.

[135]   Yancovitz M, Finelt N, Warycha MA, et al. Role of radiologic imaging at the time of initial diagnosis of stage T1b-T3b melanoma. Cancer 2007; 110(5): 1107-14.
[http://dx.doi.org/10.1002/cncr.22868] [PMID: 17620286]

[136]   Gamo R, Pampín A, Floristán U. Reflectance confocal microscopy in lentigo maligna. Actas dermo-sifiliográficas 2016; Vol. S0001-7310.

[137]   Pellacani G, Guitera P, Longo C, Avramidis M, Seidenari S, Menzies S. The impact of in vivo reflectance confocal microscopy for the diagnostic accuracy of melanoma and equivocal melanocytic lesions. J Invest Dermatol 2007; 127(12): 2759-65.
[http://dx.doi.org/10.1038/sj.jid.5700993] [PMID: 17657243]

[138]   Lorber A, Wiltgen M, Hofmann-Wellenhof R, et al. Correlation of image analysis features and visual morphology in melanocytic skin tumours using in vivo confocal laser scanning microscopy. Skin Res Technol 2009; 15(2): 237-41.
[http://dx.doi.org/10.1111/j.1600-0846.2009.00361.x] [PMID: 19622133]

[139]   Pellacani G, De Pace B, Reggiani C, et al. Distinct melanoma types based on reflectance confocal microscopy. Exp Dermatol 2014; 23(6):

414-8.
[http://dx.doi.org/10.1111/exd.12417] [PMID: 24750486]

[140]   Stanganelli I, Longo C, Mazzoni L, *et al.* Integration of reflectance confocal microscopy in sequential dermoscopy follow-up improves melanoma detection accuracy. Br J Dermatol 2015; 172(2): 365-71.
[http://dx.doi.org/10.1111/bjd.13373] [PMID: 25154446]

[141]   Calzavara-Pinton P, Longo C, Venturini M, Sala R, Pellacani G. Reflectance confocal microscopy for in vivo skin imaging. Photochem Photobiol 2008; 84(6): 1421-30.
[http://dx.doi.org/10.1111/j.1751-1097.2008.00443.x] [PMID: 19067964]

[142]   Stevenson AD, Mickan S, Mallett S, Ayya M. Systematic review of diagnostic accuracy of reflectance confocal microscopy for melanoma diagnosis in patients with clinically equivocal skin lesions. Dermatol Pract Concept 2013; 3(4): 19-27.
[http://dx.doi.org/10.5826/dpc.0304a05] [PMID: 24282659]

[143]   Pellacani G, Cesinaro AM, Seidenari S. Reflectance-mode confocal microscopy of pigmented skin lesions--improvement in melanoma diagnostic specificity. J Am Acad Dermatol 2005; 53(6): 979-85.
[http://dx.doi.org/10.1016/j.jaad.2005.08.022] [PMID: 16310058]

[144]   de Carvalho N, Farnetani F, Ciardo S, *et al.* Reflectance confocal microscopy correlates of dermoscopic patterns of facial lesions help to discriminate lentigo maligna from pigmented nonmelanocytic macules. Br J Dermatol 2015; 173(1): 128-33.
[http://dx.doi.org/10.1111/bjd.13546] [PMID: 25413382]

[145]   Nori S, Rius-Díaz F, Cuevas J, *et al.* Sensitivity and specificity of reflectance-mode confocal microscopy for *in vivo* diagnosis of basal cell carcinoma: A multicenter study. J Am Acad Dermatol 2004; 51(6): 923-30.
[http://dx.doi.org/10.1016/j.jaad.2004.06.028] [PMID: 15583584]

[146]   Que SKT, Grant-Kels JM, Longo C, Pellacani G. Basics of confocal microscopy and the complexity of diagnosing skin tumors: New imaging tools in clinical practice, diagnostic workflows, cost-estimate, and New trends. Dermatol Clin 2016; 34(4): 367-75.
[http://dx.doi.org/10.1016/j.det.2016.05.001] [PMID: 27692444]

[147]   Que SKT, Grant-Kels JM, Rabinovitz HS, Oliviero M, Scope A. Application of handheld confocal microscopy for skin cancer diagnosis: Advantages and limitations compared with the wide-probe confocal. Dermatol Clin 2016; 34(4): 469-75.
[http://dx.doi.org/10.1016/j.det.2016.05.009] [PMID: 27692452]

[148]   Song E, Grant-Kels JM, Swede H, *et al.* Paired comparison of the sensitivity and specificity of multispectral digital skin lesion analysis and reflectance confocal microscopy in the detection of melanoma *in vivo*: A cross-sectional study. J Am Acad Dermatol 2016; 75(6): 1187-1192.e2.
[http://dx.doi.org/10.1016/j.jaad.2016.07.022] [PMID: 27693007]

[149]   Holder WD Jr, White RL Jr, Zuger JH, Easton EJ Jr, Greene FL. Effectiveness of positron emission tomography for the detection of melanoma metastases. Ann Surg 1998; 227(5): 764-9.
[http://dx.doi.org/10.1097/00000658-199805000-00017] [PMID: 9605668]

[150]   Perng P, Marcus C, Subramaniam RM. (18)F-FDG PET/CT and Melanoma: Staging, Immune Modulation and Mutation-Targeted Therapy Assessment, and Prognosis. AJR Am J Roentgenol 2015; 205(2): 259-70.
[http://dx.doi.org/10.2214/AJR.14.13575] [PMID: 26204273]

[151]   Bronstein Y, Ng CS, Rohren E, *et al.* PET/CT in the management of patients with stage IIIC and IV metastatic melanoma considered candidates for surgery: Evaluation of the additive value after conventional imaging. AJR Am J Roentgenol 2012; 198(4): 902-8.
[http://dx.doi.org/10.2214/AJR.11.7280] [PMID: 22451559]

[152]   Strobel K, Dummer R, Husarik DB, Pérez Lago M, Hany TF, Steinert HC. High-risk melanoma: accuracy of FDG PET/CT with added CT morphologic information for detection of metastases. Radiology 2007; 244(2): 566-74.
[http://dx.doi.org/10.1148/radiol.2442061099] [PMID: 17641374]

[153]   Reinhardt MJ, Joe AY, Jaeger U, *et al.* Diagnostic performance of whole body dual modality 18F-FDG PET/CT imaging for N- and M-staging of malignant melanoma: Experience with 250 consecutive patients. J Clin Oncol 2006; 24(7): 1178-87.
[http://dx.doi.org/10.1200/JCO.2005.03.5634] [PMID: 16505438]

[154]   Danielsen M, Højgaard L, Kjær A, Fischer BM. Positron emission tomography in the follow-up of cutaneous malignant melanoma patients: A systematic review. Am J Nucl Med Mol Imaging 2013; 4(1): 17-28.
[PMID: 24380042]

[155]   Veit-Haibach P, Vogt FM, Jablonka R, *et al.* Diagnostic accuracy of contrast-enhanced FDG-PET/CT in primary staging of cutaneous malignant melanoma. Eur J Nucl Med Mol Imaging 2009; 36(6): 910-8.
[http://dx.doi.org/10.1007/s00259-008-1049-x] [PMID: 19156409]

[156]   Huang D, Swanson EA, Lin CP, *et al.* Optical coherence tomography. Science 1991; 254(5035): 1178-81.
[http://dx.doi.org/10.1126/science.1957169] [PMID: 1957169]

[157]   Boppart SA, Brezinski ME, Pitris C, Fujimoto JG. Optical coherence tomography for neurosurgical imaging of human intracortical melanoma. Neurosurgery 1998; 43(4): 834-41.
[http://dx.doi.org/10.1097/00006123-199810000-00068] [PMID: 9766311]

[158]   Fujimoto JG, Pitris C, Boppart SA, Brezinski ME. Optical coherence tomography: an emerging technology for biomedical imaging and optical biopsy. Neoplasia 2000; 2(1-2): 9-25.

        [http://dx.doi.org/10.1038/sj.neo.7900071] [PMID: 10933065]

[159]   Welzel J. Optical coherence tomography in dermatology: A review. Skin Res Technol 2001; 7(1): 1-9.
        [http://dx.doi.org/10.1034/j.1600-0846.2001.007001001.x] [PMID: 11301634]

[160]   Schuh S, Kaestle R, Sattler E, Welzel J. Comparison of different optical coherence tomography devices for diagnosis of non-melanoma skin
        cancer. Skin Res Technol 2016; 22(4): 395-405.
        [http://dx.doi.org/10.1111/srt.12277] [PMID: 26804618]

[161]   Olsen J, Themstrup L, Jemec GB. Optical coherence tomography in dermatology. G Ital Dermatol Venereol 2015; 150(5): 603-15.
        [PMID: 26129683]

[162]   Marx HF, Colletti PM, Raval JK, Boswell WD Jr, Zee C-S. Magnetic resonance imaging features in melanoma. Magn Reson Imaging 1990;
        8(3): 223-9.
        [http://dx.doi.org/10.1016/0730-725X(90)90093-H] [PMID: 2366635]

[163]   Takahashi M, Kohda H. Diagnostic utility of magnetic resonance imaging in malignant melanoma. J Am Acad Dermatol 1992; 27(1): 51-4.
        [http://dx.doi.org/10.1016/0190-9622(92)70155-9] [PMID: 1619076]

[164]   Zemtsov A, Dixon L. Magnetic resonance in dermatology. Arch Dermatol 1993; 129(2): 215-8.
        [http://dx.doi.org/10.1001/archderm.1993.01680230099015] [PMID: 8434981]

[165]   Patwardhan SV, Dai S, Dhawan AP. Multi-spectral image analysis and classification of melanoma using fuzzy membership based partitions.
        Comput Med Imaging Graph 2005; 29(4): 287-96.
        [http://dx.doi.org/10.1016/j.compmedimag.2004.11.001] [PMID: 15890256]

[166]   Elbaum M, Kopf AW, Rabinovitz HS, et al. Automatic differentiation of melanoma from melanocytic nevi with multispectral digital
        dermoscopy: a feasibility study. J Am Acad Dermatol 2001; 44(2): 207-18.
        [http://dx.doi.org/10.1067/mjd.2001.110395] [PMID: 11174377]

[167]   Kuzmina I, Diebele I, Jakovels D, Spigulis J, Valeine L, Kapostinsh J, et al. Towards noncontact skin melanoma selection by multispectral
        imaging analysis J Biomed Opt 2011; 16
        [http://dx.doi.org/10.1117/1.3584846]

[168]   Tomatis S, Carrara M, Bono A, et al. Automated melanoma detection with a novel multispectral imaging system: results of a prospective
        study. Phys Med Biol 2005; 50(8): 1675-87.
        [http://dx.doi.org/10.1088/0031-9155/50/8/004] [PMID: 15815089]

[169]   Zhou Y, Wang LV. Chapter 24 - Photoacoustic Tomography in the Diagnosis of Melanoma In: Imaging in Dermatology, P. Avci and G. K.
        Gupta, Eds., ed Boston: Academic Press, 2016, pp. 341-356.

[170]   Bourgeois AC, Pasiak AS, Bradley YC. Chapter 32 - The role of positron emission tomography/computed tomography in cutaneous
        melanoma In: imaging in dermatology, P. Avci and G. K. Gupta, Eds., ed Boston: Academic Press, 2016, pp. 455-466.

[171]   Sánchez-Sánchez R, Serrano-Falcón C, Rebollo Aguirre A C. Diagnostic imaging in dermatology: Utility of PET-CT in cutaneous melanoma
        Actas Dermosifiliogr 2015; 106(4): 29-34.

[172]   Gambichler T, Regeniter P, Bechara FG, et al. Characterization of benign and malignant melanocytic skin lesions using optical coherence
        tomography in vivo. J Am Acad Dermatol 2007; 57(4): 629-37.
        [http://dx.doi.org/10.1016/j.jaad.2007.05.029] [PMID: 17610989]

[173]   Wang Y, Xu D, Yang S, Xing D. Toward in vivo biopsy of melanoma based on photoacoustic and ultrasound dual imaging with an integrated
        detector. Biomed Opt Express 2016; 7(2): 279-86.
        [http://dx.doi.org/10.1364/BOE.7.000279] [PMID: 26977339]

[174]   Hoffmann K, Jung J, el Gammal S, Altmeyer P. Malignant melanoma in 20-MHz B scan sonography. Dermatology (Basel) 1992; 185(1):
        49-55.
        [http://dx.doi.org/10.1159/000247403] [PMID: 1638071]

[175]   Chami L, Lassau N, Chebil M, Robert C. Imaging of melanoma: Usefulness of ultrasonography before and after contrast injection for
        diagnosis and early evaluation of treatment. Clin Cosmet Investig Dermatol 2011; 4: 1-6.
        [PMID: 21673868]

[176]   Mandava A, Ravuri PR, Konathan R. High-resolution ultrasound imaging of cutaneous lesions. Indian J Radiol Imaging 2013; 23(3): 269-77.
        [http://dx.doi.org/10.4103/0971-3026.120272] [PMID: 24347861]

[177]   Wortsman X. Sonography of the Primary Cutaneous Melanoma: A Review. In: Radiol Res Pract 2012; Vol. 2012.

[178]   Samimi M, Perrinaud A, Naouri M, et al. High-resolution ultrasonography assists the differential diagnosis of blue naevi and cutaneous
        metastases of melanoma. Br J Dermatol 2010; 163(3): 550-6.
        [http://dx.doi.org/10.1111/j.1365-2133.2010.09903.x] [PMID: 20545694]

[179]   Serrone L, Solivetti FM, Thorel MF, Eibenschutz L, Donati P, Catricalà C. High frequency ultrasound in the preoperative staging of primary
        melanoma: A statistical analysis. Melanoma Res 2002; 12(3): 287-90.
        [http://dx.doi.org/10.1097/00008390-200206000-00013] [PMID: 12140386]

[180]   Blum A, Schmid-Wendtner MH, Mauss-Kiefer V, Eberle JY, Kuchelmeister C, Dill-Müller D. Ultrasound mapping of lymph node and
        subcutaneous metastases in patients with cutaneous melanoma: results of a prospective multicenter study. Dermatology (Basel) 2006; 212(1):

47-52.
[http://dx.doi.org/10.1159/000089022] [PMID: 16319474]

[181]   Vasefi F, MacKinnon N, Farkas DL. Chapter 16 - hyperspectral and multispectral imaging in dermatology In: Imaging in Dermatology, P. Avci and G. K. Gupta, Eds., ed Boston: Academic Press, 2016, pp. 187-201.

[182]   Ho D, Kraeva E, Jagdeo J, Levenson RM. Chapter 18 - spectral imaging in dermatology In: Imaging in Dermatology, P. Avci and G. K. Gupta, Eds., ed Boston: Academic Press, 2016, pp. 217-239.

[183]   Bonmarin M, Le Gal FA. Chapter 31 - thermal imaging in dermatology In: Imaging in Dermatology, P. Avci and G. K. Gupta, Eds., ed Boston: Academic Press, 2016, pp. 437-454.

[184]   Shada AL, Dengel LT, Petroni GR, Smolkin ME, Acton S, Slingluff CL Jr. Infrared thermography of cutaneous melanoma metastases. J Surg Res 2013; 182(1): e9-e14.
[http://dx.doi.org/10.1016/j.jss.2012.09.022] [PMID: 23043862]

[185]   Herman C. The role of dynamic infrared imaging in melanoma diagnosis. Expert Rev Dermatol 2013; 8(2): 177-84.
[http://dx.doi.org/10.1586/edm.13.15] [PMID: 23745131]

[186]   Cristofolini M, Boi S, Perani B, Recchia G, Zumiani G. Value of thermography in the diagnosis of malignant melanomas of the skin In: recent advances in medical thermology, E. F. J. Ring and B. Phillips, Eds., ed Boston, MA: Springer New York, 1984, pp. 631-634.

[187]   Doukas C, Stagkopoulos P, Maglogiannis I. Skin lesions image analysis utilizing smartphones and cloud platforms. Methods Mol Biol 2015; 1256: 435-58.
[http://dx.doi.org/10.1007/978-1-4939-2172-0_29] [PMID: 25626556]

[188]   Janda M, Loescher LJ, Banan P, Horsham C, Soyer HP. Lesion selection by melanoma high-risk consumers during skin self-examination using mobile teledermoscopy. JAMA Dermatol 2014; 150(6): 656-8.
[http://dx.doi.org/10.1001/jamadermatol.2013.7743] [PMID: 24522284]

[189]   Xing Y, Bronstein Y, Ross MI, et al. Contemporary diagnostic imaging modalities for the staging and surveillance of melanoma patients: A meta-analysis. J Natl Cancer Inst 2011; 103(2): 129-42.
[http://dx.doi.org/10.1093/jnci/djq455] [PMID: 21081714]

[190]   Malvehy J, Puig S. Follow-up of melanocytic skin lesions with digital total-body photography and digital dermoscopy: A two-step method. Clin Dermatol 2002; 20(3): 297-304.
[http://dx.doi.org/10.1016/S0738-081X(02)00220-1] [PMID: 12074871]

[191]   Mohr P, Eggermont AMM, Hauschild A, Buzaid A. Staging of cutaneous melanoma. Ann Oncol 2009; 20(Suppl. 6): vi14-21.
[http://dx.doi.org/10.1093/annonc/mdp256] [PMID: 19617293]

[192]   He J, Wang N, Tsurui H, Kato M, Iida M, Kobayashi T. Noninvasive, label-free, three-dimensional imaging of melanoma with confocal photothermal microscopy: Differentiate malignant melanoma from benign tumor tissue. Sci Rep 2016; 6: 30209.
[http://dx.doi.org/10.1038/srep30209] [PMID: 27445171]

[193]   Gómez DD, Butakoff C, Ersbøll BK, Stoecker W. Independent histogram pursuit for segmentation of skin lesions. IEEE Trans Biomed Eng 2008; 55(1): 157-61.
[http://dx.doi.org/10.1109/TBME.2007.910651] [PMID: 18232357]

[194]   Okuboyejo DA, Olugbara OO, Odunaike SA. Unsupervised Restoration of Hair-Occluded Lesion in Dermoscopic Images 18th Conference on Medical Image Understanding and Analysis. London, United Kingdom. 2014; pp. 91-6.

[195]   Abbas Q, Garcia IF, Emre Celebi M, Ahmad W, Mushtaq Q. A perceptually oriented method for contrast enhancement and segmentation of dermoscopy images. Skin Res Technol 2013; 19(1): e490-7.
[http://dx.doi.org/10.1111/j.1600-0846.2012.00670.x] [PMID: 22882675]

[196]   Garnavi R, Aldeen M, Celebi ME, Bhuiyan A, Dolianitis C, Varigos G. Automatic segmentation of dermoscopy images using histogram thresholding on optimal color channels. IEEE J Transl Eng Health Med 2010; 1: 126-34.

[197]   Hoshyar AN, Al-Jumaily A, Hoshyar AN. The Beneficial Techniques in Preprocessing Step of Skin Cancer Detection System Comparing. Procedia Comput Sci 2014; 42: 25-31.
[http://dx.doi.org/10.1016/j.procs.2014.11.029]

[198]   Rahman MM, Bhattacharya P, Desai BC. A multiple expert-based melanoma recognition system for dermoscopic images of pigmented skin lesions 8th IEEE International Conference on BioInformatics and BioEngineering (BIBE). 1-6.
[http://dx.doi.org/10.1109/BIBE.2008.4696799]

[199]   Quigley EA, Tokay BA, Jewell ST, Marchetti MA, Halpern AC. Technology and technique standards for camera-acquired digital dermatologic images: A systematic review. JAMA Dermatol 2015; 151(8): 883-90.
[http://dx.doi.org/10.1001/jamadermatol.2015.33] [PMID: 25970844]

[200]   Quintana J, Garcia R, Neumann L. A novel method for color correction in epiluminescence microscopy. Comput Med Imaging Graph 2011; 35(7-8): 646-52.
[http://dx.doi.org/10.1016/j.compmedimag.2011.03.006] [PMID: 21531539]

[201]   Iyatomi H, Celebi ME, Schaefer G, Tanaka M. Automated color calibration method for dermoscopy images. Comput Med Imaging Graph 2011; 35(2): 89-98.
[http://dx.doi.org/10.1016/j.compmedimag.2010.08.003] [PMID: 20933366]

[202]   Glaister J, Amelard R, Wong A, Clausi DA. MSIM: multistage illumination modeling of dermatological photographs for illumination-corrected skin lesion analysis. IEEE Trans Biomed Eng 2013; 60(7): 1873-83.
        [http://dx.doi.org/10.1109/TBME.2013.2244596] [PMID: 23380843]

[203]   Glaister J, Wong A, Clausi DA. Illumination Correction in Dermatological Photographs using Multi-stage Illumination Modeling for Skin Lesion Analysis 34th Annual International Conference of the IEEE Engineering in Medicine and Biology Society (EMBS). San Diego, California USA. 2012; pp. 102-5.
        [http://dx.doi.org/10.1109/EMBC.2012.6345881]

[204]   Grana C, Pellacani G, Seidenari S. Practical color calibration for dermoscopy, applied to a digital epiluminescence microscope. Skin Res Technol 2005; 11(4): 242-7.
        [http://dx.doi.org/10.1111/j.0909-725X.2005.00127.x] [PMID: 16221140]

[205]   Wighton P, Lee TK, Lui H, McLean D, Atkins MS. Chromatic aberration correction: An enhancement to the calibration of low-cost digital dermoscopes. Skin Res Technol 2011; 17(3): 339-47.
        [http://dx.doi.org/10.1111/j.1600-0846.2011.00504.x] [PMID: 21338405]

[206]   Schaefer G, Rajab MI, Celebi ME, Iyatomi H. Colour and contrast enhancement for improved skin lesion segmentation. Comput Med Imaging Graph 2011; 35(2): 99-104.
        [http://dx.doi.org/10.1016/j.compmedimag.2010.08.004] [PMID: 21035303]

[207]   Okuboyejo DA, Olugbara OO, Odunaike SA. CLAHE Inspired Segmentation of Dermoscopic Images Using Mixture of Methods In: Transactions on Engineering Technologies, H. K. Kim, S.-I. Ao, and M. A. Amouzegar, Eds., ed: Springer Netherlands, 2014, pp. 355-365.

[208]   Premaladha J, Ravichandran KS. Novel approaches for diagnosing melanoma skin lesions through supervised and deep learning algorithms. J Med Syst 2016; 40(4): 96.
        [http://dx.doi.org/10.1007/s10916-016-0460-2] [PMID: 26872778]

[209]   Abbas Q, Garcia IF, Emre Celebi M, Ahmad W. A feature-preserving hair removal algorithm for dermoscopy images. Skin Res Technol 2013; 19(1): e27-36.
        [http://dx.doi.org/10.1111/j.1600-0846.2011.00603.x] [PMID: 22211360]

[210]   Kiani K, Sharafat AR. E-shaver: An improved DullRazor(®) for digitally removing dark and light-colored hairs in dermoscopic images. Comput Biol Med 2011; 41(3): 139-45.
        [http://dx.doi.org/10.1016/j.compbiomed.2011.01.003] [PMID: 21316042]

[211]   Abbas Q, Fondón I, Rashid M. Unsupervised skin lesions border detection via two-dimensional image analysis. Comput Methods Programs Biomed 2011; 104(3): e1-e15.
        [http://dx.doi.org/10.1016/j.cmpb.2010.06.016] [PMID: 20663582]

[212]   Nguyen NH, Lee TK, Atkins MS. Segmentation of light and dark hair in dermoscopic images: A hybrid approach using a universal kernel. In: Proceedings of SPIE 7623. Medical Imaging 2010; pp. 76234N-76234N, 8.

[213]   Lee T, Ng V, Gallagher R, Coldman A, McLean D. DullRazor: a software approach to hair removal from images. Comput Biol Med 1997; 27(6): 533-43.
        [http://dx.doi.org/10.1016/S0010-4825(97)00020-6] [PMID: 9437554]

[214]   Xie F-Y, Qin S-Y, Jiang Z-G, Meng R-S. PDE-based unsupervised repair of hair-occluded information in dermoscopy images of melanoma. Comput Med Imaging Graph 2009; 33(4): 275-82.
        [http://dx.doi.org/10.1016/j.compmedimag.2009.01.003] [PMID: 19261439]

[215]   Zhou H, Rehg JM, Chen M. Exemplar-Based Segmentation of Pigmented Skin Lesions from Dermoscopy Images International Symposium on Biomedical Imaging (ISBI).
        [http://dx.doi.org/10.1109/ISBI.2010.5490372]

[216]   Wighton P, Lee TK, Atkins MS. Dermascopic hair disocclusion using inpainting.Proceeding of SPIE 6914. Medical Imaging 2008.
        [http://dx.doi.org/10.1117/12.770776]

[217]   Koehoorn J, Sobiecki A, Rauber P, Jalba A, Telea A. Efficient and effective automated digital hair removal from dermoscopy images. mathematical morphology - theory and Applications 2015; Vol. 1: pp. 1-17.

[218]   Criminisi A, Pérez P, Toyama K. Region filling and object removal by exemplar-based image inpainting. IEEE Trans Image Process 2004; 13(9): 1200-12.
        [http://dx.doi.org/10.1109/TIP.2004.833105] [PMID: 15449582]

[219]   Chung DH, Sapiro G. Segmenting skin lesions with partial-differential-equations-based image processing algorithms. IEEE Trans Med Imaging 2000; 19(7): 763-7.
        [http://dx.doi.org/10.1109/42.875204] [PMID: 11055791]

[220]   Fiorese M, Peserico E, Silletti A. VirtualShave: Automated hair removal from digital dermatoscopic images Annual International Conference of the IEEE Engineering in Medicine and Biology Society (EMBC). 5145-8.
        [http://dx.doi.org/10.1109/IEMBS.2011.6091274]

[221]   Oliveira RB, Filho ME, Ma Z, Papa JP, Pereira AS, Tavares JMRS. Computational methods for the image segmentation of pigmented skin lesions: A review. Comput Methods Programs Biomed 2016; 131: 127-41.
        [http://dx.doi.org/10.1016/j.cmpb.2016.03.032] [PMID: 27265054]

[222] Sumithra R, Suhil M, Guru DS. Segmentation and classification of skin lesions for disease diagnosis In: Procedia Comput Sci. 2015; 45: pp. 76-85.

[223] Mehta P, Shah B. Review on techniques and steps of computer aided skin cancer diagnosis. Procedia Comput Sci 2016; 85: 309-16.
[http://dx.doi.org/10.1016/j.procs.2016.05.238]

[224] Giotis I, Molders N, Land S, Biehl M, Jonkman MF, Petkov N. MED-NODE: A computer-assisted melanoma diagnosis system using non-dermoscopic images. Expert Syst Appl 2015; 42: 6578-85.
[http://dx.doi.org/10.1016/j.eswa.2015.04.034]

[225] Xie F, Li Y, Meng R, Jiang Z. No-reference hair occlusion assessment for dermoscopy images based on distribution feature. Comput Biol Med 2015; 59: 106-15.
[http://dx.doi.org/10.1016/j.compbiomed.2015.01.023] [PMID: 25701625]

[226] Wang H, Moss RH, Chen X, et al. Modified watershed technique and post-processing for segmentation of skin lesions in dermoscopy images. Comput Med Imaging Graph 2011; 35(2): 116-20.
[http://dx.doi.org/10.1016/j.compmedimag.2010.09.006] [PMID: 20970307]

[227] Afonso A, Silveira M. Hair detection in dermoscopic images using Percolation 34th Annual International Conference of the IEEE Engineering in Medisine and Biology Society (EMBS). San Diego, California USA. 2012.
[http://dx.doi.org/10.1109/EMBC.2012.6346936]

[228] Toossi MTB, Pourreza HR, Zare H, Sigari M-H, Layegh P, Azimi A. An effective hair removal algorithm for dermoscopy images. Skin Res Technol 2013; 19(3): 230-5.
[http://dx.doi.org/10.1111/srt.12015] [PMID: 23560826]

[229] Suer S, Kockara S, Mete M. An improved border detection in dermoscopy images for density based clustering. BMC Bioinformatics 2011; 12(Suppl. 10): S12.
[http://dx.doi.org/10.1186/1471-2105-12-S10-S12] [PMID: 22166058]

[230] Mete M, Kockara S, Aydin K. Fast density-based lesion detection in dermoscopy images. Comput Med Imaging Graph 2011; 35(2): 128-36.
[http://dx.doi.org/10.1016/j.compmedimag.2010.07.007] [PMID: 20800995]

[231] Celebi ME, Iyatomi H, Schaefer G, Stoecker WV. Lesion border detection in dermoscopy images. Comput Med Imaging Graph 2009; 33(2): 148-53.
[http://dx.doi.org/10.1016/j.compmedimag.2008.11.002] [PMID: 19121917]

[232] Silletti A, Peserico E, Mantovan A, Zattra E, Peserico A, Belloni Fortina A. Variability in human and automatic segmentation of melanocytic lesions 31st Annual International Conference of the IEEE Engineering in Medicine and Biology Society (EMBS). Minneapolis, Minnesota, USA. 2009; pp. 5789-92.
[http://dx.doi.org/10.1109/IEMBS.2009.5332543]

[233] Abbas Q, Celebi ME, Fondón García I, Rashid M. Lesion border detection in dermoscopy images using dynamic programming. Skin Res Technol 2011; 17(1): 91-100.
[http://dx.doi.org/10.1111/j.1600-0846.2010.00472.x] [PMID: 21226876]

[234] Abbas Q, Celebi ME, Fondón García I. Skin tumor area extraction using an improved dynamic programming approach. Skin Res Technol 2012; 18(2): 133-42.
[http://dx.doi.org/10.1111/j.1600-0846.2011.00544.x] [PMID: 21507072]

[235] Cudek P, Grzymala-Busse JW, Hippe ZW. Melanocytic Skin Lesion Image Classification. Part I: Recognition of Skin Lesion International Conference on Human System Interactions (HSI). Rzeszow, Poland. 2010.
[http://dx.doi.org/10.1109/HSI.2010.5514558]

[236] Barhoumi W, Dhahbi S, Zagrouba E. A Collaborative System for Pigmented Skin Lesions Malignancy Tracking IEEE International Workshop on Imaging Systems and Techniques (IST). Krakow, Poland. 2007.May 4-5, 2007;
[http://dx.doi.org/10.1109/IST.2007.379576]

[237] Joel G, Schmid-Saugeon P, Guggisberg D, et al. Validation of segmentation techniques for digital dermoscopy. Skin Res Technol 2002; 8(4): 240-9.
[http://dx.doi.org/10.1034/j.1600-0846.2002.00334.x] [PMID: 12423543]

[238] Zhou H, Schaefer G, Sadka AH, Celebi ME. Anisotropic Mean Shift Based Fuzzy C-Means Segmentation of Dermoscopy Images. IEEE J Sel Top Signal Process 2009; 3: 26-34.
[http://dx.doi.org/10.1109/JSTSP.2008.2010631]

[239] Chang W-Y, Huang A, Chen Y-C, et al. The feasibility of using manual segmentation in a multifeature computer-aided diagnosis system for classification of skin lesions: a retrospective comparative study. BMJ Open 2015; 5(4): e007823.
[http://dx.doi.org/10.1136/bmjopen-2015-007823] [PMID: 25941190]

[240] Abbas AA, Guo X, Tan WH, Jalab HA. Combined Spline and B-spline for an improved automatic skin lesion segmentation in dermoscopic images using optimal color channel. J Med Syst 2014; 38(8): 80.
[http://dx.doi.org/10.1007/s10916-014-0080-7] [PMID: 24957396]

[241] Messadi M, Bessaid A, Taleb-Ahmed A. Extraction of specific parameters for skin tumour classification. J Med Eng Technol 2009; 33(4): 288-95.

[http://dx.doi.org/10.1080/03091900802451315] [PMID: 19384704]

[242]   Fischer S, Schmid P, Guillod J. Analysis of skin lesions with pigmented networks Proceedings, International Conference on Image Processing. 323-6.
[http://dx.doi.org/10.1109/ICIP.1996.559498]

[243]   Taouil K, Romdhane NB. Automatic Segmentation and classification of Skin Lesion Images The 2nd International Conference on Distributed Frameworks for Multimedia Applications. 1-12.
[http://dx.doi.org/10.1109/DFMA.2006.296918]

[244]   Glaister J, Wong A, Clausi DA. Segmentation of skin lesions from digital images using joint statistical texture distinctiveness. IEEE Trans Biomed Eng 2014; 61(4): 1220-30.
[http://dx.doi.org/10.1109/TBME.2013.2297622] [PMID: 24658246]

[245]   Dhawan AP, Sicsu A. Segmentation of images of skin lesions using color and texture information of surface pigmentation. Comput Med Imaging Graph 1992; 16(3): 163-77.
[http://dx.doi.org/10.1016/0895-6111(92)90071-G] [PMID: 1623492]

[246]   Serrano C, Acha B. Pattern analysis of dermoscopic images based on Markov random fields. Pattern Recognit 2009; 42: 1052-7.
[http://dx.doi.org/10.1016/j.patcog.2008.07.011]

[247]   Xu L, Jackowski M, Goshtasby A, Roseman D, Bines S, Yu C, et al. Segmentation of skin cancer images. Image Vis Comput 1999; 17: 65-74.
[http://dx.doi.org/10.1016/S0262-8856(98)00091-2]

[248]   Hwang S, Celebi ME. Texture segmentation of dermoscopy images using Gabor filters and g-means clustering Proceedings of the International Conference on Image Processing, Computer Vision, and Pattern Recognition (IPCV). 882-6.

[249]   Flores E, Scharcanski J. Segmentation of melanocytic skin lesions using feature learning and dictionaries. Expert Syst Appl 2016; 56: 300-9.
[http://dx.doi.org/10.1016/j.eswa.2016.02.044]

[250]   Ming D, Wen Q, Chen J, Liu W. A generalized fusion approach for segmenting dermoscopy images using Markov random field 6th International Congress on Image and Signal Processing (CISP). 532-7.
[http://dx.doi.org/10.1109/CISP.2013.6744054]

[251]   Maeda J, Kawano A, Yamauchi S, Suzuki Y, Marçal A, Mendonça T. Perceptual image segmentation using fuzzy-based hierarchical algorithm and its application to dermoscopy images IEEE Conference on Soft Computing in Industrial Applications (SMCia/08). Muroran, Japan. 2008; pp. 66-71.
[http://dx.doi.org/10.1109/SMCIA.2008.5045937]

[252]   Madhankumar K, Kumar P. Characterization of skin lesions International Conference on Pattern Recognition, Informatics and Medical Engineering (PRIME). 302-6.
[http://dx.doi.org/10.1109/ICPRIME.2012.6208362]

[253]   Parolin A, Herzer E, Jung CR. Semi-automated diagnosis of melanoma through the analysis of dermatological images 23rd Conference on Graphics, Patterns and Images (SIBGRAPI). 71-8.
[http://dx.doi.org/10.1109/SIBGRAPI.2010.18]

[254]   Barcelos CAZ, Pires VB. An automatic based nonlinear diffusion equations scheme for skin lesion segmentation. Appl Math Comput 2009; 215: 251-61.
[http://dx.doi.org/10.1016/j.amc.2009.04.081]

[255]   Pires VB, Barcelos CAZ. Edge detection of skin lesions using anisotropic diffusion seventh international conference on intelligent systems design and applications.
[http://dx.doi.org/10.1109/ISDA.2007.139]

[256]   Canny J. A Computational Approach to Edge Detection In: IEEE Trans Pattern Anal Mach Intell. 1986; vol. PAMI-8.

[257]   Prewitt JMS. Object enhancement and extraction In: Picture Processing and Psychopictorics, B. Lipkin and A. Rosenfeld, Eds., ed New York: Academic Press, 1970, pp. 75-49.

[258]   Sobel I, Feldman G. A 3x3 isotropic gradient operator for image processing In: Pattern Classification and Scene Analysis,, R. Duda and P. Hart, Eds., ed: John Wiley & Sons, 1968, pp. 271-272.

[259]   Kirsch RA. Computer determination of the constituent structure of biological images. Comput Biomed Res 1971; 4(3): 315-28.
[http://dx.doi.org/10.1016/0010-4809(71)90034-6] [PMID: 5562571]

[260]   Yasmin JHJ, Sathik MM, Beevi SZ. Robust Segmentation Algorithm using LOG Edge Detector for Effective Border Detection of Noisy Skin Lesions International Conference on Computer, Communication and Electrical Technology. 60-5.

[261]   Cavalcanti PG, Scharcanski J. A coarse-to-fine approach for segmenting melanocytic skin lesions in standard camera images. Comput Methods Programs Biomed 2013; 112(3): 684-93.
[http://dx.doi.org/10.1016/j.cmpb.2013.08.010] [PMID: 24075079]

[262]   Celebi ME, Aslandogan YA, Bergstresser PR. Unsupervised Border Detection of Skin Lesion Images International Conference on Information Technology: Coding and Computing (ITCC).
[http://dx.doi.org/10.1109/ITCC.2005.283]

[263]   Nourmohamadi M, Pourghassem H. Dermoscopy Image Segmentation Using a Modified Level S*et al*gorithm 4th International Conference on Computational Intelligence and Communication Networks. 286-90.
[http://dx.doi.org/10.1109/CICN.2012.80]

[264]   Silveira M, Marques JS. Level Set Segmentation of Dermoscopy Images The International Symposium on Biomedical Imaging (ISBI). 173-6.

[265]   Situ N, Yuan X, Zouridakis G, Mullani N. Automatic Segmentation of Skin Lesion Images Using Evolutionary Strategy The International Conference on Image Processing (ICIP).
[http://dx.doi.org/10.1109/ICIP.2007.4379575]

[266]   Wong A, Scharcanski J, Fieguth P. Automatic skin lesion segmentation via iterative stochastic region merging. IEEE Trans Inf Technol Biomed 2011; 15(6): 929-36.
[http://dx.doi.org/10.1109/TITB.2011.2157829] [PMID: 21622078]

[267]   Jaworek-Korjakowska J. Novel method for border irregularity assessment in dermoscopic color images. Comput Math Methods Med 2015; 2015: 496202.
[http://dx.doi.org/10.1155/2015/496202] [PMID: 26604980]

[268]   Emre Celebi M, Alp Aslandogan Y, Stoecker WV, Iyatomi H, Oka H, Chen X. Unsupervised border detection in dermoscopy images. Skin Res Technol 2007; 13(4): 454-62.
[http://dx.doi.org/10.1111/j.1600-0846.2007.00251.x] [PMID: 17908199]

[269]   Celebi ME, Kingravi HA, Iyatomi H, *et al.* Border detection in dermoscopy images using statistical region merging. Skin Res Technol 2008; 14(3): 347-53.
[http://dx.doi.org/10.1111/j.1600-0846.2008.00301.x] [PMID: 19159382]

[270]   Celebi ME, Kingravi HA, Iyatomi H, Lee J, Aslandogan YA, Van Stoecker W, *et al.* Fast and accurate border detection in dermoscopy images using statistical region merging. In: Proceeding of SPIE 6512. Medical Imaging 2007; pp. 65123V-65123V, 10.
[http://dx.doi.org/10.1117/12.709073]

[271]   Wang H, Chen X, Moss RH, *et al.* Watershed segmentation of dermoscopy images using a watershed technique. Skin Res Technol 2010; 16(3): 378-84.
[PMID: 20637008]

[272]   Pennisi A, Bloisi DD, Nardi D, Giampetruzzi AR, Mondino C, Facchiano A. Skin lesion image segmentation using Delaunay Triangulation for melanoma detection. Comput Med Imaging Graph 2016; 52: 89-103.
[http://dx.doi.org/10.1016/j.compmedimag.2016.05.002] [PMID: 27215953]

[273]   Ma Z, Tavares JMRS. A novel approach to segment skin lesions in dermoscopic images based on a deformable model. IEEE J Biomed Health Inform 2016; 20(2): 615-23.
[http://dx.doi.org/10.1109/JBHI.2015.2390032] [PMID: 25585429]

[274]   Euijoon Ahn , Lei Bi , Jinman Kim , Changyang Li , Fulham M, Feng DD. Automated saliency-based lesion segmentation in dermoscopic images. Conf Proc IEEE Eng Med Biol Soc 2015; 2015: 3009-12.
[PMID: 26736925]

[275]   Olugbara OO, Taiwo TB, Heukelman D. Segmentation of melanoma skin lesion using perceptual color difference saliency with morphological analysis. Math Probl Eng 2018.
[http://dx.doi.org/10.1155/2018/1524286]

[276]   Mendonça T, Marçal ARS, Vieira A, Nascimento JC, Silveira M, Marques JS, *et al.* Comparison of Segmentation Methods for Automatic Diagnosis of Dermoscopy Images In: Conference of the IEEE Engineering in Medicine and Biology Society (EMBS), Cité Internationale, Lyon, France. 2007; pp. 6572-5.
[http://dx.doi.org/10.1109/IEMBS.2007.4353865]

[277]   Tang J. A multi-direction GVF snake for the segmentation of skin cancer images. Pattern Recognit 2009; 42: 1172-9.
[http://dx.doi.org/10.1016/j.patcog.2008.09.007]

[278]   Erkol B, Moss RH, Stanley RJ, Stoecker WV, Hvatum E. Automatic lesion boundary detection in dermoscopy images using gradient vector flow snakes. Skin Res Technol 2005; 11(1): 17-26.
[http://dx.doi.org/10.1111/j.1600-0846.2005.00092.x] [PMID: 15691255]

[279]   Zhou H, Li X, Schaefer G, Celebi ME, Miller P. Mean shift based gradient vector flow for image segmentation. Comput Vis Image Underst 2013; 117: 1004-16.
[http://dx.doi.org/10.1016/j.cviu.2012.11.015]

[280]   Zhou H, Schaefer G, Celebi ME, Lin F, Liu T. Gradient vector flow with mean shift for skin lesion segmentation. Comput Med Imaging Graph 2011; 35(2): 121-7.
[http://dx.doi.org/10.1016/j.compmedimag.2010.08.002] [PMID: 20832242]

[281]   Zhou H, Schaefer G, Celebi ME, Iyatomi H, Norton K-A, Liu T, *et al.* Skin lesion segmentation using an improved snake model 32nd Annual International Conference of the IEEE Engineering in Medicine and Biology Society (EMBS). 1974-7.
[http://dx.doi.org/10.1109/IEMBS.2010.5627556]

[282]   Sultana A, Ciuc M, Radulescu T, Liu W, Petrache D. Preliminary work on dermatoscopic lesion segmentation 20th European Signal Processing Conference (EUSIPCO). Bucharest, Romania. 2012; pp. 2273-7.

[283]   Silveira M, Nascimento JC, Marques JS, Marçal ARS, Mendonça T, Yamauchi S, *et al.* Comparison of segmentation methods for melanoma diagnosis in dermoscopy images. IEEE J Sel Top Signal Process 2009; 3: 35-45.
        [http://dx.doi.org/10.1109/JSTSP.2008.2011119]

[284]   Yuan X, Situ N, Zouridakis G. A narrow band graph partitioning method for skin lesion segmentation. Pattern Recognit 2009; 42: 1017-28.
        [http://dx.doi.org/10.1016/j.patcog.2008.09.006]

[285]   Zhang Z, Stoecker WV, Moss RH. Border detection on digitized skin tumor images. IEEE Trans Med Imaging 2000; 19(11): 1128-43.
        [http://dx.doi.org/10.1109/42.896789] [PMID: 11204850]

[286]   Golston JE, Moss RH, Stoecker WV. Boundary detection in skin tumor images: An overall approach and a radial search algorithm. Pattern Recognit 1990; 23: 1235-47.
        [http://dx.doi.org/10.1016/0031-3203(90)90119-6]

[287]   Mete M, Sirakov NM. Lesion detection in demoscopy images with novel density-based and active contour approaches. BMC Bioinformatics 2010; 11(Suppl. 6): S23.
        [http://dx.doi.org/10.1186/1471-2105-11-S6-S23] [PMID: 20946607]

[288]   Ivanovici M, Stoica D. Color Diffusion Model for Active Contours - An Application to Skin Lesion Segmentation 34th Annual International Conference of the IEEE Engineering in Medicine and Biology Society (EMBS). San Diego, California USA. 2012; pp. 5347-50.
        [http://dx.doi.org/10.1109/EMBC.2012.6347202]

[289]   Kasmi R, Mokrani K, Rader RK, Cole JG, Stoecker WV. Biologically inspired skin lesion segmentation using a geodesic active contour technique. Skin Res Technol 2016; 22(2): 208-22.
        [http://dx.doi.org/10.1111/srt.12252] [PMID: 26403797]

[290]   Gioi RGv, Jakubowicz J, Morcel J-M, Randall G. LSD: A Line Segment Detectot. In: Image Processing On Line. 2012.

[291]   Capdehourat G, Corez A, Bazzano A, Alonso R, Musé P. Toward a combined tool to assist dermatologists in melanoma detection from dermoscopic images of pigmented skin lesions. Pattern Recognit Lett 2011; 32: 2187-96.
        [http://dx.doi.org/10.1016/j.patrec.2011.06.015]

[292]   Dalal A, Moss RH, Stanley RJ, *et al.* Concentric decile segmentation of white and hypopigmented areas in dermoscopy images of skin lesions allows discrimination of malignant melanoma. Comput Med Imaging Graph 2011; 35(2): 148-54.
        [http://dx.doi.org/10.1016/j.compmedimag.2010.09.009] [PMID: 21074971]

[293]   Humayun J, Malik AS, Kamel N. Multilevel Thresholding for segmentation of pigmented skin lesions IEEE International Conference on Imaging Systems and Techniques (IST).
        [http://dx.doi.org/10.1109/IST.2011.5962214]

[294]   Norton K-A, Iyatomi H, Celebi ME, Schaefer G, Tanaka M, Ogawa K. Development of a Novel Border Detection Method for Melanocytic and Non-Melanocytic Dermoscopy Images 32nd Annual International Conference of the IEEE Engineering in Medicine and Biology Society (EMBS). Buenos Aires, Argentina. 2010.
        [http://dx.doi.org/10.1109/IEMBS.2010.5626499]

[295]   Sarrafzade O, Miran MH, Ghassemi P. Skin Lesion Detection in Dermoscopy Images Using Wavelet Transform and Morphology Operations 17th Iranian Conference of Biomedical Engineering (ICBME).
        [http://dx.doi.org/10.1109/ICBME.2010.5704944]

[296]   Supot S. Border detection of skin lesion images based on fuzzy C-Means thresholding 3rd International Conference on Genetic and Evolutionary Computing. 777-80.

[297]   Yuksel ME, Borlu M. Accurate segmentation of dermoscopic images by image thresholding based on Type-2 fuzzy logic. IEEE Trans Fuzzy Syst 2009; 17: 976-82.
        [http://dx.doi.org/10.1109/TFUZZ.2009.2018300]

[298]   Oliveira RB, Marranghello N, Pereira AS, Tavares JMRS. A computational approach for detecting pigmented skin lesions in macroscopic images. Expert Syst Appl 2016; 61: 53-63.
        [http://dx.doi.org/10.1016/j.eswa.2016.05.017]

[299]   Rahman MM, Bhattacharya P. An integrated and interactive decision support system for automated melanoma recognition of dermoscopic images. Comput Med Imaging Graph 2010; 34(6): 479-86.
        [http://dx.doi.org/10.1016/j.compmedimag.2009.10.003] [PMID: 19942406]

[300]   Sezgin M, Sankur B. Survey over image thresholding techniques and quantitative performance evaluation. J Electron Imaging 2004; 13: 146-65.
        [http://dx.doi.org/10.1117/1.1631315]

[301]   Otsu N. A threshold selection method from gray-level histograms. IEEE Trans Syst Man Cybern 1979; 9: 62-6.
        [http://dx.doi.org/10.1109/TSMC.1979.4310076]

[302]   Premaladha J, Priya ML, Sujitha S, Ravichandran KS. Normalised otsu's segmentation. Indian J Sci Technol 2015; 8: 1-6.
        [http://dx.doi.org/10.17485/ijst/2015/v8i22/79140]

[303]   Abbas Q, Garcia IF, Emre Celebi M, Ahmad W, Mushtaq Q. Unified approach for lesion border detection based on mixture modeling and local entropy thresholding. Skin Res Technol 2013; 19(3): 314-9.
        [http://dx.doi.org/10.1111/srt.12047] [PMID: 23573804]

[304]   Celebi ME, Hwang S, Iyatomi H, Schaefer G. Robust border detection in dermoscopy images using threshold fusion IEEE International Conference on Image Processing. Hong Kong. 2010; pp. 2541-4.
[http://dx.doi.org/10.1109/ICIP.2010.5653514]

[305]   Celebi ME, Iyatomi H, Schaefer G, Stoecker WV. Approximate lesion localization in dermoscopy images. Skin Res Technol 2009; 15(3): 314-22.
[http://dx.doi.org/10.1111/j.1600-0846.2009.00357.x] [PMID: 19624428]

[306]   Cavalcanti PG, Yari Y, Scharcanski J. Pigmented Skin Lesion Segmentation on Macroscopic Images 25th International Conference of Image and Vision Computing New Zealand (IVCNZ).
[http://dx.doi.org/10.1109/IVCNZ.2010.6148845]

[307]   Lee H, Chen Y-PP. Skin cancer extraction with optimum fuzzy thresholding technique. Appl Intell 2014; 40: 415-26.
[http://dx.doi.org/10.1007/s10489-013-0474-0]

[308]   Wighton P, Sadeghi M, Lee TK, Atkins MS. A Fully Automatic Random Walker Segmentation for Skin Lesions in a Supervised Setting International Conference on Medical Image Computing and Computer Assisted Intervention (MICCAI). 1108-15.
[http://dx.doi.org/10.1007/978-3-642-04271-3_134]

[309]   Kapur JN, Sahoo PK, Wong AKC. A new method for gray-level picture thresholding using the entropy of the histogram In: Comput Vis Graph Image Process. 1985; vol. 29: pp. 273-85.

[310]   Kittler J, Illingworth J. On threshold selection using clustering criteria. IEEE Trans Syst Man Cybern 1985; SMC-15: 652-5.
[http://dx.doi.org/10.1109/TSMC.1985.6313443]

[311]   Ridler TW, Calvard S. Picture Thresholding Using an Iterative Selection Method. IEEE Trans Syst Man Cybern 1978; 8: 630-2.
[http://dx.doi.org/10.1109/TSMC.1978.4310039]

[312]   Sahoo P, Wilkins C, Yeager J. Threshold selection using Renyi's entropy. Pattern Recognit 1997; 30: 71-84.
[http://dx.doi.org/10.1016/S0031-3203(96)00065-9]

[313]   Castillejos H, Ponomaryov V, Nino-de-Rivera L, Golikov V. Wavelet transform fuzzy algorithms for dermoscopic image segmentation. Comput Math Methods Med 2012; 2012: 578721.
[http://dx.doi.org/10.1155/2012/578721] [PMID: 22567042]

[314]   Schmid P. Segmentation of digitized dermatoscopic images by two-dimensional color clustering. IEEE Trans Med Imaging 1999; 18(2): 164-71.
[http://dx.doi.org/10.1109/42.759124] [PMID: 10232673]

[315]   Liu Z, Sun J, Smith M, Smith L, Warr R. Unsupervised sub-segmentation for pigmented skin lesions. Skin Res Technol 2012; 18(1): 77-87.
[http://dx.doi.org/10.1111/j.1600-0846.2011.00534.x] [PMID: 21545650]

[316]   Zhou H, Chen M, Zou L, Gass R, Ferris L, Drogowski L, et al. Spatially Constrained Segmentation of Dermoscopy Images International Symposium on Biomedical Imaging (ISBI).

[317]   Khakabi S, Wighton P, Lee TK, Atkins MS. Multilevel feature extraction for skin lesion segmentation in dermoscopic images In: SPIE Medical Imaging. 2012. pp. 83150E-83150E-7.

[318]   Celebi ME, Guo W, Aslandogan YA, Bergstresser PR. Skin Lesion Segmentation Using Clustering Techniques The Florida Artificial Intelligence Research Society Conference (FLAIRS). Florida, USA. 2005.

[319]   Møllersen K, Kirchesch HM, Schopf TG, Godtliebsen F. Unsupervised segmentation for digital dermoscopic images. Skin Res Technol 2010; 16(4): 401-7.
[http://dx.doi.org/10.1111/j.1600-0846.2010.00455.x] [PMID: 20923456]

[320]   Lemon J, Kockara S, Halic T, Mete M. Density-based parallel skin lesion border detection with webCL. BMC Bioinformatics 2015; 16(Suppl. 13): S5-5.
[http://dx.doi.org/10.1186/1471-2105-16-S13-S5] [PMID: 26423836]

[321]   Khalid S, Jamil U, Saleem K, et al. Segmentation of skin lesion using Cohen-Daubechies-Feauveau biorthogonal wavelet. Springerplus 2016; 5(1): 1603.
[http://dx.doi.org/10.1186/s40064-016-3211-4] [PMID: 27652176]

[322]   Sadri AR, Zekri M, Member S. segmentation of dermoscopy images using wavelet networks In: IEEE Trans Biomed Eng. 2013; 60: pp. 1134-41.

[323]   Kockara S, Mete M, Yip V, Lee B, Aydin K. A soft kinetic data structure for lesion border detection. Bioinformatics 2010; 26(12): i21-8.
[http://dx.doi.org/10.1093/bioinformatics/btq178] [PMID: 20529909]

[324]   Melli R, Grana C, Cucchiara R. Comparison of color clustering algorithms for segmentation of dermatological images.Proceedings of SPIE 6144. San Diego, CA, USA: Medical Imaging 2006; pp. 61443S-61443S, 9.
[http://dx.doi.org/10.1117/12.652061]

[325]   Kockara S, Mete M, Chen B, Aydin K. Analysis of density based and fuzzy c-means clustering methods on lesion border extraction in dermoscopy images. BMC Bioinformatics 2010; 11(Suppl. 6): S26.
[http://dx.doi.org/10.1186/1471-2105-11-S6-S26] [PMID: 20946610]

[326]   Kwasnicka H, Paradowski M. Melanocytic Lesion Images Segmentation Enforcing by Spatial Relations Based Declarative Knowledge 5th International Conference on Intelligent Systems Design and Applications (ISDA).
[http://dx.doi.org/10.1109/ISDA.2005.63]

[327]   Pereyra M, Dobigeon N, Batatia H, Tourneret J-Y. Segmentation of Skin Lesions in 2-D and 3-D Ultrasound Images Using a Spatially Coherent Generalized Rayleigh Mixture Model In: IEEE Trans Med Imaging. 2012; vol. 31: pp. 1509-20.

[328]   Zhou Y, Smith M, Smith L, Warr R. Segmentation of Clinical Lesion Images Using Normalized Cut 10th Workshop on Image Analysis for Multimedia Interactive Services (WIAMIS).
[http://dx.doi.org/10.1109/WIAMIS.2009.5031442]

[329]   Zortea M, Skrøvseth SO, Schopf TR, Kirchesch HM, Godtliebsen F. Automatic segmentation of dermoscopic images by iterative classification. Int J Biomed Imaging 2011; 2011: 972648.
[http://dx.doi.org/10.1155/2011/972648] [PMID: 21811493]

[330]   Schaefer G, Rajab MI, Celebi ME, Iyatomi H. Skin lesion segmentation using co-operative neural network edge detection and colour normalisation 9th International Conference on Infomation Technology and Applications in Biomedicine (ITAB). Larnaca, Cyprus. 2009.
[http://dx.doi.org/10.1109/ITAB.2009.5394389]

[331]   Xie F, Bovik AC. Automatic segmentation of dermoscopy images using self-generating neural networks seeded by genetic algorithm. Pattern Recognit 2013; 46: 1012-9.
[http://dx.doi.org/10.1016/j.patcog.2012.08.012]

[332]   Vennila GS, Suresh LP, Shunmuganathan KL. Dermoscopic Image Segmentation and Classification using Machine Learning Algorithms International Conference on Computing, Electronics and Electrical Technologies (ICCEET). 1122-7.
[http://dx.doi.org/10.1109/ICCEET.2012.6203834]

[333]   Garnavi R, Aldeen M, Celebi ME, Varigos G, Finch S. Border detection in dermoscopy images using hybrid thresholding on optimized color channels. Comput Med Imaging Graph 2011; 35(2): 105-15.
[http://dx.doi.org/10.1016/j.compmedimag.2010.08.001] [PMID: 20832992]

[334]   Emre Celebi M, Wen Q, Hwang S, Iyatomi H, Schaefer G. Lesion border detection in dermoscopy images using ensembles of thresholding methods. Skin Res Technol 2013; 19(1): e252-8.
[http://dx.doi.org/10.1111/j.1600-0846.2012.00636.x] [PMID: 22676490]

[335]   Cavalcanti PG, Scharcanski J, Persia LED, Milone DH. An ICA-Based Method for the Segmentation of Pigmented Skin Lesions in Macroscopic Images 33rd Annual International Conference of the IEEE Engineering in Medicine and Biology Society (EMBS). Boston, Massachusetts USA. 2011; pp. 5993-6.
[http://dx.doi.org/10.1109/IEMBS.2011.6091481]

[336]   Kreutz M, Anschutz M, Grunendick T, Rick A, Gehlen S, Hoffmann K. Automated Diagnosis of Skin Cancer Using Digital Image Processing and Mixture-of-Experts. In: Heidelberg SB, Ed. Bildverarbeitung fur die Medizin. 2001; Vol. 46: pp. 357-61.
[http://dx.doi.org/10.1007/978-3-642-56714-8_66]

[337]   Ganster H, Pinz A, Röhrer R, Wildling E, Binder M, Kittler H. Automated melanoma recognition. IEEE Trans Med Imaging 2001; 20(3): 233-9.
[http://dx.doi.org/10.1109/42.918473] [PMID: 11341712]

[338]   Celebi ME, Schaefer G, Iyatomi H, Stoecker WV, Malters JM, Grichnik JM. An improved objective evaluation measure for border detection in dermoscopy images. Skin Res Technol 2009; 15(4): 444-50.
[http://dx.doi.org/10.1111/j.1600-0846.2009.00387.x] [PMID: 19832956]

[339]   Schmid-Saugeon P. Lesion detection in dermatoscopic images using anisotropic diffusion and morphological flooding International Conference on Image Processing (ICIP). 449-53.

[340]   Celebi ME, Quan W, Hitoshi I, Kouhei S, Huiyu Z, Gerald S. A State-of-the-Art Survey on Lesion Border Detection in Dermoscopy Images In: Dermoscopy Image Analysis, M. E. Celebi, T. Mendonca, and J. S. Marques, Eds., ed: CRC Press, 2015, pp. 97-129.
[http://dx.doi.org/10.1201/b19107-5]

[341]   Chan T F, Sandberg B Y, Vese L A. Active Contours without Edges for Vector-Valued Images J Vis Commun Image Represent, vol. 11, pp. 130-141, 2000/06/01 2000.

[342]   Garnavi R, Aldeen M, Celebi ME. Weighted performance index for objective evaluation of border detection methods in dermoscopy images. Skin Res Technol 2011; 17(1): 35-44.
[http://dx.doi.org/10.1111/j.1600-0846.2010.00460.x] [PMID: 20923454]

[343]   Garnavi R, Aldeen M. Optimized weighted performance index for objective evaluation of border-detection methods in dermoscopy images. IEEE Trans Inf Technol Biomed 2011; 15(6): 908-17.
[http://dx.doi.org/10.1109/TITB.2011.2170083] [PMID: 22113339]

[344]   Ramezani M, Karimian A, Moallem P. Automatic detection of malignant melanoma using macroscopic images. J Med Signals Sens 2014; 4(4): 281-90.
[PMID: 25426432]

[345]   Marques JS, Barata C, Mendonça T. On the Role of Texture and Color in the Classification of Dermoscopy Images 34th Annual International Conference of the IEEE Engineering in Medicine and Biology Society (EMBS). San Diego, California USA. 2012; pp. 4402-5.

[http://dx.doi.org/10.1109/EMBC.2012.6346942]

[346] Stanley RJ, Stoecker WV, Moss RH, *et al.* A basis function feature-based approach for skin lesion discrimination in dermatology dermoscopy images. Skin Res Technol 2008; 14(4): 425-35.
[http://dx.doi.org/10.1111/j.1600-0846.2008.00307.x] [PMID: 18937777]

[347] Stoecker WV, Wronkiewiecz M, Chowdhury R, *et al.* Detection of granularity in dermoscopy images of malignant melanoma using color and texture features. Comput Med Imaging Graph 2011; 35(2): 144-7.
[http://dx.doi.org/10.1016/j.compmedimag.2010.09.005] [PMID: 21036538]

[348] Haralick RM. Statistical and structural approaches to Texture. Proc IEEE 1979; 67: 786-804.
[http://dx.doi.org/10.1109/PROC.1979.11328]

[349] Mitra S, Shankar BU. Medical image analysis for cancer management in natural computing framework. Inf Sci (Ny) 2015; 306: 111-31.
[http://dx.doi.org/10.1016/j.ins.2015.02.015]

[350] Lillesand TM, Keifer RW, Chipman JW. Remote Sensing and Image Interpretation In: No. Ed. 5 ed. New York: John Wiley & Sons Ltd, 2004.

[351] Ruiz D, Berenguer V, Soriano A, Sánchez B. A decision support system for the diagnosis of melanoma: A comparative approach. Expert Syst Appl 2011; 38: 15217-23.
[http://dx.doi.org/10.1016/j.eswa.2011.05.079]

[352] Salah B, Alshraideh M, Beidas R, Hayajneh F. Skin cancer recognition by using a neuro-fuzzy system. Cancer Inform 2011; 10: 1-11.
[http://dx.doi.org/10.4137/CIN.S5950] [PMID: 21340020]

[353] Jaleel JA, Salim S, Aswin RB. Computer Aided Detection of Skin Cancer International Conference on Circuits, Power and Computing Technologies (ICCPCT). 1137-42.
[http://dx.doi.org/10.1109/ICCPCT.2013.6528879]

[354] Chiem A, Al-Jumaily A, Khushaba RN. A Novel Hybrid System for Skin Lesion Detection International Conference on Intelligent Sensors, Sensor Networks and Information Processing (ISSNIP).
[http://dx.doi.org/10.1109/ISSNIP.2007.4496905]

[355] Patwardhan SV, Dhawan AP, Relue PA. Classification of melanoma using tree structured wavelet transforms. Comput Methods Programs Biomed 2003; 72(3): 223-39.
[http://dx.doi.org/10.1016/S0169-2607(02)00147-5] [PMID: 14554136]

[356] Legesse FB, Medyukhina A, Heuke S, Popp J. Texture analysis and classification in coherent anti-Stokes Raman scattering (CARS) microscopy images for automated detection of skin cancer. Comput Med Imaging Graph 2015; 43: 36-43.
[http://dx.doi.org/10.1016/j.compmedimag.2015.02.010] [PMID: 25797604]

[357] Maglogiannis I, Delibasis KK. Enhancing classification accuracy utilizing globules and dots features in digital dermoscopy. Comput Methods Programs Biomed 2015; 118(2): 124-33.
[http://dx.doi.org/10.1016/j.cmpb.2014.12.001] [PMID: 25540998]

[358] Rubegni P, Burroni M, Cevenini G, *et al.* Digital dermoscopy analysis and artificial neural network for the differentiation of clinically atypical pigmented skin lesions: a retrospective study. J Invest Dermatol 2002; 119(2): 471-4.
[http://dx.doi.org/10.1046/j.1523-1747.2002.01835.x] [PMID: 12190872]

[359] Sheha M A, Mabrouk M S, Sharawy A. Automatic detection of melanoma skin cancer using texture analysis 2012. J Comput Appl, vol. 42, pp. 22-26, March 2012.

[360] Maglogiannis I, Doukas CN. Overview of Advanced Computer Vision Systems for Skin Lesions Characterization In: IEEE Trans Inf Technol Biomed. 2009; vol. 13.

[361] Garnavi R, Aldeen M, Bailey J. Classification of Melanoma Lesions Using Wavelet-Based Texture Analysis International Conference on Digital Image Computing: Techniques and Applications (DICTA). Sydney, NSW. 2010; pp. 75-81.
[http://dx.doi.org/10.1109/DICTA.2010.22]

[362] Ballerini L, Fisher RB, Aldridge B, Rees J. Non-Melanoma Skin Lesion Classification Using Colour Image Data in a Hierarchical K-NN Classifier 9th IEEE International Symposium on Biomedical Imaging (ISBI). 358-61.
[http://dx.doi.org/10.1109/ISBI.2012.6235558]

[363] Doukas C, Stagkopoulos P, Keranoudis CT, Maglogiannis I. Automated Skin Lesion Assessment Using Mobile Technologies and Cloud Platforms 34th Annual International Conference of the IEEE Engineering in Medicine and Biology Society (EMBS). San Diego, California, USA. 2012.
[http://dx.doi.org/10.1109/EMBC.2012.6346458]

[364] Noroozi N, Zakerolhosseini A. Computerized measurement of melanocytic tumor depth in skin histopathological images. Micron 2015; 77: 44-56.
[http://dx.doi.org/10.1016/j.micron.2015.05.007] [PMID: 26102548]

[365] White RG, Perednia DA, Schowengerdt RA. Automated feature detection in digital images of skin. Comput Methods Programs Biomed 1991; 34(1): 41-60.
[http://dx.doi.org/10.1016/0169-2607(91)90081-4] [PMID: 2036789]

[366]   Andreassi L, Perotti R, Rubegni P, *et al.* Digital dermoscopy analysis for the differentiation of atypical nevi and early melanoma: A new quantitative semiology. Arch Dermatol 1999; 135(12): 1459-65.
        [http://dx.doi.org/10.1001/archderm.135.12.1459] [PMID: 10606050]

[367]   Maglogiannis I, Pavlopoulos S, Koutsouris D. An Integrated Computer Supported Acquisition, Handling, and Characterization System for Pigmented Skin Lesions in Dermatological Images In: IEEE Trans Inf Technol Biomed. 2005; 9: pp. 86-98.

[368]   Salerni G, Carrera C, Lovatto L, *et al.* Characterization of 1152 lesions excised over 10 years using total-body photography and digital dermatoscopy in the surveillance of patients at high risk for melanoma. J Am Acad Dermatol 2012; 67(5): 836-45.
        [http://dx.doi.org/10.1016/j.jaad.2012.01.028] [PMID: 22521205]

[369]   Jaworek-Korjakowska J, Kłeczek P. Automatic classification of specific melanocytic lesions using artificial intelligence. BioMed Res Int 2016; 2016: 8934242.
        [http://dx.doi.org/10.1155/2016/8934242] [PMID: 26885520]

[370]   Ferris LK, Harkes JA, Gilbert B, *et al.* Computer-aided classification of melanocytic lesions using dermoscopic images. J Am Acad Dermatol 2015; 73(5): 769-76.
        [http://dx.doi.org/10.1016/j.jaad.2015.07.028] [PMID: 26386631]

[371]   Leo GD, Liguori C, Paolillo A, Sommella P. An improved procedure for the automatic detection of dermoscopic structures in digital ELM images of skin lesions IEEE International Conference on Virtual Environments, Human-Computer Interfaces, and Measurement Systems.

[372]   Celebi ME, Iyatomi H, Stoecker WV, *et al.* Automatic detection of blue-white veil and related structures in dermoscopy images. Comput Med Imaging Graph 2008; 32(8): 670-7.
        [http://dx.doi.org/10.1016/j.compmedimag.2008.08.003] [PMID: 18804955]

[373]   García Arroyo JL, García Zapirain B. Detection of pigment network in dermoscopy images using supervised machine learning and structural analysis. Comput Biol Med 2014; 44: 144-57.
        [http://dx.doi.org/10.1016/j.compbiomed.2013.11.002] [PMID: 24314859]

[374]   Carli P, Giorgi Vd, Chiarugi A, Nardini P, Weinstock MA, Crocetti E, *et al.* Addition of dermoscopy to conventional nakedeye examination in melanoma screening: A randomized study. J Dermatol 2003; 50: 683-9.

[375]   Rastgoo M, Garcia R, Morel O, Marzani F. Automatic differentiation of melanoma from dysplastic nevi. Comput Med Imaging Graph 2015; 43: 44-52.
        [http://dx.doi.org/10.1016/j.compmedimag.2015.02.011] [PMID: 25797605]

[376]   Barata C, Ruela M, Mendonça T, Marques JS. A bag-of-features approach for the classification of melanomas in dermoscopy images: The role of color and texture descriptors In: Computer vision techniques for the diagnosis of skin cancer, series in BioEngineering, J. Scharcanski and M. E. Celebi, Eds., ed: Springer-Verlag Berlin Heidelberg, 2014, pp. 49 - 69.

[377]   Abedini M, Codella N C F, Connell J H, Garnavi R, Merler M, Pankanti S, *et al.* A generalized framework for medical image classification and recognition IBM J Res Dev 2015; vol. 59
        [http://dx.doi.org/10.1147/JRD.2015.2390017]

[378]   Li K, Wang F, Zhang L. A new algorithm for image recognition and classification based onimproved Bag of Features algorithm. Optik (Stuttg) 2016; 127: 4736-40.
        [http://dx.doi.org/10.1016/j.ijleo.2015.08.219]

[379]   Ruela M, Barata C, Marques JS, Rozeira J. A system for the detection of melanomas in dermoscopy images using shape and symmetry features. Comput Methods Biomech Biomed Engin 2015.

[380]   Abbas Q, Celebi ME, Serrano C, Garcı'a IFn, Ma G. Pattern classification of dermoscopy images: A perceptually uniform model. Pattern Recognit 2013; 46: 86-97.
        [http://dx.doi.org/10.1016/j.patcog.2012.07.027]

[381]   Dreiseitl S, Ohno-Machado L, Kittler H, Vinterbo S, Billhardt H, Binder M. A comparison of machine learning methods for the diagnosis of pigmented skin lesions. J Biomed Inform 2001; 34(1): 28-36.
        [http://dx.doi.org/10.1006/jbin.2001.1004] [PMID: 11376540]

[382]   Celebi ME, Kingravi HA, Uddin B, *et al.* A methodological approach to the classification of dermoscopy images. Comput Med Imaging Graph 2007; 31(6): 362-73.
        [http://dx.doi.org/10.1016/j.compmedimag.2007.01.003] [PMID: 17387001]

[383]   Wazaefi Y, Paris S, Fertil B. Contribution of a classifier of skin lesions to the dermatologist's decision 3rd International Conference on Image Processing Theory, Tools and Applications (IPTA).
        [http://dx.doi.org/10.1109/IPTA.2012.6469560]

[384]   Tabatabaie K, Esteki A. Independent Component Analysis as an Effective Tool for Automated Diagnosis of Melanoma IEEE Cairo International Biomedical Engineering Conference (CIBEC).
        [http://dx.doi.org/10.1109/CIBEC.2008.4786081]

[385]   Jukić A, Kopriva I, Cichocki A. Noninvasive diagnosis of melanoma with tensor decomposition-based feature extraction from clinical color image. Biomed Signal Process Control 2013; 8: 755-63.
        [http://dx.doi.org/10.1016/j.bspc.2013.07.001]

[386]   D'Alessandro B, Dhawan AP, Mullani N. Computer Aided Analysis of Epi-illumination and Transillumination Images of Skin Lesions for Diagnosis of Skin Cancers 33rd Annual International Conference of the IEEE EMBS. Boston, Massachusetts USA. 2011.
        [http://dx.doi.org/10.1109/IEMBS.2011.6090929]

[387]   Stoecker WV, Li WW, Moss RH. Automatic detection of asymmetry in skin tumors. Comput Med Imaging Graph 1992; 16(3): 191-7.
        [http://dx.doi.org/10.1016/0895-6111(92)90073-I] [PMID: 1623494]

[388]   Ng VTY, Fung BYM, Lee TK. Determining the asymmetry of skin lesion with fuzzy borders. Comput Biol Med 2005; 35(2): 103-20.
        [http://dx.doi.org/10.1016/j.compbiomed.2003.11.004] [PMID: 15567181]

[389]   Cascinelli N, Ferrario M, Bufalino R, et al. Results obtained by using a computerized image analysis system designed as an aid to diagnosis of cutaneous melanoma. Melanoma Res 1992; 2(3): 163-70.
        [http://dx.doi.org/10.1097/00008390-199209000-00004] [PMID: 1450670]

[390]   Cavalcanti PG, Scharcanski J, Baranoski GVG. A two-stage approach for discriminating melanocytic skin lesions using standard cameras. Expert Syst Appl 2013; 4054-64.
        [http://dx.doi.org/10.1016/j.eswa.2013.01.002]

[391]   Shimizu K, Iyatomi H, Norton K-A, Celebi ME. Extension of automated melanoma screening for non-melanocytic skin lesions 19th International Conference on Mechatronics and Machine Vision in Practice (M2VIP). 16-9.

[392]   Iyatomi H, Oka H, Celebi M E, Ogawa K, Argenziano G, Soyer H P, et al. Computer-Based Classification of Dermoscopy Images of Melanocytic Lesions on Acral Volar Skin J Invest Dermatol 2008; 1-6.
        [http://dx.doi.org/10.1038/jid.2008.28]

[393]   Tasoulis SK, Doukas CN, Maglogiannis I, Plagianakos VP. Classification of Dermatological Images Using Advanced Clustering Techniques 32nd Annual International Conference of the IEEE EMBS. Buenos Aires, Argentina. 2010.
        [http://dx.doi.org/10.1109/IEMBS.2010.5626242]

[394]   Lee TK, McLean DI, Atkins MS. Irregularity index: A new border irregularity measure for cutaneous melanocytic lesions. Med Image Anal 2003; 7(1): 47-64.
        [http://dx.doi.org/10.1016/S1361-8415(02)00090-7] [PMID: 12467721]

[395]   Stanley RJ, Moss RH, Van Stoecker W, Aggarwal C. A fuzzy-based histogram analysis technique for skin lesion discrimination in dermatology clinical images. Comput Med Imaging Graph 2003; 27(5): 387-96.
        [http://dx.doi.org/10.1016/S0895-6111(03)00030-2] [PMID: 12821032]

[396]   Sanchez I, Agaian S. Computer Aided Diagnosis of Lesions Extracted From Large Skin Surfaces IEEE International Conference on Systems, Man, and Cybernetics.
        [http://dx.doi.org/10.1109/ICSMC.2012.6378186]

[397]   Stanley RJ, Stoecker WV, Moss RH. A relative color approach to color discrimination for malignant melanoma detection in dermoscopy images. Skin Res Technol 2007; 13(1): 62-72.
        [http://dx.doi.org/10.1111/j.1600-0846.2007.00192.x] [PMID: 17250534]

[398]   Choi JW, Park YW, Byun SY, Youn SW. Differentiation of benign pigmented skin lesions with the aid of computer image analysis: A Novel Approach. In: Ann Dermatol. 2013; Vol. 25.

[399]   Sadeghi M, Razmara M, Lee TK, Atkins MS. A novel method for detection of pigment network in dermoscopic images using graphs. Comput Med Imaging Graph 2011; 35(2): 137-43.
        [http://dx.doi.org/10.1016/j.compmedimag.2010.07.002] [PMID: 20724109]

[400]   Braun RP, Rabinovitz HS, Oliviero M, Kopf AW, Saurat J-H. Dermoscopy of pigmented skin lesions. J Am Acad Dermatol 2005; 52(1): 109-21.
        [http://dx.doi.org/10.1016/j.jaad.2001.11.001] [PMID: 15627088]

[401]   Anantha M, Moss RH, Stoecker WV. Detection of pigment network in dermatoscopy images using texture analysis. Comput Med Imaging Graph 2004; 28(5): 225-34.
        [http://dx.doi.org/10.1016/j.compmedimag.2004.04.002] [PMID: 15249068]

[402]   Šitum M, Buljan M, Kolić M, Vučić M. Melanoma--clinical, dermatoscopical, and histopathological morphological characteristics. Acta Dermatovenerol Croat 2014; 22(1): 1-12.
        [PMID: 24813835]

[403]   Garbe C, Peris K, Hauschild A, et al. Diagnosis and treatment of melanoma. European consensus-based interdisciplinary guideline - Update 2016. Eur J Cancer 2016; 63: 201-17.
        [http://dx.doi.org/10.1016/j.ejca.2016.05.005] [PMID: 27367293]

[404]   Nowak LA, Ogorzałek MJ, Pawłowski MP. Pigmented Network Structure Detection Using Semi-Smart Adaptive Filters IEEE 6th International Conference on Systems Biology.
        [http://dx.doi.org/10.1109/ISB.2012.6314155]

[405]   Carli P, de Giorgi V, Palli D, Giannotti V, Giannotti B. Preoperative assessment of melanoma thickness by ABCD score of dermatoscopy. J Am Acad Dermatol 2000; 43(3): 459-66.
        [http://dx.doi.org/10.1067/mjd.2000.106518] [PMID: 10954657]

[406]   Stolz W, Schiffner R, Pillet L, *et al.* Improvement of monitoring of melanocytic skin lesions with the use of a computerized acquisition and
         surveillance unit with a skin surface microscopic television camera. J Am Acad Dermatol 1996; 35(2 Pt 1): 202-7.
         [http://dx.doi.org/10.1016/S0190-9622(96)90324-2] [PMID: 8708021]

[407]   Ferrara G, Argenziano G, Zgavec B, *et al.* "Compound blue nevus": A reappraisal of "superficial blue nevus with prominent intraepidermal
         dendritic melanocytes" with emphasis on dermoscopic and histopathologic features. J Am Acad Dermatol 2002; 46(1): 85-9.
         [http://dx.doi.org/10.1067/mjd.2002.117858] [PMID: 11756951]

[408]   Mendonça T, Ferreira PM, Marques JS, Marcal ARS, Rozeira J. PH^2 - A dermoscopic image database for research and benchmarking. In:
         IEEE Engineering in Medicine and Biology Society. 2013.

[409]   Khan A, Gupta K, Stanley RJ, *et al.* Fuzzy logic techniques for blotch feature evaluation in dermoscopy images. Comput Med Imaging Graph
         2009; 33(1): 50-7.
         [http://dx.doi.org/10.1016/j.compmedimag.2008.10.001] [PMID: 19027266]

[410]   Higgins HW II, Lee KC, Galan A, Leffell DJ. Melanoma in situ: Part I. Epidemiology, screening, and clinical features. J Am Acad Dermatol
         2015; 73(2): 181-90.
         [http://dx.doi.org/10.1016/j.jaad.2015.04.014] [PMID: 26183967]

[411]   Krähn G, Gottlöber P, Sander C, Peter RU. Dermatoscopy and high frequency sonography: Two useful non-invasive methods to increase
         preoperative diagnostic accuracy in pigmented skin lesions. Pigment Cell Res 1998; 11(3): 151-4.
         [http://dx.doi.org/10.1111/j.1600-0749.1998.tb00725.x] [PMID: 9730322]

[412]   Prayer L, Winkelbauer H, Gritzmann N, Winkelbauer F, Helmer M, Pehamberger H. Sonography versus palpation in the detection of regional
         lymph-node metastases in patients with malignant melanoma. Eur J Cancer 1990; 26(7): 827-30.
         [http://dx.doi.org/10.1016/0277-5379(90)90163-N] [PMID: 2145905]

17

Synthesis and Evaluation of Herbal Based Hair Dye

Rashmi Saxena Pal[*], Yogendra Pal, A.K Rai, Pranay Wal and Ankita Wal

Department of Pharmacy, Pranveer Singh Institute of Technology, NH-2, Bhauti, Kanpur (U.P), 209305, India

Abstract:

Background:

Herbal based hair dyes are being preferred on large scale, due to the vast number of advantages it exerts to overcome the ill-effects of a chemical based hair dye. We have attempted to prepare and standardize this preparation to ensure its quality as well as stability aspects.

Objective:

The current research was aimed at the preparation of herbal hair dye and the evaluation of its various parameters as organoleptic, physico-chemical, phytoconstituents, rheological aspects, patch test and stability testing for its efficacy and shelf life.

Materials and Methods:

The herbal dye was prepared in-house according to the proposed composition, using all the natural ingredients. The dye was evaluated for its organoleptic, physico-chemical and stability parameters.

Results:

The parameters were found to be comparable and sufficient for the evaluation of herbal dye. The values of different evaluations justified the usage of the hair dye.

Conclusion:

Herbal based hair dye has been prepared and evaluated using the various parameters. It offers a natural alternate, which can be used, irrespective of any side effects. The results can be incorporated while developing the pharmacopoeial standards.

Keywords: Herbal hair dye, Patch test, Organoleptic, Physico- chemical evaluation, Herbal drugs, Chemical hair dye.

1. INTRODUCTION

As compared to the chemical based hair dyes, which cause skin and other skin related diseases, natural herbal dyes are being preferred nowadays [1]. Today most of the human beings are very careful about their beauty and hairs play an important role in this. Herbal drugs without any adverse effects are used for healthy hair. Nearly 70% of human beings above 50 years struggle with the problem of balding and graying of hair. In few cases, these symptoms of ageing occur earlier. Graying starts on the skin of head at about 40 years, starting initially from the temples, followed by beard, moustache and finally up to the chest. The age at which graying starts is deeply influenced by heredity. But premature depigmentation in adults is mainly due to variety of other factors, as illness, some specific drugs, shock *etc.* [2, 3]. People have been using natural dyes since ancient times for the purpose of dyeing carpets, rugs and clothings by the use of roots, stems, barks, leaves, berries and flowers of various dye yielding plants [4]. The need of herbal based natural medicines is increasing fastly due to their natural goodness and lack of side effects. Amla, Bhringraj, Henna,

* Address correspondence to this author at the Department of Pharmacy, Pranveer Singh Institute of Technology, NH-2, Bhauti, Kanpur (U.P), 209305, India, Tel: 9129126459; E-mail: rashmisaxenapal@gmail.com

Mandara, Jatamansi, Reetha, Sariva, Curry leaves and Methi seeds are well - known ayurvedic herbal drugs traditionally used as hair colorant and for hair growth [5]. Many different extracts from plant were used for the purpose of hair dyeing in Europe and Asia before the invention of modern dyes. Indigo, known as initial fabric dye, could be mixed with henna to make different light brown to black shades of hair dye [6]. Use of these chemicals can result in unpleasant side effects, such as skin irritation, allergy, hair breakage, skin discoloration, unexpected hair color *etc.* [7 - 9]. Continuous application of such compounds on natural hair causes multiple side effects such as skin irritation, allergy, hair fall, dry scalp, erythrema and also skin cancer [10, 11]. In India, henna has been used traditionally for colouring palms and hairs. There are so many herbs like Kikar, Bihi, Bhringraj, Patnag, Akhrot, Narra, Jaborandi, Jatamansi, Amla, Kuth, Giloe, Behera which are used as a major constituents in hair care preparations mainly meant for dyeing hair [12 - 15]. Henna has been used traditionally for colouring women's bodies during marriage and other social celebrations since the times of Bronze Age. It is a part of Islamic and Hindu cultures as a hair coloring and dyeing agent for the purpose of decorating the nails or for the formation of temporary skin tattoos [16, 17]. Drugs from the plant sources are easily available, are less expensive, safe, and efficient and rarely have side effects [18]. In the present era of eco- conservation, the use of natural dyes has been revived and reviewed for the coloration of textiles and food materials [19, 20].

2. ROLE OF INGREDIENTS USED IN THE FORMULATION

2.1. Henna

its principle coloring ingredient of is lawsone, a red orange colored compound present in dried leaves of the plant in a concentration of 1 1.5% w/w. Lawsone acts as a non oxidizing hair coloring agent at a maximum concentration of 1.5% in the hair dyeing product. Other constituents in henna such as flavonoids and gallic acid act as organic mordants to the process of colouring. Carbohydrates give the henna paste a suitable consistency for adherence to the hair [21, 22]. Natural henna is usually hypoallergenic but allergic reactions occurred in mixed types including black henna. This occurs due to chemical compounds consisting of para-phenylenediamine, 2-nitro-4- phenylenediamine, 4-aminophenol and 3-aminophenol [23]. Henna has also antifungal activity against Malassezia species (causative organism of dandruff). Henna prevents premature hair fall by balancing the pH of the scalp and graying of hair. Henna leaf paste used for alleviating Jaundice, Skin diseases, Smallpox, *etc.* Extract of Henna leaves with ethanol (70%) showed significant hypoglycaemic and hypolipidaemic activities in diabetic mice [24, 25].

2.2. Amla

Berries obtained from amla enhances the absorption of calcium, helping to make healthier bones, teeth, nails, and hair. It maintains the hair color and prevents premature graying, strengthens the hair follicles [26]. Amla is the most rich and concentrated form of Vitamin C along with tannins found among the plants. Whole fruit is used as an active ingredient of the hair care preparations. The Vitamin C found in the fruit binds with tannins that protect it from being lost by heat or light [27, 28]. This fruit is also rich in tannins, minerals such as Calcium, Phosphorus, Fe and amino acid. The fruit extract is useful for hair growth and reduce hair loss [29]. Amla has antibacterial and antioxidant properties that can help promote the growth of healthy and lustrous hair [30].

2.3. Reetha

Its fruit is rich in vitamin A, D, E, K, saponin, sugars, fatty acids and mucilage. Reetha extract is useful for the promotion of hair growth and reduced dandruff [31]. Extract of fruit coat acts as a natural shampoo, therefore is used in herbal shampoos in the form of hair cleanser [32]. Reetha as soapnuts or washing nuts, play an important role as natural hair care products since older times. This plant is enriched with saponins, which makes the hair healthy, shiny, and lustrous when used on regular basis [33].

2.4. Shikakai

It contains Lupeol, Spinasterol, Lactone, Hexacosanol, Spinasterone, Calyctomine, Racimase-A Oleanolic acid, Lupenone, Betulin, Betulinic acid, Betulonic acid. The extract obtained from its pods is used as a hair cleanser and for the control of dandruff [34]. Shikakai or acacia concinna, has rich amount of vitamin C, which is beneficial for hair. Shikakai naturally lowers the pH value and retains the natural oils of the hair and keeps them lustrous and healthy. It is also effective in strengthening and conditioning hair. Amla, reetha and shikakai compliments each other, therefore, they are mixed together to have healthy and lustrous hair. All of these ingredients come in two forms, one as a dried fruit and other in powdered form. Amla, Reetha and Shikakai suit all hair types and help prevent split ends, hair fall, dandruff, greying of hair and other hair related problems, to make hair soft and silky [35].

2.5. Coffee

In hair colorants, herbs can be used in the form of powder [36], aqueous extract [37]or their seed oil to impart shades of different colour varying from reddish brown to blackish brown [38]. The herbal drugs like coffee powder [39, 40] obtained from its seeds are used as hair colorants [41, 42].

2.6. Tea

Being rich in polyphenols, selenium, copper, phytoestrogens, melatonin [43], tea also has been used in traditional Chinese medicine [44] and in Ayurvedic medicine has been used since long as hair colourant [45].

2.7. Hibiscus

It is excellent for increase in hair growth activity. Hibiscus is naturally enriched with Calcium, Phosphorus, Iron, Vitamin B1, Vitamin C, Riboflavin and Niacin, which help to promote thicker hair growth and decreases premature graying of hair [46]. This flower is used for controlling dandruff. Hibiscus exhibits antioxidant properties by producing flavonoids such as anthocyanins and other phenolic compounds. It can be used to rejuvenate the hair by conditioning it [47].

2.8. Bhringraj

Treatment with 5% of petroleum ether extract of bhringraj initiates greater number of hair follicles [48]. The oil based extract of leaves has been used traditionally for improving hair growth and for imparting natural colour to grey hair. Neelibhringaadi Tailam, mentioned in Ayurveda is suitable for promoting hair growth and for providing natural colour to grey hair [49]. Bhringraj is used in the preparation of various oil, shampoo, hair dye *etc.* [50 - 52].

2.9. Jatamansi

Nardostachys jatamansi is an important drug of Ayurveda and is used in different traditional systems of medicine such as Ayurveda, Unani, Siddha, *etc.* [53]. Its rhizomes and roots are used as a tranquilizer, laxative, cardiac tonic, for curing vertigo, nervous headache, low and high blood pressure, *etc.* [54]. The rhizomes as well as roots of the plant are medicinally rich and therefore, have been the focus of chemical studies [55].

3. MATERIALS AND METHODS

For the preparation of herbal hair dye, we have selected nine important ingredients such as Henna, Reetha, Coffee, Tea, Shikakai, Amla, Hibiscus, Bhringraj and Jatamansi. Henna leaves and flowers of hibiscus were collected from the herbal garden of PSIT. They were authenticated for their quality in the Pharmacognosy lab of the Institute. Reetha, coffee, tea, shikakai, amla, bhringraj and jatamansi all in the powdered forms were procured from the authorized stores of the local market in the powdered form. Henna leaves and the flowers of Hibiscus were shade dried and coarsely powdered. Then all the ingredients were mixed uniformly to prepare a homogenous formulation. The composition of the formulation is reflected in the Table **1**.

Table 1. Ingredients of the prepared herbal hair dye.

S. No	Ingredient	Quantity
1.	Henna	100 gms
2.	Amla	60 gms
3.	Reetha	20 gms
4.	Shikakai	20 gms
5.	Hibiscus	20 gms
6.	Coffee	20 gms
7.	Jatamansi	20 gms
8.	Bhringraj	20 gms
9.	Tea	20 gms

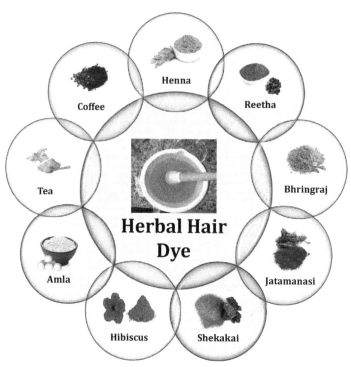

Fig. (1). Ingredients of the herbal hair dye.

3.1. Application of Hair Dye

The pack, which is in the form of powder, should be used weekly on wet hair, forming a paste of in water with optimum consistency. It should be applied evenly on the hair with the help of a brush, covering the roots to the hair tip. The scalp should be covered. It should be left for 2-3 hours on the scalp for complete drying. Then it should be removed by washing with plain water [56].

3.2. Evaluation of the Herbal Hair Dye

The prepared herbal hair dye was evaluated for its various parameters, such as organoleptic, physico-chemical, phytoconstituents and the rheological aspects.

3.2.1. Organoleptic Evaluation

Organoleptic characteristics for various sensory characters like color, taste, odour *etc.* was carefully noted down [57 - 59]. as illustrated in Table **2** The raw drugs and powders were separately studied by organoleptic and morphological characters like colour, odour, texture and appearance.

Table 2. Organoleptic evaluation of herbal dye.

S.No	Parameters	Results
1.	Colour	Greenish brown
2.	Odour	Characteristic
3.	Texture	Fine
4.	appearance	Powder

3.2.2. Physico-Chemical Evaluation

The physical and chemical features of the herbal hair dye were evaluated to determine the pH, its moisture content and its ash value for the purpose of stability, compatibility and the amount of inorganic matter present in it. Table **3** reflects the above findings.

Table 3. Physico-chemical evaluation of herbal dye.

S.No	Parameter	Results
1.	pH	6.7

(Table 3) contd.....

S.No	Parameter	Results
2.	L.O.D	1.9%
3.	Ash value	0.19

3.2.3. Phytochemical Evaluation

Prepared herbal hair dye was subjected to Phytochemical screening to reveal the presence or absence of various phytoconstituents as Carbohydrates, Lipids, Alkaloids, Sugars *etc*. The formulation when dissolved individually in 5 ml of water and filtered; the filtrates were used to test the presence of carbohydrates [60]. The aqueous extract of the formulated herbal face pack was evaluated for the presence or absence of different phytoconstituents as per the standard procedures and norms [61]. The results of phytochemical screening are highlighted in Table **4**.

Table 4. Phytochemical evaluation of herbal dye.

S.No	Parameter	Results
1.	Foam test	Present
2.	Molisch test	Present
3.	Fehling test	Absent
4.	Hager test	Present
5.	Volatile oil	Absent

3.2.4. Rheological Evaluation

Physical parameters like untapped or bulk density, tapped density, the angle of repose, Hausner's ratio, and carr's index were observed and calculated for the inhouse formulation. Bulk density symbolizes the adjustment of particles or granules collectively in the packed form. The formula for determination of bulk Density (D) is D = M/ V where M is the mass of particles and V the total volume occupied by them. This is determined by taking graduated cylinder. 100 grams of weighed formulation was added to the cylinder with the help of a funnel. The initial volume was noted and the sample was then tapped fully. The bulk density value was obtained from the initial volume and after tapping the volume noticed, from which tapped density was calculated. The angle of repose quantifies the flow properties of powder as it affects cohesion among the different particles. The fixed funnel cone method employs the calculation of Height (H) above the paper that is placed on a flat surface. The pack was carefully poured through the funnel till the formation of the peak. Here, R denotes the radius of the conical heap, tan a = H/R or a = arc tan H/R, where 'a' is the angle of repose. Hausner's ratio is linked with the interparticle friction and influences the powder flow properties. The Hausner's ratio is calculated as D /D' where D' is the tapped density and D, the bulk density. Carr's index helps to measure powder flow from bulk density [62, 63] as shown in Table **5**.

Table 5. Rheological evaluation of herbal dye.

S.No	Parameters	Results
1.	Bulk density	0.35
2.	Tapped density	0.471
3.	Angle of repose	1.04
4.	Carrs index	34.2
5.	Hausners ratio	1.34

3.3. Patch Test

This usually involves dabbing a small amount of the aqueous solution of hair dye behind the ear or on inner elbow in an area of 1sq.cm and leaving it to dry. Signs of irritation or feeing of non wellness is noted, if any.Measured and small quantities of prepared hair pack were applied to the specified area for a fixed time. Irritancy, redness, and swelling were checked and noticed for regular intervals up to 24 hours if any [64]. The results of tests for the signs of irritation are displayed in Table **6**.

Table 6. Patch test.

S.No	Parameters	Result
1.	Swelling	Negative
2.	Redness	Negative
3.	Irritation	Negative

3.4. Stability Test

Stability testing of the prepared formulation was performed by storing it at different temperature conditions for the time period of one month. The packed glass *vials* of formulation were stored at different temperature conditions *viz.*, room temperature and 35°C and were evaluated for the physical parameters like colour, odour, pH, texture, and smoothness as highlighted in Table 7 [65].

Table 7. Stability test.

S.No	Parameters	Room temperature	35C
1.	Colour	no change	no change
2.	Odour	no change	no change
3.	pH	6.7	6.8
4.	Texture	fine	fine
5.	Smoothness	smooth	smooth

4. RESULTS AND DISCUSSIONS

4.1. Uses of Hair Dye

The prepared herbal hair dye contains all the goodness of natural ingredients. Apart from acting as a hair dye, this formulation, because of the perfect blend of herbals, also acts as a hair growth promoter, hair nourisher, conditioner and anti-dandruff agent as well. Henna acting as the base powder, acts as the universal hair dye as it used for its colouring properties throughout the globe. It is also beneficial in the removal of excess oil from the scalp and conditions the hair well. Reetha restores the health of dull, dry, and damaged hair. Bhringraj aids in improving the circulation of blood flow at the root of the hair by providing more nutrients to support hair growth. The extract of jatamansi is helpful in the growth of hair. It is beneficial for smooth, silky and healthy hair too. Shikakai is packed with vitamins A, C, D and K, which together form a powerful antioxidant. This antioxidant is probably the only thing your hair needs to cleanse the scalp of the sebum buildup, unclog pores, kill infection-causing bacteria and stimulate hair growth. Regular using of hibiscus flower juice can easily restrict hair fall control, dandruff and graying of hair even when you are touching 50 years of age. This is an age-old remedy for all those people who have been struggling for healthy hair that is free from grey hair. It also contains essential fatty acids, which strengthen hair follicles and provides shine and new life. The sufficient amount of vitamin C in amla helps to halt pre-mature greying. It is a great hair conditioner and also remover of dandruff. Tea imparts perfect colour to the hair in combination with other herbs. It is good for the growth of hair and fights against dandruff. Coffee for hair strengthens hair by improving the overall quality and texture of it. It is absorbed by the follicles, making them softer and shinier, instantly. Organoleptic evaluation findings revealed that the pack is smooth and pleasant smelling powder. Physicochemical parameters reflected that the moisture content was as minimal as 1.9%. pH was found neutral to suit the requirements of different scalp types. Ash value was found to be nominal, signifying the presence of inorganic radicals in appropriate amounts. It shows the presence of major phytoconstituents, which acts as true nourisher for the scalp as well as hair. Irritancy test revealed negative results for irritancy, redness and swelling as the herbals in their natural form without use of artificial additives were found to be compatible with the proteins of hair Stability tests performed at different temperatures over a regular period of one month disclosed the inert nature of the pack in the terms of colour, odour, appearance, texture, and pH. From the above observations, it has been signified that since the formulation is constituted with naturally occurring dried herbal ingredients, there are almost minimal possibilities of the deterioration of the formulation, as there is no moisture containing substance in either raw or processed form. The formulation was kept for one month at room temperature to observe the changes in its color, odour,texture and appearance. The pH was also noticed before and after one month. The formulation was found to be stable. It can be easily stored and used at any temperature, at any place. Since it is a natural herbal based formulation, it is free from the ill-effects of ammonia based chemical dyes. However, the regular use of it provides voluminous, smooth and well coloured hair. Its continuous use shows superb effects later on. Since natural ingredients are known for their non-toxic, non-habit forming properties and no chemicals, preservatives, artificial colors or perfumes has been incorporated in the pack, the chances of its degradation are almost close to the minimal. This leads to an increased shelf life with stable ingredients.

CONCLUSION

A herbal hair pack colours the hair in an utmost gentle manner. The advantages of herbal based cosmetics are their nontoxic nature. It nutrifies the skin of the scalp and hair. This hair formulation provides vital nourishment to the skin. It helps to treat dandruff by removal of excess oil from scalp. Frequent use of this pack leads to manageable, frizz free coloured hair. Pollution, ageing, stress and harsh climates badly affect the quality of hair. In this research, we found effective properties of the herbal hair pack and further studies are needed to be performed to explore more useful benefits of this herbal hair pack. Natural remedies are widely accepted with open hands nowadays as they are safer with minimal side effects as compared to the chemical based products. Herbal formulations are in great demand to fulfill the needs of the growing world market. It is a noticeable attempt to formulate the herbal hair pack containing the goodness of powders of different plants, which are excellent for hair care.

HUMAN AND ANIMAL RIGHTS

No Animals/Humans were used for studies that are base of this research.

CONFLICT OF INTEREST

The authors declare no conflict of interest, financial or otherwise.

ACKNOWLEDGEMENTS

Declared none.

REFERENCES

[1]   Natural colorants and dye In: Pharmacognosy and phytochemistry. 1st Ed. India: Career publication 2004; 1: pp. 98-117.

[2]   Kumar S, Akhila A, Naqvi AA, Farooqi AH, Singh AK, Uniyal GC, et al. Medicinal plants in skin care. Lucknow, India: CIMAP 1994; pp. 425-30.

[3]   Orfanos CE, Happle R. Hair and hair diseases. Germany: Spring-veriang berlin heidelberg 1990; pp. 19-44.
        [http://dx.doi.org/10.1007/978-3-642-74612-3]

[4]   Gulrajani ML. Natural dyes and their applications to textiles. India: IIT New Delhi 1992; pp. 1-2.

[5]   Ashok D, Vaidya B, Devasagayam T. Current status of herbal drugs in India: An overview. J Clin Biochem Nutr 2007; 41(1): 1-11.

[6]   Khare CP. Indian herbal remedies: Rational western therapy, ayurvedic, and other traditional usage. Botany Springer 2003; p. 89.

[7]   Brown K. Hair colourants. J Soc Cosmet Chem 1982; 33: 375-83.

[8]   Madhusudan RY, Sujatha P. Formulation and evaluation of commonly used natural hair colorants. Nat Prod Rad 2008; 7(1): 45-8.

[9]   Mielke H. Lead-based hair products: Too hazardous for household use. J Am Pharm Assoc 1997.
        [http://dx.doi.org/10.1016/S1086-5802(16)30183-8]

[10]   Balsam MS. Edward sagarin, cosmetics science and technology. John Wiley & Sons 1972.

[11]   Koutros S, Silverman DT, Baris D, et al. Hair dye use and risk of bladder cancer in the New England bladder cancer study. Int J Cancer 2011; 129(12): 2894-904.
        [http://dx.doi.org/10.1002/ijc.26245] [PMID: 21678399]

[12]   Kalia AN. Text book of industrial pharmacognosy. New Delhi: CBS Publishers 2005; p. 264.

[13]   Kumar S, Akhila A, Naqvi AA, Forooqi AHA, Singh AK, Singh D. Medicinal plants in skin care. Lucknow: CIMAP 1994; pp. 51-62.

[14]   Baran R, Maibah HI. Cosmetic dermatology in children Text book of cosmetic dermatology. 2nd ed. London: CRC Press 1998; pp. 507-8.

[15]   Nadkarni KM. Indian materia medica. Popular Prakashan 1976; pp. 630-, 680, 1202.

[16]   Al-Suwaidi A, Ahmed H. Determination of para-phenylenediamine (PPD) in henna in the United Arab Emirates. Int J Environ Res Public Health 2010; 7(4): 1681-93.
        [http://dx.doi.org/10.3390/ijerph7041681] [PMID: 20617053]

[17]   Polat M, Dikilitaş M, Oztaş P, Alli N. Allergic contact dermatitis to pure henna. Dermatol Online J 2009; 15(1): 15.
        [PMID: 19281720]

[18]   Kumar KS, Begum A, Shashidhar B, *et al.* Formulation and evaluation of 100% herbal hair dye. International Journal of Advanced Research
        In Medical & Pharmaceutical Sciences 2016; (2):

[19]   Mac Dougall Color in food woodhead publishing Ltd 1st Ed.. 2002.

[20]   Ali NF, El-Mohamedy RSR. Eco-friendly and protective natural dye from red prickly pear (Opuntia lasiacantha Pfeiffer) plant. J Saudi Chem
        Soc 2010; 15: 257-61.
        [http://dx.doi.org/10.1016/j.jscs.2010.10.001]

[21]   Patel MM, Solanki BR, Gurav NC, Patel PH, Verma SS. Method development for Lawsone estimation in Trichup herbal hair powder by high-
        performance thin layer chromatography. J Adv Pharm Technol Res 2013; 4(3): 160-5.
        [http://dx.doi.org/10.4103/2231-4040.116780] [PMID: 24083204]

[22]   S.G. DESIGN AND EVALUTION OF HERBAL HAIR OIL FORMULATIONS BY USING ETHANOLIC EXTRACT OF Ziziphus jujuba
        Mill. LEAVES Int J Pharma Bio Sci 2017; 8(3): 322-7.

[23]   Saif FA. Henna beyond skin arts: Literatures review. J Pak Assoc Dermatol 2016; 26(1): 58-65.

[24]   Grabley S, Thiericke R. Bioactive agents from natural sources: Trends in discovery and application. Adv Biochem Eng Biotechnol 1999; 64:
        101-54.
        [http://dx.doi.org/10.1007/3-540-49811-7_4] [PMID: 9933977]

[25]   Chaudhary G,. Lawsonia inermis Linnaeus: A phytopharmacological review. Int J Pharm Sci Drug Res 2013; 2(2): 91-8.

[26]   Singh E, Sharma S, Pareek A, Dwivedi J, Yadav S, Sharma S. Phytochemistry, traditional uses and cancer chemopreventive activity of amla
        (Phyllanthus emblica): The sustainer. J Appl Pharm Sci 2011; 2: 176-83.

[27]   Nisha P, Singhal RS, Pandit AB. A study on degradation kinetics of ascorbic acid in amla (Phyllanthus emblica L.) during cooking. Int J Food
        Sci Nutr 2004; 55(5): 415-22.
        [http://dx.doi.org/10.1080/09637480412331321823] [PMID: 15545050]

[28]   Gopalan C, Sastri BV, Balasubramaniam SC. Nutritive value of indian foods. Hyderabad, India: NIN 1991.

[29]   Dahanukar S, Thatte U. Ayurveda Revisited. 3rd ed. Mumbai: Popular Prakashan 2000.

[30]   Turner DM. Natural product source material use in the pharmaceutical industry: The Glaxo experience. J Ethnopharmacol 1996; 51(1-3):
        39-43.
        [http://dx.doi.org/10.1016/0378-8741(95)01348-2] [PMID: 9213629]

[31]   Anjali J,. Hair care formulations. World J Pharm Pharm Sci 2016; 5(6): 630-48.

[32]   Fatima A,. Int J Pharm Sci Res 2013; 4(10): 3746-60.

[33]   Wonderful benefits and uses Of soapnuts (Reetha). Home, health and wellness, ingredients and uses http://www.stylecraze.com/articles/
        benefits-of-soapnuts-for-skin-hair-and-health/#gref

[34]   Fatima A, Alok S, Agarwal P, Singh P, Verma A. Benefits of herbal extracts in cosmetics: A review. Int J Pharm Sci Res 2013; 4(10):
        3746-60.

[35]   Haircare: Include amla, reetha and Shikakai for healthy and happy hair. NDTV FOOD. Anusha Singh updated: May 10, 2018 Available from:
        https://food.ndtv.com/beauty/haircare-include-amla-reetha-and-shikakai-for-healthy-and-happy-hair-1848507

[36]   Upadhyay VP, Mishra AK. Workshop on selected medicinal plants. In: Ministry of Commerce, Chemexcil; Bombay. 1985.

[37]   Upadhyay VP. Current research in ayurvedic medicine (International Seminar). In: Himalayan Institute; Chicago, USA. 1980.

[38]   Upadhyay VP. International Seminar on Medicinal Plants. Plants as cosmetics. In: Mungpoo, Govt. of West Bengal: Publication and
        Information Directorate, CSIR,; New Delhi. 1985.

[39]   Wealth of India. Raw materials. In: Anonymus. New Delhi: Mungpoo, Govt. of West Bengal: Publication and Information Directorate, CSIR,
        1997; 1.

[40]   Kitrikar K, Basu BD. Indian Medicinal Plants. 2nd ed. Allahabad: L. M. Basu 1993; Vol. I: pp. 335-6.

[41]   Chopra RN, Nayar SL, Chopra IC. Glossary of indian medicinal plant. New Delhi: CSIR 1956.

[42]   Ambasta ST. Useful plants of india. New Delhi: PID, CSIR; 1986.

[43]   Trüeb RM. Pharmacologic interventions in aging hair. Clin Interv Aging 2006; 1(2): 121-9.
        [http://dx.doi.org/10.2147/ciia.2006.1.2.121] [PMID: 18044109]

[44]   Chein E. Age reversal, from hormones to telomeres. WorldLink Med Pub 1998.

[45]   Lurie R, Ben-Amitai D, Laron Z. Laron syndrome (primary growth hormone insensitivity): a unique model to explore the effect of insulin-like
        growth factor 1 deficiency on human hair. Dermatology (Basel) 2004; 208(4): 314-8.
        [http://dx.doi.org/10.1159/000077839] [PMID: 15178913]

[46]   Banerjee PS. Spectrophotometric methods for the determination of selected drugs in pharmaceutical formulations. J Chem Pharm Res 2009;

1(1): 261-7.

[47]   Dweck AC. On the Centella asicatica trail. Soap. Perfumery and Cosmetics Asia 1996; 1: 41-2.

[48]   Khare CP. Encyclopedia of indian medicinal plants. New york: Springerverlag Berlin Heidelberg 2004; pp. 197-8.

[49]   Williamson EM. Major herbs Of ayurveda. China: Churchill Livigstone 2002; pp. 126-8.

[50]   Porwal P, Sharma A, Gupta SP. Henna based cream preparation, characterization and its comparison with marketed hair dyes. J Herbal Med Tech 2011; 5(1): 55-61.

[51]   Banerjee P, Sharma M. Preparation, evaluation and hair growth stimulating activity of herbal oil. J Chem Pharm Res 2009; 1(1): 261-7.

[52]   Baziga KA, Heyan SA. Formulation and evaluation of herbal shampoo from zizyphus spine leaves extract. Int J Res Ayurveda Pharm 2011; 2(6): 1802-6.

[53]   Subedi BP, Shrestha R. Plant profile: Jatamansi (nardostachys grandiflora). Himalayan Bioresources 1999; 3: 14-5.

[54]   Chaudhary S, Chandrashekar KS, Pai KS, et al. Evaluation of antioxidant and anticancer activity of extract and fractions of Nardostachys jatamansi DC in breast carcinoma. BMC Complement Altern Med 2015; 15: 50.
        [http://dx.doi.org/10.1186/s12906-015-0563-1] [PMID: 25886964]

[55]   Purnima BM. Kothiyal P. A review article on phytochemistry and pharmacological profiles of Nardostachys jatamansi DC-medicinal herb. Journal of pharmacognosy and phytochemistry 2015; 3(5): 102-6.

[56]   Pal RS, Pal Y, Wal P. In-house preparation and standardization of herbal face pack. Open Dermatol J 2017; 11: 72-80.
        [http://dx.doi.org/10.2174/1874372201711010072]

[57]   Wallis TE. Text book of Pharmacognosy. 5th Ed.. New Delhi: CBS publishers & distributors, 2002; 123: pp. (132)210-5.

[58]   Rajpal V. Standardization of botanicals. New Delhi. Eastern Publishers 2002; 1: 39-44.

[59]   Tandon N, Sharma M. Quality standards of indian medicinal plants. New Delhi. Indian Council of Medical Research 2010; 8: 161-3.

[60]   Kokate CK, Purohit AP, Gokhale SB. Pharmacognosy. 42nd ed.. Pune: India: Nirali Prakashan 2008; 6: pp. 1-A1.

[61]   Khandelwal KR. Practical pharmacognosy. 12th ed. 2004.

[62]   Lachman L, Lieberman HA, Kanig JL. The Theory and practice of industrial pharmacy. 3rd ed. 1987.

[63]   Aulton ME. Pharmaceutics, The science of dosage forms design. 2nd ed. 2002.

[64]   Mandeep S, Shalini S, Sukhbir LK, Ram KS, Rajendra J. Preparation and evaluation of herbal cosmetic cream. Pharmacologyonline 2011; 1258-64.

[65]   Rani S, Hiremanth R. Formulation & evaluation of poly-herbal face wash gel. World J Pharm Pharm Sci 2015; 4(6): 585-8.

Permissions

All chapters in this book were first published in TODJ, by Bentham Open; hereby published with permission under the Creative Commons Attribution License or equivalent. Every chapter published in this book has been scrutinized by our experts. Their significance has been extensively debated. The topics covered herein carry significant findings which will fuel the growth of the discipline. They may even be implemented as practical applications or may be referred to as a beginning point for another development.

The contributors of this book come from diverse backgrounds, making this book a truly international effort. This book will bring forth new frontiers with its revolutionizing research information and detailed analysis of the nascent developments around the world.

We would like to thank all the contributing authors for lending their expertise to make the book truly unique. They have played a crucial role in the development of this book. Without their invaluable contributions this book wouldn't have been possible. They have made vital efforts to compile up to date information on the varied aspects of this subject to make this book a valuable addition to the collection of many professionals and students.

This book was conceptualized with the vision of imparting up-to-date information and advanced data in this field. To ensure the same, a matchless editorial board was set up. Every individual on the board went through rigorous rounds of assessment to prove their worth. After which they invested a large part of their time researching and compiling the most relevant data for our readers.

The editorial board has been involved in producing this book since its inception. They have spent rigorous hours researching and exploring the diverse topics which have resulted in the successful publishing of this book. They have passed on their knowledge of decades through this book. To expedite this challenging task, the publisher supported the team at every step. A small team of assistant editors was also appointed to further simplify the editing procedure and attain best results for the readers.

Apart from the editorial board, the designing team has also invested a significant amount of their time in understanding the subject and creating the most relevant covers. They scrutinized every image to scout for the most suitable representation of the subject and create an appropriate cover for the book.

The publishing team has been an ardent support to the editorial, designing and production team. Their endless efforts to recruit the best for this project, has resulted in the accomplishment of this book. They are a veteran in the field of academics and their pool of knowledge is as vast as their experience in printing. Their expertise and guidance has proved useful at every step. Their uncompromising quality standards have made this book an exceptional effort. Their encouragement from time to time has been an inspiration for everyone.

The publisher and the editorial board hope that this book will prove to be a valuable piece of knowledge for researchers, students, practitioners and scholars across the globe.

List of Contributors

Rashmi Saxena Pal, Yogendra Pal and Pranay Wal
Department of Pharmacy, PSIT, NH-2, Bhauti, Kanpur (U.P), 209305, India

Tesfaye Gabriel
Department of Pharmaceutics and Social Pharmacy, School of Pharmacy, College of Health Sciences, Addis Ababa University, Addis Ababa, Ethiopia

N. V. Deeva, Yu. M. Krinitsyna, S. V. Musta ina, O. D. Rymar and I. G. Sergeeva
Novosibirsk State University, Institute of Molecular Pathology and Pathomorphology, Research Institute of Internal and Preventive Medicine – Branch of the Institute of Cytology and Genetics, Novosibirsk, Russia

Vivek Choudhary and Wendy B. Bollag
Charlie Norwood VA Medical Center, One Freedom Way, Augusta, GA 30904, USA
Department of Physiology, 1120 15th Street, Medical College of Georgia at Augusta University (formerly Georgia Regents University), Augusta, GA 30912, USA

Lakiea J. Bailey
Department of Physiology, 1120 15th Street, Medical College of Georgia at Augusta University (formerly Georgia Regents University), Augusta, GA 30912, USA

Shiro Iino, Suguru Sato, Natsuki Baba, Naoki Maruta, Wataru Takashima, Noritaka Oyama and Minoru Hasegawa
Department of Dermatology, Division of Medicine, Faculty of Medical Sciences, University of Fukui, Fukui, Japan

Takahiro Kiyohara
Department of Dermatology, Kansai Medical University, Osaka, Japan

Masato Yasuda
Department of Plastic Surgery, University of Saga, Saga, Japan

Haneen Hamada, Erik Zimerson, Magnus Bruze, Marléne Isaksson and Malin Engfeldt
Department of Occupational and Environmental Dermatology, Lund University, Skåne University Hospital, Malmö, Sweden

Eve Lebas, Charlotte Castronovo, Florence Libon, Nazli Tassoudji and Arjen F. Nikkels
Dermatology (Dermato-oncology unit), University Hospital Centre, CHU du Sart Tilman, Liège, Belgium

Jorge E. Arrese
Dermatopathology, University Hospital Centre, CHU du Sart Tilman, Liège, Belgium

Laurence Seidel
Biostatistics University Hospital Centre, CHU du Sart Tilman, Liège, Belgium

Magdalena Krajewska–Włodarczyk
Department of Rheumatology of Municipal Hospital in Olsztyn, Olsztyn, Poland

Agnieszka Owczarczyk-Saczonek and Waldemar Placek
Department of Dermatology, Sexually Transmitted Diseases and Clinical Immunology, The University of Warmia and Mazury in Olsztyn, Olsztyn, Poland

Damilola A Okuboyejo and Oludayo O Olugbara
ICT and Society Research Group, Durban University of Technology, Durban, South Africa

Ayman Abdelmaksoud
Dermatology and Leprology Hospital, Elsamanoudy street, 5, Mansoura, Egypt

Domenico Bonamonte and Angela Filoni
Section of Dermatology, Department of Biomedical Science and Human Oncology, University of Bari, 11, Piazza Giulio Cesare, Bari, 70124, Italy

Michelangelo Vestita
Section of Dermatology, Department of Biomedical Science and Human Oncology, University of Bari, 11, Piazza Giulio Cesare, Bari, 70124, Italy
Unit of Plastic and Reconstructive Surgery, Department of Emergency and Organ Transplantation, University of Bari, 11, Piazza Giulio Cesare, Bari, 70124, Italy

Giuseppe Giudice
Unit of Plastic and Reconstructive Surgery, Department of Emergency and Organ Transplantation, University of Bari, 11, Piazza Giulio Cesare, Bari, 70124, Italy

Julia Shah, Lorie Gottwald, Ashley Sheskey and Craig Burkhart
Department of Dermatology, University of Toledo College of Medicine, Toledo, USA

Khitam Al-Refu
Department of Internal Medicine, Mutah University, Karak, Jordan

Carnero Gregorio M
Efficiency, quality and costs in Health Services Research Group (EFISALUD), Galicia Sur Health Research Institute (IIS Galicia Sur). SERGAS-UVIGO Postdoctoral Researcher, University of Vigo, Vigo, Spain

Elga Sidhom and Mara Pilmane
Institute of Anatomy and Anthropology, Riga Stradins University, Riga, Latvia

Carmen Rodríguez Cerdeira
Efficiency, quality and costs in Health Services Research Group (EFISALUD), Galicia Sur Health Research Institute (IIS Galicia Sur). SERGAS-UVIGO Dermatology Service, Hospital do Meixoeiro and University of Vigo, Vigo, Spain

Sánchez Blanco E
Dermatology Service, Hospital do Meixoeiro and University of Vigo, Vigo, Spain

Sánchez Blanco B
Postdoctoral Researcher, Conselleria de Educación, Xunta Galicia, Vigo. Spain
Predoctoral Researcher, Family Physician, EOXI, Vigo. Spain

Ryan S. Sefcik
University of Toledo, College of Medicine, Toledo, Ohio, OH, USA

Craig G. Burkhart
Department of Medicine, University of Toledo College of Medicine, Toledo; Department of Medicine, Ohio University of Osteopathic Medicine, Athens, Ohio, OH, USA

Mallory K. Smith
Wayne State University School of Medicine, Detroit, MI, USA

Tasneem F. Mohammad and Iltefat H. Hamzavi
Department of Dermatology, Henry Ford Hospital, Detroit, MI, USA

A. K Rai and Ankita Wal
Department of Pharmacy, Pranveer Singh Institute of Technology, NH-2, Bhauti, Kanpur (U.P), 209305, India

Index